THE WELLNESS ZONE

THE WELLNESS ZONE
Your Guide
for Optimal Wellness

Third Edition

Dominique Livkamal

AEON

First edition published in Australia in 2005,
by DOM Montville, Queensland
Second edition published in Australia in 2008,
by DOM Montville, Queensland

This edition published in 2021 by
Aeon Books
PO Box 76401
London W5 9RG

British Library Cataloguing in Publication Data

A C.I.P. for this book is available from the British Library

ISBN-13: 978-1-91280-794-9

Typeset by Medlar Publishing Solutions Pvt Ltd, India
Printed in Great Britain

www.aeonbooks.co.uk

CONTENTS

CHAPTER ONE

Introduction

T he poem below is a vision I have of health care and the path of
medicines. Wishing you health, joy and vibrancy.

Healings for everyone

The aroma of a highland rose pulsating against the wind
A warm bowl of ginger and lentil soup, carrot juice or a dram
of whisky
Pharmaceuticals
Hormonal and emotional support
Meditating by the ocean, diving in its deep cool calm
Sipping Lemon water, so cleansing on more levels than one
Mind having its Healing place over matter
We can all be strong and thrive
The needle that holds life
The emergency, another life saved
Freshly picked comfrey tea from my organic garden
The sages use sage
Past regressions, opening doors, easing the pain that gently
slips away
Feeling the blissful moment, consciousness in transformation
Channelling, breathing freely, we ritualise the oracles, toss the
coins, the flick of a card
We change patterns of our making, the conscious decision to
heal and to refresh our soul
Visualisation of our beauty within
Awareness is just awareness
These things are all medicine

The highest energy we can muster from above, coming down like a cascading sensation of completeness. Are we grounded?

We chant, meditate, rebirth, reiki and sling crystals across our beings

All for healing

We eat, drink and breathe our medicine

Lighting a candle to the flame of gratefulness

Yogic, tantric, meditative, art therapies, elevated and surreal

The giving of our Doctor's learnings, ritual is cultural

The surgeons have their preciseness of skill, trusting and complete

Wherever it comes from? Herbalism, traditional cultural remedies, Western biomedicines, Chinese traditional, Ayurvedic, early vedic, siddha, reiki, yunani, crystal healing, spiritual, shamanism, witchery, religious, homeopathy, cellularopathy, nutritional, orthodox, avatar, fox, a prescription from your trusted practitioner, or a pebble on the beach.

The aim is the same… to cure

Or to circumvent the tragedy of dis-ease

Healing our Earth and her sacred spirits

Our Universe and all that resides under and around her umbrella

Whatever your bent or belief

In the name of survival, growth, understanding, personal indulgences or scientific advance

We eat, drink and breathe our medicines

Never before have we had so much access to knowledge and learning

The secrets of the medics are freely available to all, for the asking

The golden key has unlocked past exclusiveness creating a kaleidoscope of healings and medicines

No more can we close our minds

Every way is a way

Every healing is a success

Every Potion that cures is a medicine

Isolated in the lab with billions of dollars in backing

Channelled in the snow-capped caves of a rare and elusive mountain top

Or randomly mixed in the alchemist's kitchen

Our medicines are evolving.

We can only be grateful that we have the resources available to gain the skills and healings we need

Always the answer comes

Always at the right time and way

The future of the medicines are exciting and frightening

Where does it lead us?

Do we allow the huge advances to work for us or against the good of everyone? There are serious environmental and ethical conflicts

Exploitations and abuses that cloud the Hippocratic Oath

As individuals we can only be honest in our work, share the information we have and create good medicines. Respect the healer and the medicine that works within

I would love to see everyone work together for the common good

For the alternative ways to blend harmoniously with the orthodox ways

A professional respect created between the different beliefs

Educational, spiritual, physical and emotional status of practitioners

With the governing bodies recognising these differences

Allowing medicine and science to grow to its true potential

Eliminating the greed and fulfilling the planets medical needs with sustainability, ecology, indigenous, new age sciences

… and Together we grow

Dominique Livkamal (1999)

CHAPTER TWO

Your Wellness Zone

Welcome to the Wellness Zone

My original comments in the first edition in 2005 still hold true today, and I have decided to keep them in print for your information. The Wellness Zone is a timeless health zone. There are some basic truths and simple techniques in natural health care that need to be passed on, and that could help you immensely if you chose to follow folk tradition and make time to put your health first. I trust that by publishing the third edition of this book, I have contributed to your ongoing health care needs and services.

Take a few minutes every day to think about your health; think about what you do to make your body well or unwell. Think and act. Exercise, eat well and mitigate any unhealthy lifestyle choices as much as you can.

Keep your body clean, which means keeping the acidity out of your cells and replacing toxins with good clean blood. Do what you can today to have a healthier tomorrow in every way. Too many people are mindless of their health care. Treat your body like the temple it is and give it the respect it deserves. Just a small amount of effort can bring about great results.

It's easy to take good health for granted and that's a real danger in today's over-polluted, toxic and chemically damaged world. Even if you think you are eating well and aren't exposed to many poisons, you are probably wrong. Most of us are exposed to too many pollutants; we need to look after ourselves and treat our health as our highest priority, ensuring that we don't just become statistics in an over-subscribed public health care system.

Accept that we are not perfect, we are human and part of being human involves making mistakes with our health. If you think you are taking inappropriate medications, drugs or supplements, then talk with

5

your Health Care Practitioner and make the necessary changes. Often there is no need to be on multiple medications as they can cause unnecessary side effects; there are usually alternatives and your practitioner can help you with this.

I hope this book can help you too. I have tried to outline the best the natural health care industry has to offer as I know it, from my experiences and studies. There is always a wealth of new information available and I enjoy attending conferences, reading research and exploring the world online to read, listen, understand and then interpret this information for my patients.

If you are unwell, sick, upset, diseased, uncomfortable, depressed, irritable, hormonal or just too stressed and too tired to cope, then I hope you will pick up this book, open it to the section that relates to you and read what I have to contribute to the subject. I want to inspire you in the knowledge that you will be okay again. I want to add positive aspects to your health care and I want you to know that your body is the most amazing self-healing organism if you can just stop, rest, relax, breathe, stretch, drink water, let the world go on outside your door and allow yourself to get better. Take the time your body needs to make yourself well again. Eat simple foods, take natural medicines, leave the fear behind you and trust that you will be okay. Also, research, communicate and find out as much as you can about your illness and take the best options available to get well.

Sometimes all we need to get well is a dark room, a comfortable bed, fresh water and silence. Other times it's not quite that simple. But consider this, if we took the first option of rest when we felt the initial signs of any illness, do you think a deeper illness would follow? Possibly not. Perhaps if we lived simpler lives and didn't get so mentally, emotionally and physically caught up in the busyness of the world, then we could conceivably enjoy optimal health.

The information presented in the third edition of *The Wellness Zone* is all my original work, most of it is reprinted from the previous editions which have sold out and are no longer in print. I have also added some updated information to this new edition.

I hope you enjoy this book as much as the last. I also trust that you will take the information and add it to your own research and experiences. Each system of medicine has its strengths and weaknesses. Folk, herbal and nutritional medicines are my passion, interest and career base. These medicines are what I write about and what I believe should be used as your first option for home remedies and healing simple illnesses.

Keep your immunity strong, your mind focused, your body clean and flexible, and your heart filled with love, and you will have optimal health.

Dominique Livkamal

Master of Public Health (Health Promotion)
Graduate Diploma in Health Science
Bachelor of Health Science (Complementary Medicine)
Advanced Diploma Naturopathy
Diploma in Journalism
Diploma in Zen Thai Shiatsu and Zen Thai Shiatsu teacher
Kundalini yoga teacher as taught by yogi Bhajan
Qualified; public health advocate, naturopath, nutritionist, herbalist and journalist
In 2012, was awarded 'Australian Herbalist of the Year' by the Naturopathic Herbalist Association of Australia
In 2015, was made a Fellow of the Naturopathic Herbalist Association of Australia

What is the Wellness Zone?

The Wellness Zone is developed to help you have a healthy lifestyle, living within any physical boundaries that you experience. You will find your own level of wellness where you know what triggers good health and what triggers ill health. Understand you have a choice; yes, you do have a choice every minute of every day to create optimal wellness in your life.

Each of us is already living in our own Wellness Zone. But are you aware of that? Are you aware of the ability that you have to alter the state of your health through simple daily lifestyle choices?

Please use the below as a check list, whenever you need confirmation about whether you are in your Wellness Zone or not.

How do you know if you are in your Wellness Zone?

You will know by assessing these indicators and addressing any areas that need your attention. If you are uncomfortable about all or any of these points then think about how you can adjust your attitude or lifestyle so that you feel more comfortable and know that you are doing your best to maintain your Wellness Zone. It is natural and normal for people to live in comfort and to be reasonably happy with their lifestyle choices.

- You feel healthier
- You are in less pain or your illness is less inhibiting
- You are comfortable with the choices you make
- You have improved energy levels
- You are capable of focusing on your priorities
- You are feeling emotionally in control
- Your stress levels are in control
- You are acting on the decisions you have made to improve your health
- You know you are making wise lifestyle choices
- You are able to minimalise negative habits and addictions
- You are thinking more positively
- You feel like your body is operating as well as it can including digestion, cardiovascular, hormonal, libido, immunity, mental function and nervous system
- You are making the effort to eat healthy foods that nourish your body
- Your life is moving in the direction that meets your goals
- You know you are doing your best under the current circumstances
- You are reasonably happy

How do you know if you are out of your Wellness Zone?

You will know that you have compromised your Wellness Zone by assessing these indicators and addressing any areas that need your attention. If you are uncomfortable about all or any of these points then you will need to adjust your attitude or lifestyle to bring yourself back into your Wellness Zone. If you think that any of points listed below are natural and normal states of health then you really do need to address your health care regime. It is not natural or normal for a person to live in pain or discomfort. If you are in this position then you may gain a lot of information from this book to help bring your body into balance and wellness.

- You are feeling upset or depressed
- You are not coping with daily challenges in a balanced manner

- You are feeling pain or illness intensely
- You know that your health needs improving
- You are eating for emotional reasons
- You are not feeling in control of your lifestyle or circumstances
- You know that you are making unwise choices for your Wellness Zone
- You are not able to stay focused on tasks or keep to plans
- You are not thinking clearly
- You are bending to bad habits or addictions
- Your stress levels are high
- You do not care what happens with your health care plan
- You find excess fault with people or circumstances and tend to blame others
- You are feeling emotionally unbalanced
- You feel that your body is not operating optimally and that there needs to be some improvement
- You are not trying to do your best under the current circumstances
- You are not feeling reasonably happy
- You know you are sick in some way

Get started on your Wellness Zone today! The choice is yours!

Take a few minutes to write down your priorities in life, or you can mentally reflect on these if you do not want to make notes. What are your preferred choices in your home, work, study and all the things that you know are important and essential for your happiness? This is the starting point for adapting your current Wellness Zone. Figure out for yourself what choices you want to make for your own health. Look at the positives and the negatives in your life. Take a few minutes to make note of all the positive aspects of your life that you wish to maintain. Then once you have completed this list start a new list of all the things you would like to change if you could. This is a great starting point towards better health and wellness, as you will look back on these thoughts in the future and see how much you have altered your view on wellness. You will also be proud of yourself as you start to see clearly where you need to look for better health in the future. You are able to change your priorities and your desires for different aspects of your Wellness Zone at any time depending upon your current circumstances. As time goes by you will need to make adjustments and this is necessary for good health as change is inevitable.

What do you personally want from your Wellness Zone?

Finding your way through the maze of choices today can be daunting. So, it's best to look at where you are now. After all, everything that is happening in your life today has happened because, whether consciously or unconsciously, you did something to put it there. You made a choice somewhere in the past that has led you to the place where you are now.

These choices can be spontaneous, or they can be well planned. You are the one who decides what you want and how you will achieve it. If not, then you are just drifting along and it's time you made some decisions for yourself that will benefit you and those you love.

The emotional aspects of our lives that reside in the depths of our hearts and minds with injustices, abuses and traumas can limit us from reaching our potential. In order to achieve optimal health, you need to eliminate the voice in your mind that remembers every past failure and reconnect with the good voice that is willing to take a risk on good health and get positive.

Don't compromise your good health. Think about your highest priorities and what you want for your body today and in the future. Then take steps to improve your health until you are satisfied with the results.

Each of us has different priorities. Some basic factors can help you become healthy much faster. These are: fresh air, clean water, fresh unprocessed foods, a good nutritional profile, and herbal preventative and supporting medicines as required; minimal unnecessary stresses, lots of love, laughter and friendship; minimal conflict; a passionate career and a desire to be as healthy as you can. This is what you need to have a healthy body and to have your optimal Wellness Zone. Anything less than this is a compromise and can be improved upon in the fullness of time.

Keep your personal environment as clean as possible with the minimal use of any chemicals that may change their structure once exposed to your body. These chemicals are everywhere from the toiletries you purchase, the environment you live in and the food you eat that has been sprayed with pesticides and insecticides long before it has reached your plate! Chemicals are everywhere. Be aware of your own exposure as much as possible and take healthy countermeasures to avoid any damage to your body. These countermeasures include keeping your body and your environment as clean as possible.

The positive factors

Think of the aspects of your average day that you really enjoy and that add to the personal health you wish to maintain. These are the desirable aspects that need to be included in your Wellness Zone. These are the elements that make your life feel rich and complete. The list can be as long or as short as you want to make it (e.g. yoga, fitness, surfing, etc.).

Once you have written this list read it back and see whether there is anything else to add.

What needs some improvement?

Make a list/note/vision board to look at the aspects of your life where you need work! Are you self-sabotaging? Do you need some more discipline in areas that you want to make better in your life? What needs developing?

This aspect, like the positives list can be as long or short as you want to make it, but remember that these are the aspects of yourself that you could transform into positives to enhance your Wellness Zone. The negatives are aspects of your Wellness Zone that are holding you back from being the person you wish to be. You can look at the developing list in a very positive light; the growth list is the bridge between your current self and your future self. It's the bridge that you can build simply by looking at your weaknesses and habits and adjusting them. Turn them around through time and effort to become your strengths and positives!

We all need to honestly address the blocks that stop us from moving forward and living in our Wellness Zone. Be honest when writing this list and keep it personal. Look at yourself objectively to get the most out of it... and be kind to yourself; remember you are already doing a great job.

The fixed aspects

The fixed aspects of your life are those that are not changeable at this point in time. They are the factors that you need to live with irrespective of what you want to change. This is the list that must be incorporated into your Wellness Zone and must be a core to the Wellness Zone. If there are any parts to the fixed list that you are not happy about, then what you need to do is make the most of the situation and try to make your life as comfortable as possible around these fixed aspects. Ideas for this list are things that you cannot change at this point in time through commitment, habit or environment.

Nothing is ever permanent. Even what we consider a fixed aspect is only transitory anyway. There is a saying: 'This too shall pass', and it shall. Anyone familiar with the *I Ching* and the book of changes will recognise that life is all change, and it is constant change. So, it doesn't really matter how much routine you can put into routine, or how much emphasis you put into the fixed list, the fixed list is only fixed as long as something doesn't change to unfix it. So, make the most of it and try to enjoy the journey along the way. Make the decision today to be as well as you can be, make the commitment to your future health. Don't let yourself become another statistic of the health system.

Creating your wellness wish list

The wellness wish list is your guide to help you decide what is acceptable and necessary for your Wellness Zone. This list is compiled of the desires you have for your life at this point in time. It must be realistic and needs to fit into your life in a practical and achievable way. Very simply we all need to accept the present and move to make changes for the future; this can be done in your own way in the comfort of your Wellness Zone. The Wellness Zone is a place that is as flexible as you are. It can take you a day, a week, a month, or even a year to decide on the boundaries of your Wellness Zone. You may change and alter the aspects of your Wellness Zone many times over many years until one day you will realise that you don't need to alter anything anymore, and that you truly are living in your Wellness Zone. The Wellness Zone is an acceptability zone. It is you saying, 'I accept my life, I accept the way it is and I am well; however, I am making my future Wellness Zone a little more like the way I dream life to be'. This is about meeting your personal dreams, if we were all the same, this world would be very boring. Cherish and applaud your individuality … remember 'everyone else is taken' (Yogi Bhajan*)*. You are in control of yourself being healthy, in control of yourself being the best person you can be in the moment, whatever the situation, you need to find your centre and discover your Wellness Zone.

This list is one where you can look at ways of turning your life around. Write down your wildest dreams next and see what stuff you're really made of!

Go on, dream big, it's certainly one way to keep your mind positive and your feet firmly anchored to the wish list, the dream wheel of life. Once you have looked at this list again, you can add information, take away information or simply laugh at yourself! Why not have a good laugh; it's one of the best medicines.

Don't undervalue your health

At the end of the day, it's all that truly belongs to you. Be aware of how you are using your energy and keep your body well-nourished, strong and healthy.

Do not work yourself into the ground now for the ideal that one day you will retire and you can then enjoy all the fruits (money) of your labour that you have so tirelessly worked for. No, this is a mistake, because unless you find your Wellness Zone whilst you are working so hard, then you may find yourself retiring with high cholesterol, obesity, diabetes, coronary heart disease, cancer or vision problems, to name a few. Yes, your retirement years may be spent in Health Care Practitioners' waiting rooms and pharmacies waiting for your next batch of medication. And of course we shouldn't forget the anti-depressants, because you're going to need them when you realise your dream of good health and a retirement spent lounging around has been shattered.

However, good health in older age can be a reality if you plan ahead now. Find your Wellness Zone, get there and stay there. This may involve some hard work, like taking up an exercise programme now, to avoid the coronary illnesses of old age, plus you may need to make a bit of time to meditate, or do some quiet thinking with yourself. Perhaps finding your Wellness Zone will mean you need to make adaptations to the way you think about health care. Maybe you will need some nutritional supplements on a regular basis to help with certain aspects of your health, but isn't that a better option than sticking to no plan? What is your plan?

Do you have a plan for your Wellness Zone? If you answered no, then you are one of the majority. Often we go to work, expose ourselves to stress, toxins, pressures of all sorts and never give a second thought to what it may be doing to our future. Often we are so busy that we don't even give our Wellness Zone a thought. Well, those days are over, because once you have read this book you will not be able to ignore yourself any longer. You will not be able to just think everything is OK, and muddle along the road of business. No, you will have to take a long hard look at yourself and think about how you can be in your Wellness Zone? You will have to start to appreciate your good health, make notes on when it is failing you, take steps to counterbalance the negative aspects of your health care regime. This means that from today onwards you cannot undervalue your health anymore.

PART I

YOUR MIND BODY ZONE

Create a healthy body and mind

To create a healthy body and mind, you need to be aware of your own needs and the choices you make to create and maintain your Wellness Zone. It's wonderful if you can think smart for your health and each day make healthy choices.

That's what the Wellness Zone is about. It's about you being the best person you can be today; it's about making healthy food and medicine choices based on information you have researched.

Understanding herbal medicines, pharmaceutical medicines and alternative health practices and the place they can have in your medicine chest is a good way to approach your mind–body focus zone. Sometimes you may need to visit your Health Care Practitioner. Understanding your options is necessary to make informed and well-rounded choices as various incidences occur. The Wellness Zone is about you having control and being responsible for the choices you make each day. The solution to any health problem is the one that has the maximum healing benefit to your body with the least side effects. This solution can come from many avenues of health care. You may need to look at new solutions as the world changes and access to various medicines alters. The best way to find a programme to help you is to understand your choices and also understand your own body and what it requires to be in good health and to maintain optimal balance.

Know your body

How do you decide whether you are healthy? Do you need some work to improve your health? Can you see where problems are most likely to occur in the future? What countermeasures can you take to improve your Wellness Zone?

Get inspired by your Wellness Zone with some basic understanding of the different systems of your body and how they will benefit when you look after them optimally.

To understand yourself, you need to be capable of looking at each aspect of your life on a daily basis and deciding whether you are really in your Wellness Zone or whether you need to make a few adjustments which will ensure that you are having the best day possible.

Often we can be healthy and something goes wrong physically that is out of our control. This random illness can come from many sources. It's not pleasant, but it's something that happens to all of us from time to time. In many incidences you are able to help yourself with the right attitude, rest, medicines, fresh air, clean water and good environmental influences. Be inspired daily by your own health, be observant of what is going on and try to understand your own solutions. If you notice that something is not right with an area of your body, it's necessary to follow up with diagnosis and healing solutions to bring you back into balance again. Sometimes this is simply done at home with rest and natural solutions. Other times you will need professional assistance. However you choose to heal your body, you will benefit from understanding it and the functions of each organ and system. These systems all work together to create the whole body which is essentially dependent upon each system and organ functioning optimally. So, if you have a small problem in one part of your body, it's wise to repair the problem before it gets out of hand and affects other parts of your body. This is why awareness is so important for your Wellness Zone. If you miss a problem when it is minor then you may find it accelerates out of control and causes further complications that may hinder your daily activities. Often we can heal small ailments readily whilst getting on with our normal routine. However, if it grows into a larger problem, stronger medicine and some rest time may be necessary.

Genetics

You need to take into account the genetic traits that are carried through your family and through the environment. Take the time to look at what illnesses have affected what people and what ages they have had these illnesses to try to get a pattern of your genetics if you can. If you can get this information it can help you understand your potential weaknesses.

Research has shown time and again that certain diseases are genetically influenced and you can minimalise your risk of contracting these conditions if you know about them early enough to tailor your diet, health care and nutritional supplements. This will be a major factor to take into consideration with any healing regime in the future as we recognise what illnesses are likely to affect what people. Whenever you change environment, diet or lifestyle factors this may affect the way your body responds to disease and illness. You may find that you are more prone to the illnesses of the new environment where you live and your body will adjust accordingly. Human genes have not changed over time; however, during the last 100 years we have seen societal examples as diet has become more processed and many people suffer from over-consumption and under-nutrition, which can lead to a myriad of cardiovascular, inflammatory and hormonal illnesses that plague many countries today. Your genes are not designed for modern living, and if you do consume unnatural foods and medicines then you will get the expected results, as your body rebels and creates disease in an attempt to bring itself back into balance. You need to take responsibility to find out what you can about your genetics and environment and how they can affect your Wellness Zone. Some examples here are coronary heart disease, diabetes, cancer, arthritis, hemochromatosis, gout, migraines, obesity and all the complications, even the way women cope with menopause and elderly afflictions such as Parkinson's and Alzheimer's. Many common illnesses are genetically or environmentally influenced causing your body to respond with illness. The interesting fact is that many of these can be minimalised by preventative measures taken now to help you stay in optimal health to avoid this future illness.

Never take no for an answer when it comes to minimalising these genetic illnesses. Know that if you do your best now, by taking appropriate supplements and foods, you can change the effects that the environment could have on your health. Yes, one day your vigilance will pay off in your health stakes and you will be glad you did take measures to help your future health. The measures you take can be simple additions to your nutritional profile to increase your health today and tomorrow. The results will not show overnight, but with regular practise you will be doing your best for your Wellness Zone. You need to find out if there are any genetic conditions you need to be aware of, and if so research these conditions and take positive steps to help prevent them happening to you. This is what's known as preventative health care. Once you understand the condition then take nutritional medicines to help stop you from falling prey to this illness. Look at the research and find out what foods are to be avoided, what lifestyle choices minimalise your chances of getting this condition and what you can do to help yourself stay healthier for longer. This is how you will find your Wellness Zone for genetics. The Wellness Zone is important for every one of us. It's the place where we feel our best. And when you suffer from a genetic condition you need to know how to help yourself. Leave no stone unturned. Visit your Health Care Practitioner and get the lowdown on the condition from their perspective. Use the internet; it's a fabulous tool for accessing information about almost anything. You can take the best of alternative health and also work with the orthodox medical system to come up with whatever treatments are best for you. Don't ever allow yourself to close your mind off to any system of medicine. The answers may be in unexpected places and your solution may be very simple given the right treatments.

Take a look at your medicine

Herbal medicines and nutritional medicines are natural medicines. These are the medicines you may use to help prevent illness in the future. These are also the medicines you may need to bring your body into balance whilst it is sick or recovering from sickness. Herbal medicines are all plant-based and specifically targeted at assisting your body to heal itself with maximum support. Herbal medicines and nutritional medicines help your body to do what it is designed to do naturally, which is repair itself without the intervention of functionally blocking substances.

On the other hand pharmaceutical medicines can be of benefit to your body in specific circumstances. There are many differences between the way pharmaceutical medicines work compared to the natural herbal and nutritional choices. You are in control of what medicines you take for an ailment from the smallest cold to a serious illness. Make sure you research the information available and make wise choices with the medicines you take. Often you can complement the different types of medicines for optimal results. For example, various nutritional medicines can minimalise the side effects of some pharmaceutical medicines and certain herbal medicines are safer alternatives to some pharmaceutical medicines. Also you may find that some types of medicines act faster or have less side effects than others. Each person is an individual and the best approach to taking any medicine is to respect the individuality of yourself and understand that the medicines may have vastly different effects on your body than on another person's. If you take a medicine and get side effects, ensure you contact your Health Care Professional and look at alternatives. On the other hand, if a medicine is working well for you, try to get as much information as possible about the medicine and make sure that there are no long-term consequences that could be detrimental to your Wellness Zone in the future.

Herbal medicines are generally a safe option. They have varied traditional cultural histories that have proven them worthy, through human consumption, over hundreds if not thousands of years of use. Nutritional medicines are also fairly safe so long as you ensure the body is in balance and there is not an overload of specific nutrients which can swing the body into illness. Many pharmaceutical medicines are safe in small amounts and for short periods of time as they do a specific job. You then stop taking the medicine and allow your body to take over the natural process of rebalancing. However, beware of medicines that are taken for a long term, as this is when you run the risk of imbalance and side effects.

If you have a first aid kit at home make sure this is filled with healthy relief for acute symptoms. Look at homeopathic, herbal and nutritional solutions for small daily ailments. Add in some pharmaceutical relief as required and remember that when your body is balanced and healthy you only need minimal influence from medicines, except the preventative herbals and nutritional medicines that will act to help prevent future illness and disease.

Let your food be your medicine

Herbs, vitamins and health supplements are just that ... supplements. There's an old saying: 'Let your food be your medicine and your medicine be your food'. Adhere to this principle and know that it's a waste of money to keep swallowing a load of potions in the name of preventative health care unless you are specific in your selections. We read all the time about new breakthroughs as research develops and information becomes available about the active constituents in various substances that we will all benefit from. Many of us are easily persuaded by the attributes of various supplements and want to try them out. This can lead to a situation where we have a cupboard full of half-empty bottles. How do you know which ones work? Trial and error is the only way. Don't start on a large selection of new products on any one day, slowly introduce them and see for yourself if there is benefit. If you wish to change the supplements you take, eliminate one at a time, leaving a few days between the elimination of any particular supplement. Then, if you're feeling a shift in energy, for better or worse, act accordingly. Either reintroduce the supplement knowing the difference in how you feel, or keep it off the menu for a while. Often a synergistic blend of supplements is needed for optimal healing. This is prescribed by your Health Care Practitioner for a specific time frame, and will include the best nutritional and herbal supplements to aid your condition.

CHAPTER THREE

Digestive

You are what you eat

Ensure that you eat the right foods for your body's needs and that these foods are being assimilated and digested correctly in your body. You want the nutrients to circulate through your body to ensure optimal use. You must also make sure that you are eliminating unwanted toxins and waste products effectively. This is the key to good health; you are responsible for what you eat and how you treat that food once it has been swallowed.

Food is fuel, make your food your medicine and let your medicine be your food. Such a simple concept. The digestive tract is technically external to your body. It's a tubular structure that goes from your mouth to your anus, with openings at each end. It is external because this tract is not open to any other body parts. Nutrients must be absorbed through the layers to reach the organs and be utilised as fuel. The food may start off as a delicious meal, which should be chewed well so that it turns into a liquid nutrient called chyme. Technically you get the nutrients from the fuel absorbed into your small intestine so that it goes into your blood stream and becomes new cells which is your body tomorrow.

The fuel you take in determines what your future body will look like, functioning and healthy or ill, according to what you do to it. Digestive enzymes for carbohydrates start in your mouth, and there are others in your stomach for proteins. Further digestive juices are required again in the small intestine to help emulsify fats and absorb nutrients into your blood stream where they are transported to your liver for processing. From your liver the nutrients are distributed to various body parts as required. It's simple. If you eat nourishing foods your body will be nourished. If you eat unhealthy foods, your body becomes unhealthy. If you eat poisons and toxins, then you will be polluting your body. Inflammation is an unnatural state in your body and at the first sign of inflammation anywhere you need to ask what allergens you have been exposed to. You also need to ask yourself what effect this is having, firstly on your digestive tract, as there are many immunity cells in this area of your body. If there is a problem, ensure you fix it quickly as inflammation can spread into your organs and joints and this can be a precursor for many chronic illnesses. Often it's the unnatural foods eaten that can create the inflammation.

Monitor your food

Everyone would be better off if they monitored the foods eaten and the circumstances that they are eating under. Do your body a favour and treat it like it's on a health food diet every day! Only eat the best foods you can get, buy or grow the freshest produce, use the least amount of additives and keep preservatives and processed items to a minimum!

Eat when you're hungry. The messages your body and mind send to each other are important and you need to keep your metabolism boosted to be trim and terrific and avoid your body turning into an obesity statistic. If you ignore the feeling of hunger, then it's simple, your body will get the message to store its next meal.

Our bodies have ancient and perfected mechanisms that will stop you starving yourself to death. The feast and famine belief that is ingrained in every cell in your body. Have you ever noticed that you put on weight fairly quickly after the recovery of an illness or the completion of a fad weight loss programme? Our bodies like to store fat, just like we like to store things and hoard; your body has a very high intelligence.

So, if you get hungry, either have a drink, a piece of fruit or something light to eat. Hunger doesn't mean a huge meal is called for. Listen to the cravings in your mind. Are they sensory induced? (By walking past the cake shop and seeing that delicious treat?) Or are they nutritionally induced when you feel like eating something good like eggs or fresh fruit? The latter is the one to listen to as it creates good and appropriate eating habits. If you see something and want to eat it simply because you see it and it smells delicious, then you may need to do a little check with yourself and decide if it really is a good thing to consume and what benefit this food will offer you nutritionally.

Emotional eating?

Eat delicious foods. When you eat a food, make sure it's something you really love eating. Why eat it if it's not fabulous? They should be simple fresh foods. People often go for long periods of time without eating and then find themselves filling up on the nearest and often easiest options, just for the sake of eating. There are a lot of mental agendas that go hand in hand with foods. All the emotional baggage that we carry about can sometimes be seen on our bodies as pockets of fats as we consume those foods that decrease health and morale.

If you do feel angry or upset, then food is certainly not your best medicine. The best things you can do are to drink water and relax. Wait until you feel calm before having a meal. Fruit is another good alternative to a meal when you are under acute (sudden) stress. However, if the stress becomes chronic (long term) then you will need to take supplements to keep yourself boosted and feeling strong.

The fastest track to sickness is mindless neglect

Eating badly … if you mindlessly eat and think that it's safe to consume refined sugars and fatty foods, then you are on the path to sickness. Some of the worst things you can do include consuming saturated fatty acids, overdoing alcohol, ingesting toxic poisons through breathing, the skin or diet, taking excess pharmaceutical medications or other drugs, and ignoring your health care. Stay away from processed foods, sugar, carbonated drinks and excess eating. Don't eat foods you know are bad combinations for you; if you get sick or react badly to certain foods, consider eliminating them from your diet.

The fastest track to wellness is thoughtful eating

Be conscious about what you put in your mouth every time you eat. The foods you need to prioritise are the freshest and most delicious foods that are grown locally. Other than that you need to ensure there are essential fatty acids in your diet and nutritional support as and when it is needed.

The best things you can do for your health are to breathe fresh air and drink clean water. Eat unprocessed natural foods in balanced quantities.

Get adequate exercise and stay flexible in body and mind. Avoid stress whenever possible. Keep your mind and spirit positive and healthy. Keep your immunity strong. And get plenty of sleep.

Keep your body fluids flowing

If you have good digestion then you will probably be assimilating nutrients well. This means that you will be getting adequate nutrition from the foods you eat. The key to good health is eating nutrient packed foods that are readily digested. You need to be aware of digestive disturbances that involve your tract being blocked or congested in any way. The most obvious is constipation. Many health problems are caused by blocked tubes. These are not limited to your digestive tract and can be arteries, bowels, veins, lymph nodes, glands; nephrons in the kidneys, nodules in the liver, cholesterol build-up in the gall bladder. Once again it's simple. If you keep your tubes unblocked, then you will keep the energy moving in your body. And as the body fluids are flowing freely, you will experience good health.

Create your own wellness diet

You need to create food combinations that work for you

Some of us have stomachs like a cast iron pot and can eat and digest almost any food combination; that is until our body finally catches up with us and has a healing crisis in the form of a heart attack, gout, arthritis or some other condition that was created through bad living and inappropriate combinations.

You need to take note of how you feel after eating certain foods. You may feel energised, or you may feel depleted of energy. You may feel tired, hyperactive, depressed or angry. There are many emotions that can occur after eating food in certain combinations, and you need to be aware of this. See how you can alter your eating habits to achieve a Wellness Zone diet which makes you feel vibrant and strong.

How to eliminate foods that don't agree with you

If you think that a particular food is causing you grief and want to try an elimination diet, simply stop eating that food for a month. The reason to stop for a month is that you will then have removed that food's residue from your digestive tract. Hopefully, the negative allergen will have cleansed on a cellular level after four weeks of elimination. If you notice a difference straight away that is positive to your health, then this is a definite sign the food is an allergen (i.e. the sinus clears up after the elimination of dairy products from a diet). It may not always be so obvious and can take a few weeks for any benefits to show.

In severe allergy cases it can take several months before the residue is sufficiently moved along and eliminated before you notice a difference (i.e. gluten). So, after four weeks of not eating the suspected food, eat some. And eat it in rather large amounts for three days. Note how you are feeling and compare your sense of wellness to the elimination period (especially the last two weeks).

Now if you feel an effect from the food that is negative, then cut it out of your diet for another month and then try the food again and see whether there is a negative response. If there is, cut it out for two months and try again. If you are unable to tolerate the food after a two month elimination, then clearly you have a specific allergy to the food and it is best left out of your diet.

The time frames are rather important, as many people have varied diets and you need to eliminate the offending food over a longer period to take into account the daily variations in a person's diet and lifestyle. This will enable you to see whether another unsuspected aspect of the diet or environment is the true offender and not the originally suspected food.

It's a good idea to have a Health Care Practitioner work with you to eliminate foods as you need to ensure that your nutritional and calorie needs are met for your lifestyle. There are other elimination diets that you may wish to talk to your Health Care Practitioner about which may suit your personal needs.

Eat right for your body

For digestive juices to flow well, it is recommended that you don't combine carbohydrates with proteins, or fruit with vegetables. This is because different digestive enzymes are required for each group of foods. These principles of food combinations have been used very successfully. However it's unrealistic for you to take a giant leap into the unknown world of food combining with the menus generally used in our society.

Try to have a meal in the evening containing protein with green and orange vegetables. Keep the starchy type vegetables to a minimum when you eat proteins.

You need to have some bitter herbals or a drink before you eat any meal that contains fatty acids, as you require bile to emulsify the fats in your small intestine. Also when you have carbohydrates, chew your food extra well because the digestive enzymes for this food group start their secretion in your mouth.

Realistically it's better to eat what you enjoy in moderation; however, it is good to have a focus with each meal. Keep one type of food in a smaller proportion to the others when you want to combine foods for healthier assimilation. For example, have a meaty meal with lots of green and orange vegetables and only a small amount of starchy foods. Or have a starchy pasta meal with only a small amount of protein added. Green and orange non-starchy vegetables including pumpkin can be eaten with both starchy and protein meals. These are also the foods that contain lots of antioxidants and phyto-chemicals, which are good for your health. So, eat up those greens!

Food combining isn't a strict law of eating, In fact nothing is. It's *your* Wellness Zone and you do exactly as you please. However, it's something to consider if you suffer from any gastric reflux, bloating, constipation, irritable bowel syndrome, digestive disturbances or pains in your stomach.

Digestive enzymes

These are essential for the digestion and eventual assimilation of all foods eaten. You only have a limited supply of digestive enzymes and as you get older digestion is one area that tends to suffer, if you are not eating foods in appropriate combinations for your body.

Raw foods contain many necessary enzymes. Pineapple and paw paw are both high in digestive enzymes and good to eat before meals. Try this lovely digestive mix to make and keep in the fridge at home to help with any digestive problems.

Paw paw digestive blend

Take one large paw paw and blend the whole fruit including the seeds, but excluding the skin. Now add 500 ml of good naturally fermented apple cider vinegar. Mix this formula well and take 5 to 15 ml plus water before the main meals of the day such as lunch and dinner.

Increase your digestive enzymes to help relieve inflammation

Increasing the digestive enzymes in your stomach and small intestine may be a good place to start if you are concerned about inflammatory conditions such as arthritis. This will allow your body to deal with food more effectively and hopefully help eliminate chronic acidity in the system. You also need to ensure you drink plenty of water and that your body weight is as close to healthy as possible. If you are within your Wellness Zone and you think that you need to lose some weight then do it, start today, because the fastest path to many illnesses and especially inflammatory illnesses is to be overweight.

If children have any of these conditions, then look at possible reasons as to why this has occurred. Obviously, their little bodies are not processing nutrients effectively and this may even be something as simple as gluten intolerance. Leave no stone unturned. Whenever there is inflammation present, the body is responding to something that doesn't belong there.

So, if there is wear and tear then you know the solution and you know how the problem occurred. But, if there is no wear and tear then you need to readdress your whole lifestyle and find the trigger that is constantly making the situation worse. Talk with your Health Care Practitioner and find the solution. This is *your* Wellness Zone and an over-acidic body with inflammatory pain certainly isn't comfortable!

Have the power to say no to bad food choices

Say *no*. Practice saying *no*. You see, it's easier in the long run for you to say *no* when you are confronted with bad food choices. A bad food choice is one that creates an after-effect on your body, mind and emotions; this would have been avoided had you avoided that food.

Examples are: bloating from wheat-based products, candida thrush from yeast and sugars, emotional upsets from alcohol and preservatives, stomach pains from MSG, hyperactivity from some additives, allergies and mucous from some dairy foods or wheat-based products and obesity. There are many responses we can have to different foods. It's a personal decision and your personal right to say *no* to bad food choices. A bad food choice is a food that you have decided doesn't agree with you for whatever reason. You do not have to justify this decision in today's world. You have the right and the personal responsibility to say *no* to whatever foods you don't want to eat.

The biggest reason young people should be encouraged to say *no* to bad food choices is because bad food habits lead to bad food diseases and obesity, and also malnutrition, coronary heart disease, diabetes and arthritis as well as many other problems associated with continued bad food choices. Often these selections are made through a lack of understanding or knowledge of what a good food choice is.

The Wellness Zone is your own personal zone. Just because your partner or friends choose to indulge in certain foods and beverages, doesn't mean you have to go along with their choices. Just because the advertising on television has persuaded your friend to order three pizzas for the price of one, doesn't mean you need to go along with their decision and eat the pizza too. You can usually create a nutritious meal for yourself, easily and conveniently, from what is available in your fridge, providing you make sure it's stocked with some healthy basics that are ready at hand.

Start simply with changing food choices

Make simple food choices and changes that will improve your Wellness Zone now. It's easy. Just add more fresh fruit and vegetables into your diet. Try to eat a few servings of raw fruit or vegetables each day. If you are already doing this then increase the amount. Eat a raw salad with lunch or dinner and some raw fruit with breakfast each day.

You may only need one serving of high carbohydrate foods such as bread, pasta, rice and cereals. Nuts and seeds can be added to your diet. Just add a tablespoon each of sesame seeds, pumpkin seeds, flax seeds and almonds to your diet each day.

Eat lots of brightly coloured vegetables. Good quality essential cold-pressed oils such as macadamia, olive, avocado and flaxseed. Quality apple cider vinegar, lemon juice and garlic are all great to use as dressings for hot or cold vegetables. Eat tofu and tempeh, soy milk and soy cheeses, also dairy products, especially fresh cheese and yoghurt daily.

Butter is better and full cream milk is an excellent nutritious drink. Meat is good, so is offal, chicken should be free range and so should eggs. Remember, fresh is best.

Try to always eat unprocessed foods and develop a joy in cooking. Cooking is easy. Eat three to five times a day. Chew your food well. Count to 20 at least. There's an old saying 'drink your food and chew your drinks!' Mmmm. Just a thought really. But you get the message here!

The best herbs for cooking are the ones you grow in your garden. Number one is parsley: chop it up and sprinkle it over everything. Learn to love garlic, mint and ginger. These can be the basis of most evening meals combined with fresh vegetables and protein. Be moderate in your intake of food, make each meal delicious and develop the taste for chilli, sea salt and Asian greens. You probably need about 1 gram of protein for each kilo of body weight per day. So for the average adult of 70 kilos, you could eat two eggs (10 grams each), two scoops of protein powder (10 grams each) and a piece of meat the size of the palm of your hand (which will be 20 to 30 grams of protein) per day.

The most important foods are fruit, vegetables, nuts and seeds. Coffee is actually good for your gall bladder. One good coffee a day is okay. More than three coffees a day can lead to too much acidity in your body as well as terrible headaches from withdrawal when you stop. Herbal teas are delicious, develop a taste for them as you will learn to appreciate the different varieties and health giving benefits of herbal infusions.

Don't skip meals, this decreases your metabolism and makes your body want to store fat.

Don't do all this at once. Take it easy and you can be as moderate or as strict as you like with your eating regime. Keep a food diary and you will see what you are eating and become aware of what choices you are making. This is your Wellness Zone. Nobody else wins or loses but you! So make it good.

Getting healthy is something we all need to address from time to time as we start to feel less buoyant. Herbs are best used for specific conditions and only for the time needed then stopped once you are well again. Sometimes you can take a dose of a nutrient and it will accelerate the healing process, other times you can unnecessarily take nutrients and they will just be eliminated with other waste products from your system. Balance your supplement intake with your diet.

Don't always believe what you see

The supermarket is like a fast-food franchise. The idea is to present the consumer with as many tempting choices as possible and then empty their purse in the process. Go to the supermarket for limited and specific choices. Visit your local markets on the weekend and buy fresh local foods, befriend the local butcher, baker and fruit seller. Find out if there are any vineyards, cheese factories or local producers in your district, get to know the area where you live and buy ethically and locally. It's fun to shop from people you befriend as they are supplying you with the freshest local foods which are always a more delicious choice. Mass produced food is often produced as cheaply as possible with the aim of satisfying the minimal requirements of the consumer whilst maximising the profit for producer, distributor and retailer along the trail of business.

When you consider buying a food from the grower directly, then you are ensuring your body gets the food in a very fresh format. This can result in better nutrition and health without the heavy transport, distribution and packaging costs involved in mass production. This is important energetically for the foods we eat. Because if you can put fresh local produce in your cooking and enjoy the fresh enzymes, vitamins, minerals and proteins, then you will have your body vibrating on a more energetic level and your cells will be happier because they are getting cleaner and better fuel. Also you will be happier because you can support your local community, the same community you rely on to support your business and family. It's give-and-take and reciprocated relationships that contribute to your Wellness Zone!

Bulk-buying makes good sense

What is grown in your local district that you are able to purchase in bulk? Buy food in bulk and preserve it for the off-season. There are some good books around on making preserves, from stewed cherries, peaches, apples and other fruit to tomato puree, salted lemons, pickled onions, garlic extract, ginger beer and other easily produced items. Purchasing goods in bulk is excellent for saving money and also saves on packaging. Your time too is saved, which will help you to relax more and allow extra time for other tasks.

Buy flour, honey, salt, vinegar, olive oil and whatever you use a lot of, in bulk a couple of times a year, instead of racing to the supermarket regularly and buying small amounts. This will probably cost you under half what the smaller quantities would cost. Get 20 litres of raw honey from the grower, you will then have a long-term supply of honey for a fraction of the cost. Nuts, seeds, herbs and spices, not only will you have these products at your disposal, but you will also find you spend your money on necessary and healthier choices in foods, because you will not be putting yourself in the tempting supermarket environment.

Make sure you buy soaps, dishwashing liquids, detergents, cleaning products, garbage bags, laundry needs and bathroom products, such as shampoos, conditioners, toilet paper and toothpastes, in bulk buys too. You may spend more money on the day, but you will be rewarded with only attending to these tasks twice a year instead of almost weekly. The only weekly purchases you will need to make are dairy products, some meats and protein choices and fresh fruit and vegetables that you don't grow or don't have preserved. This is a smart way to shop and a way to help you make healthier choices all round. It can be expensive to set up this system if you try to do it all at once.

Find a quality and reasonably priced catering supplier or community cooperative nearby, and start to buy one or two items each week until you have built up your stocks! There are internet buying groups you can join and some health food wholesalers are happy to sell to the public in bulk. Ask if they offer special deals or if they give a discount such as a '12 plus 1' on toothpaste, etc.

Herbal medicines can help digestive disturbances

Keep your digestion comfortable and you will find that your overall health will be better. Often the solution to simple problems can be found in your kitchen.

Carminatives

Herbs that relieve discomfort associated with digestion including colic and dyspepsia are called carminatives. You probably already have these on your spice rack at home. They are common everyday herbs used in cooking in many cultures. Add them to your meals at every opportunity. We all need good digestion, and this is the group of herbals that contribute most to this area. Carminatives contain essential oils (hence the delicious smells), as well as resins, flavonoids and tannins as their main active constituents.

Most carminatives are hot and warming remedies that stimulate your digestive process. The volatile constituents help release air pockets in the digestive tract, and this can relieve dyspepsia and strengthen digestion. Be careful to keep the warming herbs warm and not too hot, as the heat may overstimulate your system and exacerbate pre-existing problems.

Carminatives are useful for dyspepsia and flatulence, nausea and vomiting, ulcers, hiatus hernia, heartburn, diarrhoea, gastritis, gastroenteritis, colitis and other irritations of the digestive tract. It's best to get a personal extract made to suit your needs when you take therapeutic doses of these herbs. But, generally speaking, you are your own Health Care Practitioner every night when you cook up a treat in your kitchen adding these delicious and essential herbs to the menu.

Carminative herbs for your digestive tract include peppermint, fennel, aniseed, melissa, myrtle leaf, coriander, cinnamon, turmeric, garlic and ginger. Some aromatic constituents can be absorbed across the blood-brain barrier where they are able to influence central nervous response. This can happen when you inhale linalool, a monoterpene alcohol found in many aromatic herbs including coriander, as a central sedative, hypnotic and anti-convulsant. In contrast to most of the aromatic compounds present in these herbs, linalool is cooling, traditionally used for hot, inflamed digestive disorders. Coriander is delicious fresh from the garden in salads and pesto. A perfect summer accompaniment.

Astringent aromatics contain essential oils and these are helpful for people with loose bowels. Tannins are binding and tone your membranes. They can decrease leakage of large molecules across the intestine wall. This helps stop auto-intoxication and can limit allergic responses. Bitter herbals help relieve digestive discomfort through increasing the secretion of bile.

Antimicrobial actives in essential oils such as eugenol and citral can help reduce the uncomfortable effects of the bacteria *Helicobacter pylori*, which can be responsible for ulceration and common viruses that attack your digestive system.

Herbs that calm your digestive tract act in many ways including stomachic, spasmolytic, anti-inflammatory, digestive, stimulant, astringent and antiemetic. Take these herbs blended synergistically for maximum benefit. Appreciate the simplicity and availability of carminatives and incorporate them into most meals when you can. Many carminatives are also delicious as herbal infusions and can be taken as beverages regularly throughout the day.

Demulcents

Other herbs you may want to use to help with digestive disturbances are the demulcents. These protect and soothe irritated mucous membranes. This includes your digestive tract and lungs. They have a lubricating effect and in large doses act as a bulk laxative, while in small doses they help prevent diarrhoea. Demulcents soothe your system when you have had too much acidic food and also when you are combining foods badly. They can reduce your sensitivity to irritants and gastric acid, and relieve muscle spasms.

Demulcents maintain their soothing, anti-inflammatory nature when they are applied as creams to your skin. These demulcents have a physical effect on your digestive tract as the active molecules are quite large and won't readily absorb into your blood stream. Demulcents can have an effect on the kidneys and lungs via pathways in the digestive tract. One of the actions of demulcent herbs is to assist you in the excretion of unwanted waste and cholesterol by dislodging it from the walls of your small and large intestines and helping to eliminate it via your bowels.

Demulcents are also used in weight loss programmes as they can be bulk fillers, which are not able to be absorbed and carry little calorific weight. They are a great source of fibre with cleansing abilities that are soothing to your digestive tract. Demulcents can decrease absorption of nutrients and medications to your blood, so make sure you take other medicines at another time in the day when these fibres won't absorb all of the goodness from your medicines, leaving you with none!

The active constituents are polysaccharides, fixed oils, gums and mucilage. Demulcents are helpful when your mucous membranes are uncomfortable, ulcerated or irritated. This includes diarrhoea, constipation and irritable bowel syndrome.

Demulcents are also beneficial for respiratory tract infections, especially those repetitive coughs and raspy throats. You can also use them as topical applications for boils, inflammations and skin rashes.

Demulcent herbs that you can incorporate in your health programme are:

- Flaxseed with the added benefits of omega-3 fatty acids.
- Comfrey (for external use only) which is an excellent binder of any broken tissue.
- Aloe Vera (mixing this herb with probiotics seems to improve healing when this combination is taken last thing at night before sleep!)
- Slippery elm is probably the most popular demulcent and can be added to foods or for external poultices. You can mix the powder of slippery elm with turmeric for a traditional digestive tract healing salve: simply mix with warm water and drink. This salve lines the inside of your digestive tract allowing healing for ulcers and other disturbances.
- Marshmallow is a good all-round digestive tract healing and soothing herb that is added to many herbal tea blends for this reason.

Herbs are an important contributor to digestive system health and you can only benefit from having an open mind and the ability to self-diagnose where applicable. Talk to your Health Care Practitioner when you want digestive tract herbals.

Dietary choices

Each of us needs to look at our dietary choices every day. You must be very selective in what you eat. The criteria is simple, the food must be as fresh as possible. This means that it's better to eat fresh garden vegetables from your own garden than it is to eat three-week-old beans from another country!

Just take the freshest and most local choice in foods when you can. Be aware of where your food is coming from and try to eat it as close to its processing and harvesting time as possible.

Food must be recognisable, i.e. as unprocessed as possible. Keep your food real! Avoid canned, frozen and dried foods whenever there is a fresh option available. Making your sauces out of fresh tomatoes instead of puree or tinned tomatoes is a good example.

The food must be plant or animal based with the least possible amount of added toxicity. Eat organic when it's available or when you can afford this option.

Ask questions about the sprays used as pesticides and insecticides for the food choices you make. The residues from these toxins can easily find their way into your body where it is not easily removed.

Food must be prepared and processed in a hygienic and caring environment. Make sure foods are kept fresher in the fridge. Make sure you don't eat food prepared by people with viruses, illnesses or unhygienic behaviour, i.e. dirty hands, dirty pans, benches, etc. Also, never cook when you are upset or angry, not only does the recipe not work as well, but also those who eat the food will pick up the energy of the angry, upset cook and this will ensure the food is not as well assimilated or enjoyed! So, cook with love and care. Send happy vibrations to your meals!

Keep your salt and sugar down

Keep your intake of salt and sugar to a minimum. Where salt goes, water follows. This is simple. You will retain fluids if you have a high sodium diet. And where sugar goes, fat follows. So, make sure you keep the sugar out of your recipes, only add small amounts and be careful with both of these ingredients as they can become almost addictive.

Often, we can develop a sweet or salty tooth and don't realise that we are adding too much of either ingredient! If you do have a meal of processed foods or feel that you have overloaded your body with rich food and alcohol, take it easy the next day and you will find you can balance your body again.

It's also important not to be fanatical in your dietary choices and lifestyle. Who wants to go out to dinner with someone who has an extremely limited diet through self-choice and not medical necessity? Who wants to spend their life wandering about and refusing simple foods and pleasures because of some fad diet that is limiting their intake of some nutritious and soulful foods?

The energy of food

Food has energy. Whether it is animal or plant-based your food will carry the energy from its processing life and you will be influenced by this energy. Have you ever noticed that different foods affect you in different ways? You feel good after one food and you feel tired after another. Perhaps you bloat after some types of foods. Is your body saying it's had enough? Do you need to eat this food anymore? You are the only one who can tell how a food affects you. You can have someone else look at you, test you for allergies or diagnose a particular food group as being bad for you externally. You will probably already know this yourself, and often these tests are just confirmations.

One of the skills you need to develop to help you create and maintain your optimal Wellness Zone is to know how different foods affect your body and your emotions. Perhaps you lose concentration while doing mental tasks after eating certain foods. Perhaps you fall asleep quickly after some meals. Or maybe you just feel like everything is too much after some types of foods. This is your personal responsibility to yourself to find out what foods affect you and how! If you ate to feel good and energised, then you would probably have stronger immunity and your body would be thankful each day as you are leaping through life with an extra buoyancy. However the reverse can be true too. If you are eating non-energised foods that depress your emotions and that don't provide adequate nutrition to your body, then the natural result will be lowered immunity and therefore vulnerability to disease and lowered energy levels.

Keeping a food diary

There are two ways to keep a food diary. The first is obviously writing down what you eat and when you eat it. This is good as it brings to your awareness the daily choices you are making with foods and you will see patterns emerge over time. For example you may not have noticed some unconscious snacking. The amount and regularity of certain foods will become obvious to you as you note how much of each food group you eat and when you eat it.

If you are watching your body weight, recovering from illness, have specific allergies or just want to be conscious of how and what you eat, keep a food diary. All you need is a note pad or your regular diary, write down what you eat and when you eat it. Then if you do notice energy changes or any illnesses, you can refer back to your food diary and see what may have been the culprit. You can even keep a record of your responses and energy levels after meals for a few weeks; this way you will know what foods are positive for your energy levels and what foods may contribute to extra stress in your day!

The second way to keep a food diary is to just write down what foods you have eaten when you have an energy shift; do this for the last two meals or so. This way you are not technically keeping a strict food diary, you are noting responses and energy shifts in your life and seeing whether there is an association to the foods you have been eating. It gets pretty obvious when a food is the culprit of your energy shifts; when consistently the same foods are provoking the same responses. As long as you are conscious of your Wellness Zone and able to recognise what foods to avoid, what foods not to avoid and what your personal threshold to any food is, then you can keep your food diary either way.

Get rid of parasites regularly

Parasites find their way into your body when you are in a foreign environment, or when you are exposed to filthy food processing in restaurants and cafes, or when you drink water, or even when you pat your friend's pooch. Parasites can be sitting waiting for you in public toilets, on park benches, train and bus seats and even on that window with the lovely view. The more you travel, the more exposure you will have to different parasites. You will be continuously exposed to parasites throughout life and you need to regularly take a cleanse to ensure that you are able to keep them at bay and eliminate them as much as possible. Parasites can become lodged in your digestive tract where they excrete their poisons making you sick with auto-intoxication as you reabsorb nutrients back into your system. One sure sign of parasites is an itchy anus. Otherwise there are often no signs at all. Sometimes you may find that parasites create illness and digestive disturbances and these can be eliminated over time. Parasites are dangerous because they can leak through your small intestine into your liver and travel to other organs from there. Yes, parasites can infuse into your whole body. One herb that gets rid of parasites when they are in your organs is black walnut hulls in extract form taken in very small doses for a long period of time. This can be taken for a year or longer. Other herbs for parasites include pumpkin seeds eaten regularly with meals, garlic, mugwort, Chinese wormwood and standard wormwood.

If you have a herbal extract of black walnut and Chinese wormwood in equal parts (a 1:2 extract), you will need to take a teaspoon of the formula mixed with a little water every night before bed for three weeks. Do this at the beginning of each season: winter, spring, summer and autumn. This is a good way to help eliminate parasites and protect your body. Children can be given half this amount if they are less than 40 kilos. Grapefruit seed extract is an excellent herb to help eliminate parasites and this can also be taken at night before bed for three weeks as described above for the other herbs. You will need 5 ml of grapefruit seed extract a day.

Tape worms are not common in many places. However they are difficult to eliminate as they can grow very long. If you have tape worms take the formula as above, but keep taking it for three months. You will also find that if you sit on a large bowl of warm milk directly after a complete bowel movement, the tape worm may come out naturally; they tend to go along with the warmth of the bowel and can be eliminated this way so long as they are able to stay in liquid such as the milk.

Ring worms can be eliminated with the use of olive leaf extract or tea tree oil as well as the herbs taken internally daily. You will need to have a good blood cleansing programme to eliminate ring worms and keep them away. You can put yourself on a parasite cleanse regularly for preventative health.

Prebiotics and probiotics

Prebiotics and probiotics are important additions to the diets of people suffering from: impaired immunity function, *Candida albicans*, high lipoprotein levels of low-density lipoprotein (LDL) cholesterol or other serious health conditions that are indicated by compromised digestion, weakness, chronic fatigue and general debilitation.

'Good' bacteria belong in our body. They are naturally occurring and help to keep us in peak physical condition. However, when we ingest other bacteria that are not so good for our body, we can open the way to ill health. There are times when we are exposed to the stripping of natural microflorae that naturally inhabit our system. These times are when we take antibiotics medicinally, or when we eat foods that have been treated with antibiotics to create weak spots in our own natural microbiome.

Microflora sites in our body

Microflora occurs in our skin in the form of fungi where the area is moist and warm. The oral and upper respiratory tract is home to many bacteria that inhabit the space between the teeth and gums. The pharynx can be inhabited by *Neisseria*, *Bordetella*, *Corynebacterium* and *Streptococcus*. Your urogenital system can be invaded by transient organisms such as candida. Conjunctiva flora includes the invasion of haemophilias and staphylococcus which can be very dangerous and has caused blindness in outback populations in Australia. Our gastrointestinal tract harbours transient, unfriendly bacteria, such as *Helicobacter pylori*, which research has shown to be a precursor of ulceration in the stomach and duodenum. The small intestine is not heavily populated with bacteria. The large intestine is home to our natural bacteria, such as acidophilus and the bifi-dobacteria, which need to stay in strong quantities to keep the baddies at bay as they pass through our body in the normal excretion processes.

The natural organisms that occur in our body are balanced. Healthy people will have mature, diverse and specific microflorae occupying little niches within the different systems of their body where they are required. For example, colonisation is found in the crypts of some organisms whilst others are found on the epithelial tissue of the villi. Some micro-organisms, such as filamentous, are found in very specific sites, such as columnar epithelium, in the small intestine.

How to use prebiotics and probiotics for good health

Remember that our body's environment will change according to diet, disease, environmental toxicity, environmental climate changes and exposure to pathogens that we are not normally exposed to. For example, drinking water in another country, food cooked or grown a certain way, or the contamination of food by filthy cooking procedures. There are many and varied ways that we require the addition of prebiotics and probiotics to our diet.

Prebiotics are taken in our diet in the form of foods that have undergone a specific fermentation process. This leads to their eventual role as micro-organisms in our bodies where they act as a macrophage to other unfriendly bacteria. They can also act as a non-digestible food ingredient that will affect the host (you) by selectively targeting the growth and activity of 'good bacteria'. They have the effect of improving your health by supporting the friendly bacteria and assisting in the growth of their population.

Fructose in a good example because it contains oligosaccharides that have the potential to stimulate bifidobacteria in the colon. Foods that can act as prebiotics in our bodies are chicory, onion, garlic, asparagus, artichoke, cabbage and bananas.

Probiotics are either a mono or mixed culture of live micro-organisms which, when taken internally, improve the properties of the indigenous microflorae. Probiotics contain live micro-organisms usually as freeze-dried cells or in a fermented product.

The most important reason for using probiotics is that they influence the good and naturally occurring microflora, resulting in the formation and reconstruction of a well-balanced system. You would consider the addition of probiotics in your diet when you are concerned that your system is out of balance and requires restoring to optimal health again.

Probiotics are known to reduce the production of carcinogens and inhibit the growth of many unfriendly bacteria. They are also reputed to help maintain optimum pH, reduce putrefaction and endotoxemia, assist with the body's self-healing mechanisms in cancer of the bladder and colon, assist with urinary tract infections (*Candida*) and are beneficial in post antibiotic therapy to restore the natural balance. Probiotics are handy when travelling to help with diarrhoea and the maintenance of normal intestinal floras.

Probiotics are available in many and varied ways. You can purchase off the shelf a dose of up to 25 billion cells of acidophilus and bifidobacteria. This is a very high dose and you can take it for post antibiotic recovery and immune system dysfunction. You will need to store this product between 2–8° Celsius in most cases, however there are some freeze-dried varieties available.

The old-fashioned and natural way to take probiotics is in the form of fresh unprocessed dairy foods, such as yoghurt and milk. Unfortunately because of tuberculosis we are unable to purchase fresh raw cow's milk, but you can still purchase goat's milk. Possibly the best way to take probiotics naturally is with yoghurt. In acute cases, however, you may need to take commercial capsules of probiotics to fast-track the restoration of healthy microflorae, such as in the case of antibiotic consumption.

Allergies

Clear your allergy now and avoid future chronic illness

Do you have an uncomfortable allergic reaction when exposed to supposedly normal environmental and dietary substances?

If you answered yes, you're not alone. Almost everyone has some kind of allergic response to a food, chemical or environmental influence. Allergies are getting very specific and very complicated. This can be confusing and the current methods of testing for allergies are not always accurate. The best way to ascertain your susceptibility to an allergen is to test your own response via elimination and time-consuming independent testing. However, anyone can do this elimination testing if committed to improving their health and living an allergy free life. It's fairly simple. If you know that you are allergic to something specific, then stay away from it as much as possible. If you are in a situation where you are forced to face this allergen, take precautions before and after to prevent or minimalise the negative effects on your body.

We live in a toxic world; our bodies are more congested and stressed than ever before. We have so many technological advances at our disposal, and some of these are clearly carcinogenic. So, what are the long-term effects on health and wellness?

The logical progression from repeated allergen exposure leads to compromise and inefficient physiology if the allergy is not eliminated from the body at the earliest opportunity. There are many illnesses that arise from allergic responses, and these include many auto-immune diseases, respiratory problems, cancer, *Candida albicans*, fatty liver, heart and circulatory failures, hormonal problems, attention disorders, migraines, arthritis, digestive disturbances, mental depressions and degenerative diseases.

The best help you give yourself as an allergy sufferer is to become responsible for your own healing process. There are certain genetically predisposed allergic conditions that are a serious threat to life if not diagnosed and treated. Visit your Health Care Practitioner and ask to be tested if you think your illness is based on a genetic allergic condition. You need to know what the triggers are to allergic response.

Keep your children well

All too often parents ignore simple allergic responses in children and then wonder why their child suffers from serious or multiple illnesses? Did you know that autism has a direct link to coeliac disease? Did you also know that attention deficit disorders could be related to the non-absorption of essential fatty acids and nutrients through the digestive tract, stopping these nutrients from reaching the brain? Many behavioural problems in children are caused because their tiny bodies cannot cope with the onslaught of preservatives, additives and artificial foods?

Allergies in children are all too common. Asthma is becoming very prevalent and many children become slow with school work and focusing ability when they are placed on medication. This could well be avoided with some clear observations and actions from vigilant parents. The simple act of moving your pets outside can have a beneficial effect on allergic children. Even keeping cleaning products well out of their range of smell can help your children to stay more healthy.

The earlier you address the symptoms of allergy and eliminate the offending items from the environment and diet, the sooner your child will be on the road to health. However if the symptoms are ignored it can lead to multiple medications. Other problems can develop into chronic illnesses. The herbs for children are basically the same as adults, except of course you need to control the doses according to body size and condition.

Elderberry is a good herb of choice for children, combined with vitamin C and some good immune boosting herbs, such as echinacea and garlic, and also reishi mushroom for added protection. Horseradish and white horehound are excellent for upper respiratory responses. Olive leaf is wonderfully gentle and a powerful antimicrobial, alterative and strengthener. If you are confident the child does not suffer from any seafood allergies, then give them omega-3 fish oil, otherwise flaxseed oil will work well to help reduce bronchial constrictions and enhance optimal metabolism.

Even very young babies can show signs of allergic reaction. Take note of these and visit your Health Care Practitioner for some support and assistance with appropriate herbs and dietary adjustments. Asthma and eczema can be treated naturally in the early stages to avoid a childhood plagued with medications and complications. Prevention is still the best medicine.

Is my allergy acute or chronic?

If you are suffering from airborne allergic reactions, they are mostly acute and you can usually pinpoint the offending substance fairly easily. Choose from herbs and supplements to help you recover from the acute situation. You may need to experiment with quantities and different combinations to get the right mix to help you quickly overcome an allergic response. Lighten the digestive load on your body and rest as often as possible. These types of allergic responses are often centred on our respiratory tract and you will need to take appropriate natural medicines targeted for this area. These are not damaging on your long-term health and pass relatively quickly, so long as you are sensible and avoid future exposure. Acute allergic responses to plants and environmental exposure need to be addressed quickly so that you do not develop further problems.

The dangerous allergies are the ones that are not so obvious and can become chronic, slowly building up toxicity in your body. These are the allergies that can lead to debilitating and even life-threatening diseases, as your body is no longer able to function optimally. To work out the cause of these chronic allergies, you will need to eliminate foods and slowly reintroduce items. You will also need to explore your environment and decide if carpets, bedding, pets, body products, clothing, air conditioning etc are to blame for your continued discomfort. This detective work, though time-consuming, is certainly worth the effort.

What's making you sick?

Look at every food you eat, every medication or perfume you use and every place you go. Find out what is triggering your allergies and then use the best of natural remedies, orthodox medicines and alternative practices to eliminate the problem. Carry a notebook and keep a record of foods eaten, places visited and times of day, etc. Then if you have an allergic response, look back in the notebook and see if there are any past connections.

Once you stop a certain action that leads to the allergy, your body may respond with withdrawal symptoms and crave the substance that causes the response. Once you have resisted going back to the old habit, your body will clear itself and hopefully you will no longer have to deal with the allergy, unless you are exposed to the allergen again. This can be as simple as being allergic to the toxins in nail polish, or perhaps a preservative in a certain food that you have always enjoyed.

Our body produces mucous as a response to pathogens entering it that are considered obtrusive. If we keep taking in these pathogens that are causing our allergy, we will continue to make more and more mucous. Mucous is insidious stuff. It is in your head cavity, your torso and your digestive tract, filtering to your organs. It can build up and form thick black straps of old mucous in your large intestine.

Allergic bodies often have so much mucous that they can feel extremely bloated. The only way to stop this cycle is to eliminate the problem. You will need to control your diet with a very restricted intake of food, you will also need to take herbs and supplements that deal specifically with the body systems that are affected by your particular allergies. Remember that if inflammation is left unchecked, it can cause havoc with your entire system.

Elimination diet is the key to healing allergies

Whenever there is a problem with allergies you can never ignore elimination and cleansing of your liver as the first step to recovery and good health. Always cleanse your elimination organs. This involves lungs, liver, kidneys, large intestine and skin. Eliminate excess mucous as quickly as possible. This is where old-fashioned lemon and honey comes in handy.

Lemon and honey drink

Take the juice of one lemon and squeeze into cup. Place in one small teaspoon of honey. Fill cup up with water. Hot for a hot drink and cold for a chilled version

Drink these three times daily. Lemon juice is excellent to help eliminate uric and lactic acid from your system as well as breaking down mucous and helping it to leave your body. Lemon juice also works to cleanse your liver and kidneys, balance hydrochloric acid secretions, tone your lungs and generally help your body operate effectively as a complete system. Apple cider vinegar can also be used for the same purpose, depending upon your taste and the seasonal availability of lemons.

Use milk thistle and dandelion for liver cleansing, gall bladder toning and kidney function. Parsley root is good for kidney function, pau d'Arco for eliminating internal pathogens and sheep sorrel for cellular health. Acidophilus powder and aloe vera both assist with digestive ailments. Support your adrenals with homeopathic DHEA tablets (available at most health food stores) and omega-3 and omega-6 fatty acids are necessary to optimise the healing.

Add loads of garlic to your cooking, along with capsicum pepper and ginger root as the main spices added to at least one meal per day.

This will stimulate the cleansing and elimination programme, ridding your body of allergens as quickly as possible. Take fibre in the form of rice bran or oat bran to clear the digestive tract. If you visit a Health Care Practitioner, they can design your elimination diet individually, depending upon every aspect of your lifestyle. Many elimination diets contain lemon juice or apple cider vinegar and beetroot which is a fabulous blood cleanser and really helps get rid of any nastiness in your system. Just remember that you need to complement medications with a health regime and consult a Health Care Practitioner who is supportive of nutritional and natural medicines if you are taking medications.

Juices are a great kick-start for your elimination programme. Salads, stir-fry vegetables and pots of vegetable soup are also a good starting point depending upon your desired outcome and health status.

It's easier to put yourself on a strict elimination diet and rebuild your body now while you are suffering an allergic response, than to ignore the problems and face deeper illness later in life. You may be busy or stressed, but what if you lose the health you enjoy altogether and find yourself with a debilitating condition that involves 100% of your attention? Allergy elimination doesn't stop you from getting up in the morning and getting on with your life. In fact after a few weeks of a strict diet, exercise programme and herbal and nutritional support you may feel lighter and healthier than you have in years. You may find that you are able to reintroduce certain foods into your diet that you were unable to eat before.

Elimination involves eating fresh, unprocessed foods. These should be eaten in specific combinations and quantities depending upon what you are trying to achieve. You will find that certain food groups will be introduced at different stages of the diet to trigger responses from your body. A good elimination diet will result in you feeling energised and aware of the foods you are unable to consume due to allergic response.

Be strong and fight off future allergic responses

Often the immune system is so compromised from years of over reactions, it can lead to further illnesses. So the importance of building your immunity is paramount. Once we have the elimination organs working well we need to boost and protect the immunity. This is done by a super strong dose of astragalus and cat's claw. Add some red clover as this is an alterative herb and will target the area that needs help. Maritime pine is wonderful at this time as it helps you feel strong, especially if you are run down from dealing with your allergy. Then of course the homeopathic DHEA for adrenal support, hormonal balancing and the feeling of well-being that DHEA offers.

Add some homeopathic melatonin to the programme if you're having difficulty sleeping under a load of external stress or generally not dreaming. Melatonin is a hormone secreted from the pineal gland and controls the night and day responses. It's interesting to note that when a body is out of sync from chronic allergic responses, they often don't have clear vivid dreams and can feel out of time with themselves. Melatonin helps put this all back in balance.

Andrographis is another herb that has broad spectrum immune boosting effects and antimicrobial effects. Gotu kola has been used in Chinese medicine for centuries as a venous decongestant, anti-inflammatory and immune support herb, and liquorice root is good generally for all allergic and immune compromised conditions.

However you would do well to talk with someone and get the right combination of herbs and supplements for you. Some herbs will not help your allergic reaction and can even make it worse. Herbs that come from the flower of the plant or other aerial parts that are picked at certain times of the year are best avoided if you have an allergic response to them. Talk with your practitioner about what herbs come from various parts of the plant and how they can benefit or hinder your healing from allergies.

Are your hormones triggering your allergic responses?

For women especially, hormones can play a monthly cyclic role in allergy responses. You are more susceptible to allergies for the first week of your menstrual cycle then as you reach ovulation you are at your strongest and have a decreased response. From there the response will increase again until you are at the lowest ebb at the beginning of your cycle again. The herbs for this hormonal fluctuation are adjusted to the hormonal cycle depending on the specifics of your symptoms. Always remember to take hormonal balancing herbs in therapeutic doses. Too often people take small amounts of herbs and wonder why they are not getting results. You need to take adequate amounts of the right herbs for your situation in the right doses depending on the symptoms, your body weight and the situation.

It can get rather complicated with hormonal herbs, as the cycle changes for your body so your programme needs to take this into account. The hormones that may be related to your allergic response are in your thyroid, adrenal and gonadal glands, these can lead to exhaustion and the natural follow-on of more chronic allergic reactions.

Stress levels can also be triggers to allergens

If you are under stress, your body will respond to allergens more than usual. There is the psychosomatic factor whereby, if you are feeling on top of the world then you may be able to blow off the occasional allergic response quickly, whereas if you are down in the dumps then you may respond excessively. This relates to emotions as well as mental stressors. If you are experiencing high stress levels, then increase your intake of omega-3 fatty acids in the form of fish or flaxseed oils. Increase your omega-6 fatty acids with spirulina or evening primrose oil (take omega-3 and omega-6 in 2:1 ratio, i.e. two parts omega-3 and one part omega-6). Get lots of sleep, and take DHEA and melatonin along with some good B group vitamins and possibly the herb hypericum.

Use flower remedies to help decrease the stress on your mind and emotions. Flower essences can be mixed specifically for your needs and often in combination. Be aware of your personal stressors and the role of specific herbs and nutrients to ensure that allergens have less effect on your body. Of course stress needs to be addressed on all levels as it may be a big contributor to your allergies. If so, slow down and change your lifestyle. Long-term health is more important than the stressed life that makes you sick.

Get positive in attitude and you will get healthy

Basically, following an elimination diet followed by boosting your body with immune support is the best approach to eliminating allergic responses. You need to be aware of what you are allergic to. Talk to your Health Care Practitioner if you think that a medication is having a negative effect and may be a trigger to an allergic response. See if this medication can be eliminated or changed to one that you do not have a response to.

Ask your practitioner to mix you the appropriate natural herbs and offer you supplements that will help you minimalise responses. It can take between six months and two years before you are cleared of an allergy and its associated response. Be patient, be kind to yourself and be vigilant about what is triggering your allergies.

Gluten intolerance

Allergies come in all shapes and forms. Often what we eat is the biggest culprit, creating havoc with body processes and leading to degenerative conditions. Gluten intolerance is becoming more prevalent in today's society. This could be because a lot of commercial foods are based on wheat products which we tend to consume a great deal of. It can also be a genetic predisposition which can start at any age from infancy onwards. Whatever the cause, gluten intolerance doesn't mean you need to miss out on the good things in life. This is one condition that is completely controlled by the foods you consume. If you have a complete intolerance, known as coeliac condition, then you will be able to heal your body and monitor your diet to ensure that good health is a close ally.

What is gluten intolerance?

Basically it is an allergy to gliadin, which is a component in gluten. Gluten is the protein found in wheat, barley, rye and suspected in oats. If you have this intolerance then you will have a negative allergic response when you eat these foods. You will have an abnormal immune response and may experience symptoms such as abdominal bloating, pains in the small intestine several hours after eating, constipation, diarrhoea, dark circles under the eyes, high fevers, fluid retention or auto-immune conditions, such as arthritis, thyroiditis and liver disease. You may also feel tired and below par much of the time such as with chronic fatigue syndrome.

Other problems experienced by people with gluten intolerance are: anaemia, dermatitis, weight loss, down's syndrome, epilepsy and hypersplenism. Also, some forms of digestive tract cancers have been suspected to be undiagnosed coeliac. These responses are diverse and vary between people. Sometimes the response is acute and you feel it soon after eating the alleged allergen, other times the response can be chronic and builds up in severity over time.

Gluten intolerance, as such, is a localised digestive tract disorder if diagnosed and responded to quickly. However it can become degenerative and extremely damaging to your whole body if left untreated by dietary changes.

There are various levels of gluten intolerance, the most severe being coeliac condition, which is a complete intolerance to gluten. We all have our individual threshold to gluten tolerance. If you have a genetic pre-disposition to coeliac condition then it's best to get the antigliadin IgA blood test that will show whether you are creating antibodies in your system to deal with gluten. It will show the levels of antigliadin anti-body (AGA) and endomysial antibody (EMA).

However, this test alone is not enough; you should really also have a small bowel biopsy which will determine the exact extent of the problem. The biopsy will show characteristic changes in the duodenum, includ-ing flattening or loss of villi and increased numbers of lymphocytes in the epithelium. This test is best done at the initial stages of suspicion regarding gluten intolerance. This is because if you put someone on a gluten-free diet, the tests may not be accurate. With very small children who have a clear genetic background for coeliac condition the biopsy is often not carried out and the blood tests are considered enough of a positive indicator of the condition. As a parent it can often be difficult to allow an undernourished and sickly child to undergo general antisep-tics when you are fairly confident of the problem. However, whatever age you are, discuss the situation with your Health Care Professional and act on your intuition and the information given.

If you have a predisposition then you may likely have a lesser degree of intolerance to gluten. Even if you don't have a genetic predisposition to coeliac, you may well have developed a threshold of tolerance to gluten. During and after menopause, women can experience intoler-ance to gluten that didn't exist in the past. They often find that bloating and fluid retention symptoms are reduced when they take gluten out of their diet.

At other times you may notice an intolerance to gluten when you are eating a regular diet containing breads, pastas and wheat products. You may feel lethargic and have dark circles under your eyes, then almost miraculously after a week or so on a gluten-free diet these symptoms disappear. Conditions such as this are called non-coeliac gluten intoler-ance and characterised by the fermentation of wheat starch in the small intestine. This can be caused by bad food combining. Gluten intol-erance can just develop over time without any specific trigger or predisposition.

What to do if you are gluten intolerant?

The first and best step is to get tested. This is because you don't want to be subjected to strict life-long eating patterns without necessity. If you find that you suffer from non-coeliac gluten intolerance then you can safely eliminate gluten foods from your diet, knowing that from time to time you can break the rules and consume small amounts of gluten without severe side effects. This means that if you eat the occasional slice of wheat bread, the results are not earth-shattering and you will recover within a few days. However if you do have coeliac condition then you must walk the straight and narrow and only consume gluten-free foods. This is basically the only solution and for coeliac condition. No wheat, no rye, no barley, and at this stage in history no oats. Oats are controversial at the moment and more research needs to be completed before it is conclusively okay to eat oats.

When you consider foods that are commercial, you will need to stay away from malt extract (although some say that maltodextrin is okay), you will also need to stay away from all '1400' starches except '1412' and '1422' which are maize derived. No beer, unless you can find a gluten-free beer. You will need to check labels vigilantly as even a minute dose of gluten will trigger the condition; it has a homeopathic effect and causes a response very quickly as the body is so sensitive to this allergen. MSG '621', '623' and '628' are also baddies to be avoided at all costs.

You must remain positive and be thankful that good health is entirely controlled by the foods you consume. There are no orthodox Western medicines that target this condition, but there are herbs and natural medicines you can consume to help heal your body and re-energise yourself.

What foods are gluten-free and where do you get them?

Bread and pasta made from rice, corn (maize) and potato make up the mainstay of your cereals. There are gluten-free bread mixes available that make good substitutes to wheat, for cakes, biscuits and many other traditional wheat products. Most good health food shops and some supermarkets stock a variety of these foods which are reasonably priced and tasty.

The hardest thing for people with gluten intolerance is to be prepared with travel foods wherever you go. You need to be organised and have a handy substitute snack or bar ready in case you are unable to purchase gluten-free foods when you go out. Most restaurants and cafes are switched-on these days and provide gluten-free options on their menus. People living on a good gluten-free diet often get frustrated that more cakes and delicious pies are not made with gluten-free flours as it is a simple exchange when cooking.

The good part of gluten intolerance is that it only affects the cereals you eat. All other unprocessed foods consumed are gluten-free. However it is a case of consistently checking with chefs, packaging and menus to ensure you are getting gluten-free foods.

Always ask to see the packaging of any processed foods as even chips and ice creams can contain gluten. Often the oil that fish and chips are cooked in can be contaminated with the batter from fish which is easily attached to the chips and can cause a rapid response in a sensitive person. Lard, used as a frying medium, tends to create this response from deep frying more than plant derived frying oils. (Just check when you order deep-fried foods.)

Herbs to help heal and lifestyle choices

Many people thrive on green chlorophyll, alfalfa and spirulina. There tends to be extra acidity in the system of chronic gluten intolerant sufferers and acidity needs to be removed. So, you would consider having a clear alkaline forming diet that is made up of mostly fresh fruit and vegetables.

Because there has been a malabsorption of foods through the small intestine for a long period of time you will definitely need to look at iron supplements and folic acid. Also, a strong and easily absorbed multi-vitamin is necessary. Nettle and withania are two good herbs for this condition as nettle is good for iron and withania is indicated for any debilitated state. If you are low in energy then Siberian ginseng and red clover can be combined with other boosting herbs.

One of the best herbs for gluten intolerance is aloe vera combined with the bifidobacteria and acidophilus friendly bacteria. You will possibly need a complete healing of the digestive tract and here you will need to consider herbs such as slippery elm and all the regular digestive tract herbs used for restoring the whole system back to optimal functioning. Add in some ganoderma mushroom to help reduce autoimmune markers.

Often juices, soups and light foods are recommended for a few months until the healing process is well under way. However you need to talk with your Health Care Practitioner about this and get an eating plan that will suit your lifestyle. You may wish to visit your nutritionist, dietitian, local pharmacist or Health Care Practitioner to discuss your eating plan. But the bottom line rule for coeliac condition is that you cannot ever eat foods containing gliadin. There is no other option if you want to heal.

There used to be a misunderstanding that you grow out of the condition and that you will be able to go back to normal wheat-based diet after a period of time. This is not true. Once diagnosed with coeliac you will have to stay on a gluten-free diet for life. If you revert to a wheat-based diet the symptoms may not become apparent for a period of time whilst your body is degenerating again. This means that you gradually become sicker and the chances of these degenerative chronic conditions associated with coeliac will become extremely high for you. The result, is always having to return to a gluten-free diet and recovering your health and energy again.

If you are worried about gluten intolerance then try an elimination diet for a few weeks and see how you feel. If you suspect that you have gluten intolerance then reintroduce wheat to your diet again and get tested. It's amazing how good you can feel on a non-allergenic gluten-free diet. No more drowsiness and no more exhaustion experienced by an overloaded, overreactive system.

Diabetes

Diabetes is another rapidly growing health epidemic. Studies indicate that for every person diagnosed, there is another person out there suffering from undiagnosed diabetes type 2. You can avoid diabetes and you can balance your blood sugar levels with herbs and nutritional supplements.

What is diabetes?

Diabetes is a metabolic disorder whereby you are not producing a sufficient balance of the hormones in your pancreas. These hormones are insulin and glucagon. These two hormones regulate sugar and fat metabolism. With diabetes, insulin is the hormone in trouble. It's required to carry glucose into your cells as fuel for your body, and when you have too much or too little sugar in your blood at any given time you may suffer from many metabolic diseases and energy fluctuations.

Diabetes is basically categorised into two types. 'Type 1', which is insulin dependent diabetes. Juvenile onset is when your pancreas beta cells do not produce insulin at all and you are required to replace this insulin constantly with each intake of food. This accounts for a little over 10% of diabetics. It is a condition commonly starting in early childhood and unfortunately requires ongoing replacement of insulin for life.

The other 90% of diabetics suffer from 'Type 2', also known as diabetes mellitus, where the beta cells in the pancreas are unable to produce sufficient amounts of insulin for your body's needs. This is also called metabolic resistant and late onset diabetes and is an escalating problem in our society. With 'Type 2' diabetes, you produce small amounts of insulin. However you need to find a healthy solution to prevent the escalating series of illnesses and side effects that tend to occur when this form of diabetes is not held in check.

The research shows that people with diabetes are three times more likely to die of cardiovascular disease than non-diabetics. Diabetes can cause kidney disease which may result in renal failure. Diabetes can cause neuropathy from the damage done to nerve cells following continually high levels of blood glucose. The retina of your eyes can also be damaged resulting in diabetic retinopathy which can result in blindness. Also diabetics often tend to be overweight and suffer from syndrome X because of the insistence of insulin to store fat instead of burning it.

Self-help for diabetes

'Type 2' Diabetes does not occur naturally when your body is in an ideal environment and your diet is nutritionally sound and meeting your requirements. Diabetes often occurs from over-consumption and under-nutrition, whereby you are not taking your body's needs into account naturally. This means that although you may think you are eating well, there is obviously an imbalance between what your body was genetically designed to do and what it is trying to deal with. This is a direct result of the environment we live in which is helping to create this diabetes epidemic.

If you look at many indigenous societies who have been introduced to the Western model of eating, then you will see that the change to white sugar, white flour, processed foods and alcohol is definitely an influencing factor to the greater incidence of diabetes.

'Type 2' Diabetes is another way for your body to say that it is out of balance and needs realigning. This can be done with changes to your environment and your dietary choices. You may need to readjust the way you think about food, you may need to take nutritional supplements and you may need to alter the way you relate to stresses and other environmental factors that could be contributing to the condition.

'Type 2' Diabetes is diagnosed after fasting for 12 hours, then blood sugar levels are measured. You can do this yourself initially with a prick test kit available from your local pharmacy. Please visit your Health Care Practitioner to discuss the situation and get them to test you again to confirm the diagnosis if diabetes is suspected. Many people get worried and upset when they suspect they have diabetes. Try to stay calm and know that it is a metabolic imbalance and that with the right care you will be able to rebalance your system again. However, be warned that with the wrong diet and continued negligence of your body's needs then the situation can worsen.

Many people who start out with a simple metabolic imbalance make the situation far worse for themselves by only adhering to medical procedures and not making the necessary shifts in perception that they need to create wellness. The biggest precursor to 'Type 2' diabetes is diet and lifestyle practices. Drugs are available to help you. However, success has been found with herbal medicine and dietary changes that can assist you in maintaining normal levels of blood glucose thereby avoiding the nasty effects of diabetes. Work closely with your Health Care Practitioner and ensure you monitor blood glucose levels regularly.

Diabetics need to keep their glucagon (fat burning hormone) levels up and their insulin (fat storing hormone) levels down within the pancreas to avoid diabetic weight gain. As with all metabolic disorders, always make sure your liver is kept in good health. Drink lemon or carrot juice and water, and eat a good raw food diet. Keep your food as simple and unprocessed as possible. Avoid all refined sugars and foods that are fast burners in your body.

Many people are able to keep diabetes 'Type 2' under control through diet, attitude, lifestyle choices and the use of magnesium, essential fatty acids, chromium and herbs.

The best herbs for balancing blood sugar levels

Bitter melon

This is one of the longest standing herbs for the treatment of diabetes. The fruit and seeds can both be used fresh and in foods. Studies of the extract from the unripe fruit of bitter melon have been shown to reduce blood glucose levels for 'Type 1' and 'Type 2' diabetes. It has also been shown to reduce the after-mealtime increase in blood sugar by as much as 50%. If you live in an area where the bitter melon grows, the fresh juice is best taken just before meals.

Bitter melon juice

Simply extract the bitter melon juice and mix 200 ml with 200 ml of fresh aloe vera juice. Keep in the fridge and sip 30 ml before meals.

Gurmar

Gurmar is also known as gymnema. In Indian medicine this herb is known to destroy the desire and taste for sugar, and it has been used as a herbal mainstay remedy by chewing the leaves to decrease the sensitivity of taste buds to sweet tastes. This is the perfect herb to get rid of your sweet tooth! The effect lasts for several hours. The extract is also known to decrease your appetite.

The active gymnemic acids help improve the function of pancreatic beta cells enabling the body to be more efficient at making insulin. Research has shown that gymnema may also decrease glucose absorption from food and improve the ability of the body to use glucose for energy.

Gymnema has been shown to work on 'Type 1' and 'Type 2' diabetes. There are no toxic side effects known to this herb. Take 2 to 5 ml of the extract before each meal depending upon your weight and type of diabetes. Talk with your Health Care Practitioner and ensure you monitor your blood glucose levels before and after meals to ensure you are taking the correct dose.

Bilberry

An old favourite, bilberry is also on the list of best herbs for diabetes. This time we extract the leaf as it contains chromium, which is excellent to help with the uptake of glucose into the blood stream. Chromium is a vital factor in the glucose tolerance factor which assists with improved insulin function. If you are deficient in chromium then you are likely to have difficulty regulating blood sugar levels. The signs of chromium deficiency are: anxiety, fatigue, sugar cravings, excess hunger, glucose intolerance and high cholesterol levels.

If you take the extract of bilberry berries combined with the leaves, then you can ensure that you are also getting the antioxidant and cardiovascular strengthening properties. The actives in bilberry also help to decrease retinal problems and cataracts that are often associated with diabetes.

You may lose weight when taking a herbal combination for diabetes that contains the leaf extract of bilberry. Like other diabetic herbal solutions, this one tends to curb your appetite and the desire for sweet treats! Also, the advantages of ensuring your chromium levels are balanced are that it helps reduce the depressed emotions that are often associated with insulin resistance.

Stevia

Side-effect free, stevia is a perfect herb of choice for those suffering from diabetes. It is an excellent sweetener and also helps to reduce blood sugar levels. Trials have shown that 5 grams of stevia extract taken before meals three times a day can reduce blood sugar levels. Research indicates that the active stevioside improves insulin secretion in the pancreas via a direct action on pancreatic beta cells.

To use stevia as a sweetener, add one to two drops of liquid to a drink and taste. It is very strong and you will only need a tiny amount as a sugar replacement.

Goats rue

The active constituent in goats rue called galegine has hypoglycaemic properties. This leads to the production of biguanide drugs such as metformin which is used to increase the efficiency and sensitivity of insulin. Research has shown that goats rue increases the number of beta cells and the size of the 'Islets of Langerhans' in the pancreas. The herb also potentates the effect of insulin and gluconeogenesis.

When goats rue extract is taken orally, patients report no nasty side effects and get the benefit of reduced serum glucose; also some weight reduction takes place. This herb has also shown to have a regenerative effect on the beta cells in the pancreas. Patients with mild diabetes 'type 2' can often take this herb alone, and combined with appropriate regular dieting, have no need for other medications. Talk to your Health Care Practitioner, but as a general rule, 5 ml of 1:2 ethanol extract can be taken three times a day before meals.

Fenugreek

Research has shown that fenugreek improves blood glucose levels in both types of diabetes. Fenugreek significantly decreases fasting blood glucose levels and improves glucose tolerance test results, as well as decreasing blood cholesterol and triglyceride levels.

Fenugreek seeds are high in fibre and this may help block the absorption of carbohydrates through the digestive tract into the blood stream, decreasing the amount of sugars absorbed. Soak 15 grams of seed in a cup of boiling water and leave covered until it cools down. Drink the liquid and add the seeds to your food during the day. Alternately you could have the herbal extract: 10 ml twice a day before meals.

Research into the avoidance of 'type 2' diabetes through the adequate intake of omega-3 has been shown to improve metabolic sequelae of insulin resistance by helping control hypertension and plasma triglycerides. You need a ratio of two omega-3 fatty acids to one omega-6 fatty acid for optimal balance in your body.

Sweeteners

A sweet tooth for celebrations
A sweet tooth when you're sad
A sweet tooth just for a treat
A sweet tooth to be bad!

Most of us have a sweet tooth naturally. Have you ever met someone who truly doesn't enjoy a delicious, sweet crème brulee, chocolate mud cake, Belgium chocolates or just a dash of sweetness in their cuppa? There are those who are hypoglycaemic and require regular energy boosts of nutrition through the day. Isn't it easier to grab a butterscotch lolly or a delicious, sweet treat instead of eating savoury foods that will take longer to kick in than the sugar-sweet buzz of energy?

There are some alternatives to sugar in your diet. These alternatives are not only healthy herbal remedies that will satisfy your cravings for sweetness, but they are also beneficial to your health in other ways as well.

Sugar

For just a little more energy ... I'm so tired today! The white crystalline granules we know of as sugar are an unnatural substance produced by industrial processes on sugar cane or sugar beets. It is refined down to pure sucrose, after stripping away all the vitamins, minerals, proteins, enzymes and other beneficial nutrients. Sugar is first pressed as a juice from the cane (or beet) and refined into molasses; it is then refined into brown sugar and finally into strange white crystals that are an alien chemical to the human system.

What is left is a concentrated unnatural substance which the human body is not able to handle, at least not in anywhere near the quantities that we now ingest due to today's lifestyle. Sugar is addictive. The average person now consumes approximately 50 kilos of sugar per year. It is considered a 'food' and ingested in massive quantities.

However not all sugars are created equal and raw cane sugar is the best pick if you need to use sugar in your diet. Unlike refined sugars, unrefined raw cane sugar has not been stripped of its nutrients and fibre even though it will still give you the same rise in blood sugar levels as white sugar.

The dangers of sugar to your health

Studies have shown that sugar is by far the leading cause of dental deterioration, cavities in teeth, tooth loss, bleeding gums and failure of bone structure. It is also a contributing factor to diabetes, hyperglycaemia and hypoglycaemia. It has the harmful effect of unbalancing the endocrine system and injuring it's components such as the adrenal glands, pancreas and liver, causing blood sugar levels to fluctuate widely. It is a contributory cause to heart disease, arteriosclerosis, mental illness, depression, senility, hypertension and cancer.

Sugar increases overgrowth of the candida yeast organism and is known to increase chronic fatigue; it can trigger binge eating in those with bulimia as well as increasing PMS symptoms. Sugar increases hyperactivity in children and contributes to existing anxiety and irritability. Sugar can make it difficult to lose weight because of constantly high insulin levels, which cause the body to store excess carbs as fat, and this is known as metabolic resistance. These are all serious health reasons to avoid sugar and there are alternative choices that you can easily incorporate into your diet.

Artificial sweeteners

The choices we have with artificial sweeteners are really quite dangerous to your health. Unfortunately, research has shown that saccharin can be a possible contributing cause to cancer and that its partner aspartame has been shown to turn into formaldehyde in your body. Now this is not a healthy sweet choice! The results of people using these artificial sweeteners over the long term are difficult to determine. How do you know whether a particular substance that you took in your diet was the contributing cause to the kidney disease or cancer that you get in 20 years from now? This is difficult to determine. However these sweeteners are surrounded by suspicion and best avoided when you can have naturally healthy choices.

Natural alternatives

Xyitol—delicious and natural, use only half the amount of sugar

Xyitol naturally occurs in fruit and vegetables. It is commercially derived from hardwood trees to make the white crystal powder that is sold as a sweetener. It has about 40% less calories than sugar and has been shown to inhibit bacterial growth, especially strep mutants which cause cavities. You will need to introduce Xyitol slowly into your diet as it can have the side effect of diarrhoea in a small number of people.

Date sugar—the less processing, the better

Date sugar doesn't cause the same sugar rush as white sugar because it is a complex sugar. Date sugar also retains its nutritional value and fibre in the same way that raw cane sugar does because of the limited processing. The problems with date sugar are that it is high in calories, and often doesn't mix well in liquids.

Brown rice syrup—the slow burning sweetener

Brown Rice syrup is a complex carbohydrate which is made by culturing brown rice with enzymes to break it down. It is then cooked to become a liquid syrup which is popular as a sweetener. Brown rice syrup contains only about 3% glucose which is easily absorbed into the blood stream quickly, giving your body a complex energy source of slow burning carbohydrates thereby a constant stream of energy over the next few hours. It's certainly a healthy choice for your pancreas, whilst also allowing your body to enjoy the quick fix of a little sweetness.

Honey—it was Winnie's favourite

Compared to other sugar sources, honey has also been found to keep levels of blood sugar fairly constant. Honey is higher in calories than sugar, however it does contain extra nutrients and is a natural healthy alternative for those who do not suffer from diabetes. Honey is a pure source of natural unrefined sugars and carbohydrates which are easily absorbed by the body, providing an instant energy boost with long-lasting effects. At traditional Indian weddings, the bridegroom is often offered honey to boost his stamina, perhaps this is why Cupid's emblem was a bee!

Honey is an all-round healing elixir which can promote general health and well-being. A daily dose of honey, whether as a sweetener in hot drinks, by the spoonful or spread on toast, will boost the body's supply of antioxidants—essential for protecting the body against free radicals.

Flush out your system and give yourself a daily boost with this cleansing tonic: mix a spoonful or two of honey and the juice of half a lemon into a cup of hot water and drink each morning before breakfast.

Herbal honey—for your health

A dash of this and a dash of that. Add it together and good health is yours! Adding herbal extracts in small quantities to your honey is a quick and delicious way to boost your health. Honey is one of my favourite carriers for herbal mixtures. These are just a few herbal honey ideas. You can also make up your own combinations depending upon your health requirements.

Happy Herbals Honey!

Dieters—add two drops of *Gymnema sylvestre* to each teaspoon of honey you use in cooking and for drinks throughout the day. This will help with the uptake of insulin and help stop sugar cravings; you won't even taste the difference.

Improve your memory—add ginkgo biloba, brahmi or gotu kola to your morning cuppa with a dash of honey. Simply add one drop of each herbal extract to three cups of tea or coffee with honey every day. Voila! Improved memory and sweet cravings satisfied!

Digestive tonic—peppermint and golden seal make a good herbal combination to aid digestion for rich foods and can be used in baking as well as in beverages to aid digestion. Add two drops of each into your beverage with honey to flavour.

Sinusitis relief—add five drops of fenugreek extract to a cup with the juice of one lemon and a teaspoon of raw honey. Drink this mixture four times a day when your symptoms are acute.

Stevia—the queen of herbal sweeteners

It's rare for there to be one choice that's perfect for everyone ... but the leaf of the stevia plant is just that. Native to Paraguay, stevia contains a variety of minerals and vitamins and can be 30 times sweeter than sugar. Hundreds of scientific studies have documented stevia's contribution to regulating blood sugar in diabetics and hypoglycaemics, lowering elevated blood pressure, aiding the healing of wounds, reducing acne and improving digestion. Stevia has a Glycaemic Index of zero, making it safe for diabetes and hypoglycaemia. It also promotes pancreatic health, improves digestion, and soothes upset stomachs. Aside from the nutritional benefits, stevia can also aid dieters as it contains no calories and reduces cravings for sweets, whereas synthetic chemical sweeteners trigger cravings. Preliminary research shows that stevia clears the communication pathway between the stomach and the brain, reducing hunger sensations faster. Use stevia sparingly as it is very sweet.

Constipation—need help to get things going?

This is a problem which can be caused by dietary habits, lifestyle choices, hormonal imbalances and environmental factors. You will see many laxatives and bowel enhancers on the market. You need to know about these agents and how they can help or hinder your health.

Basically cathartics are agents that stimulate bowel movements: they are laxatives that are divided into groups. Aperients are mild agents producing a single bowel movement, cathartics are stronger, producing a more copious bowel movement and purgatives are powerful agents causing numerous watery evacuations.

The fewer cathartics you need to use, the better it is for your health. However, if you are constipated it's healthier for you to use one of these and get a good bowel movement while you also address the underlying problem.

The best laxatives are dietary fibres such as oat bran and rice bran. Including adequate levels of these in your diet can do a lot to prevent and reverse constipation. Dietary fibre levels should be considered and increased before you consider taking any cathartic herbs. Keep in mind that most cathartic herbs contain fibres such as psyllium hulls in large proportions. Make sure you drink plenty of water as dehydration is another trigger for constipation. Magnesium can also be helpful to increase the flow of bowel movements.

The major cathartic herbs contain anthraquinone pigments and phenolic compounds, generally in glycosides or a free state. These are stimulant cathartics. Their action does not depend on the direct irritation of the colon; there is a lag time of six to eight hours between administration of anthraquinones and a bowel movement. You would usually take these at night time. Many cathartic herbs contain constituents that modify their action, especially tannins and fibres, allowing you greater comfort.

Although not as harsh as mineral and saline laxatives, herbal laxatives still have the potential to dehydrate and cause electrolyte loss when used for extended periods, so maintaining abundant fluid intake is essential. They can taint the milk of nursing mothers and extreme care is required if they are to be used during pregnancy or breastfeeding. Bulk cathartics such as psyllium are gentler in action but to be effective they require adequate intake of fluids.

You also need to remember that any agent which increases the flow of peristalsis may also decrease the absorption of nutrients in your small and large intestines. This means that you may miss out on critical nutrients that you have eaten but not assimilated. Another problem to be aware of is that the bulking agents are capable of absorbing nutrients, carried through and out of your system within the bulking agents, and your body again misses out on valuable nutrition.

You can use cathartics for constipation, irritable bowel syndrome, haemorrhoids, anal fissures, portal congestion or as preparation and support for a detox. You can take them for chronic skin disorders that refuse to clear up or before and after abdominal and rectal operations. However, don't get into the habit of taking these herbs regularly, try to look at a long-term solution. You may also take these herbs when you have an acute cold or flu and want to clear your bowels to stop auto-intoxication of the toxic illness.

The cathartic herbs you will see most often are: cascara, cassia senna, rhubarb, black walnut, and psyllium. Choose the least purgative required to create a bowel movement.

Omega fatty acids are necessary for good health

What is omega-3?

Omega-3 is a fat, but unlike other dietary fats this one is necessary for the optimal development and health of your entire body. Alpha-linoleic acid (ALA) is the parent omega-3 fatty acid. The long-chain omega-3 fatty acids, eicosapentaenoic acid (EPA) and docosahexaenoic acid (DHA) are the types of omega-3 that your body is able to synthesise from ALA taken in the diet from fish oils and flaxseed oil. These omega-3 fatty acids are polyunsaturated fatty acids (PUFAS) that are not made by your body and must be taken in through diet. Therefore they are essential.

What does omega-3 do to help my health?

- *Improves cell membrane integrity*
- *Anti-inflammatory properties*
- *Improve your mental focus and vision*
- *Reproductive health*
- *Immune protection*

What are the best forms of omega-3 and how do i take it?

Omega-3 is obtained from flaxseed oil and deep water fish. The richest species of fish are sardines, Atlantic, stock eye and pacific salmon, mackerel, pacific herring, lake trout, European anchovy, and bluefish tuna. Fish do not naturally have omega-3 in their body, they need to eat it in the form of algae which they synthesise into these essential fatty acids DHA and EPA. You will find that the oilier the fish, the more omega-3 there is in the flesh.

Eating fresh fish is best as you will get between 2.5 and 8 grams of omega-3 per 200 gram serving. People of all ages and all stages of life would do well to take omega-3 daily to help the development of all cells and body functions.

Are there any health risks associated with omega-3?

There is concern that some fish may be contaminated by carcinogenic poisons such as DDT, dieldrin, PCB's, dioxin or heptachlor as well as methyl mercury. These contaminants are present in low levels in the water and fish have the ability to bioaccumulate and biomagnify environmental contaminants. These poisons are stored in the fatty tissue of the fish and can be transferred to your fatty tissue when you eat the fish.

We are fortunate that government agencies in many countries control the sale of fish with restrictions on the levels of these contaminants. Be aware that some tinned and processed omega-3 fish sold can contain hormones and antibiotics that have been fed to the fish in commercial fish farms overseas that are not so strictly regulated as they are in Australia and New Zealand. This results in the omega-3 levels being substantially lower and there is risk of the fatty acids becoming saturated in the same way that beef fat is saturated. Research has shown that Atlantic and South Pacific salmon are not treated with hormones or antibiotics to increase their growth rate. So the fish from Australia and New Zealand are premium omega-3 quality.

There are some gastrointestinal problems that can occur when you take omega-3 capsules such as reflux and general discomfort. The best way to avoid this is to freeze the omega-3 capsule for one hour before taking it. This prevents the capsule from breaking down in your stomach and has the same effect as the enteric coated capsules which don't break down in your body until they are in the small intestine.

Other problems can occur if you are on any cardiovascular medications that thin the blood such as aspirin. You may find that you bruise easier or bleeding time increases with wounds and nose bleeds. To avoid this problem simply take your omega-3 with meals and keep the dose to a minimum so that you get the health benefits of omega-3 without this side effect.

The only other concern for omega-3 is that if you have liver disease you may need to take it in conjunction with milk thistle as this will help flush your detoxification pathways and ensure that the fatty acids leave your liver and are processed effectively.

Also, what about the environment? Fish are in the ocean and they are an important part of the eco system. As our waters are fished out there is potential to make species extinct due to abuse and over fishing. When you eat fish, or take omega fatty acids please be conscious of this potential problem and try to source your fish from ethical and local fish farms when possible.

Keep your gall bladder in good health

Your gall bladder is a small pouch that is located next to your liver. The gall bladder fills up with bile which is made in your liver and is needed by your small intestine to help emulsify fats and digest foods once they have passed through your stomach. Without good quantities of bile you will have digestive problems including constipation, malabsorption of nutrients and possibly pains in your abdominal area.

Gallstones can be formed easily when you don't have enough bile or when there is limited movement of bile through the liver to the gall bladder. Gallstones are common, especially in younger women and in those who don't eat breakfast! This is because the residues from oestrogen, minerals and bile are able to rest in the gall bladder, increasing the opportunity to create gallstones. Many people fear that they will have to have their gall bladder removed when they are diagnosed with gallstones. This is not always the case but you need to take regular preventative measures to help stop the formation of gallstones and also to help eliminate them when they are very small, preventing them from growing bigger.

The first key to gallstone prevention is to eat regular meals that allow the flow of bile to freely travel through your gall bladder on a regular basis. You also need to have bitter foods before meals or with meals to help the secretion of bile which is made in your liver. Gallstones can form when you have oestrogen travelling freely to the gall bladder, this can be arrested with the addition of turmeric to your diet. The herb globe artichoke is good to help eliminate and prevent the formation of gallstones. Magnesium taken regularly in your diet can also be of assistance. Olive oil and lemon juice in combination eaten in salads and with meals is a good preventative. Green apples contain malic acid which helps break down gallstones.

If you think that you have gallstones, be very careful in the approach you use to help remove them. You can try taking small amounts of green apple, olive oil, magnesium, globe artichoke and lemon juice to see whether these create more pain or whether they relieve the symptoms. Don't try to eliminate the gallstones without knowing how big they are and without the assistance of your Health Care Practitioner, as if the stones become lodged in the bile duct you could experience severe pain and may be in danger. Many people think that they can remove gallstones quickly. However this is only safe when they are very young, soft and small. Orange juice with olive oil, apple cider vinegar and apple juice is a good daily tonic to help prevent their formation in the first place.

CHAPTER FOUR

Respiratory

Breathe deeply for good oxygen supply

Your respiratory tract includes your head cavity and lungs. This system is crucial for passing oxygen into your body and passing toxins out. The lungs are a fine mesh of beautiful little alveoli that suck up and diffuse oxygen, carbon dioxide and chemicals across from the external environment into your body. This is for your body, the difference between life and death.

You need to keep your head cavity as free of mucous as possible, i.e. sinuses, rhinitis, etc. must be eliminated. The best herbs for this job are fenugreek, with some ginger root, lemon juice and honey taken as a beverage each day. You need to stop any post nasal drips, clear up any built-up mucous straps that are forming in your upper respiratory tract as these can become insidious and spread down to your digestive tract and interfere with your large intestine if left untreated for long periods of time.

Also, you need to keep your lungs clean and clear so smoking is off the healthy list. We've all seen pictures showing the lungs of a smoker; it certainly isn't a pretty sight. If you imagine, every good breath of oxygen that goes into your body is filtered through that messy toxic tar, so dirty lungs equal a dirty system. Every cell in your body is only as clean as the fuel you give it. Oxygen is your body's fuel, along with food and water.

If you suffer from asthma, allergies or any conditions that cause havoc to your respiratory tract, then you would do well to visit your Health Care Practitioner and talk about complementary medicines. Many people ask for alternatives to asthma medicines—essential fatty acids, a good nutritional profile, specific herbals (depending upon their medicines) and also breathing techniques are worth trying. Asthma is seasonal in many people and it can be easier to jump at the first 'cure' instead of trying to find the cause.

Emphysema, tuberculosis, bronchitis, pneumonia and pleurisy are all conditions that can be improved with extra oxygen to the system, and once again good nutrition and care. Your respiratory tract is the entrance point of many chemicals to your body and these go straight to the blood stream, feeding your heart first. Therefore, your heart is taking the good blood or the toxic blood first, if you are infusing toxins. You need to seek professional help when you are concerned about any possible lung diseases. These can become infectious and your good health depends upon you taking care of your breathing system. Learn to take care of your lungs and you have a better chance of living a healthy lifestyle.

Lung preventatives for good health

- No smoking or exposure to toxins through the lungs is a priority
- Good fresh air
- Vitamin E and antioxidants. Essential fatty acids omega-3
- Lemon juice and honey, taken as a beverage daily

A good nutritional profile, specifically targeting any preventative solutions, is essential if you are prone to any personal or genetic lung conditions.

Respiratory tract herbal solutions

There are some good herbs you can take when you want to get rid of exudates from your respiratory tract. They are good for trachea, lung and bronchial conditions. Expectorants can stimulate your system with irritants causing elimination, they can soften mucous and reduce inflammation. Anodyne expectorants work by depressing the coughing mechanism, thereby giving you relief. Bronchodilators increase the dilation of your bronchial passage, increasing elimination of mucous which relieves any breathing constriction associated with asthma. Whilst anticatarrhals relieve congestion in your respiratory tract without elimination.

Most expectorants act by stimulating the ciliated epithelium of your respiratory mucosa as herbal constituents are excreted. These are mostly essential oils and saponins. Expectorants tend to turn sputum into liquid qualities and may inhibit the offending organism. Bronchodilators either stimulate the sympathetic nervous system or block the parasympathetic nervous system. They also act as decongestants and anticatarrhals. Flavonoids such as quercetin inhibit the release of histamine from mast cells which helps reduce allergic reactions associated with asthma or allergies such as sinus and hayfever.

Use expectorant herbals when there is any sign of bronchitis, coughing, asthma, restricted breathing, whooping cough, croup, pneumonia, pleurisy, upper respiratory infections and congestion. Also, take expectorants for respiratory viruses, otitis media, tinnitus, sinusitis, rhinitis, or hayfever.

Basically, if you have difficulty with your head cavity in any way that can be associated with the build-up of mucous or allergic congestion, please consider these herbals as a good non-addictive, side-effect-free solution to your ills. The sooner you take the herbals at the onset of the problem, the easier it is to ease the tension and allow you to breathe freely again and stop coughing. Don't stop taking these herbs when the problem is solved. You need to keep them up for a good three to four days after you think you are better, for long-term results. Often we stop taking herbs when we think we are better as the symptoms have subsided. However, the vulnerability is still in your body and this is where the extra few days of therapy really works, in repair and prevention.

Many good herbal cough formulas use liquorice root as a basic ingredient. This herb is rather thick and can stick itself to the lining of your throat to help the other herbs act faster. The addition of some thyme and olive leaf extract make a good, strong, cough and cold formula, ensuring that the symptoms are not only relieved with the expectorant herbals but also that the antimicrobial action gets in and kills any bugs or nasties that are lurking in the mucous. Nettles are well known in traditional medicines as relievers of many lung conditions. This herb has been used for tuberculosis and other infectious lung diseases, repairing and strengthening the lungs. A strong and persistent cough is often relieved once and for all with the daily addition of nettle extract or nettle tea. Nettle is used as a preventative herb for cancer and other immune compromised illnesses.

If you have a cough that won't shift, combine liquorice root with some cat's claw, olive leaf, thyme, nettle and sage extracts. This will help you as it is soothing, antimicrobial and repairing. This is a good strong formula which may be invaluable with the increasing arrival of unknown strong viruses and bacteria each year. Thyme has been used traditionally for whooping cough which makes it a valuable addition to the formula. If you drink fresh thyme tea every day during the winter you may be able to avoid all coughs. Olive leaf extract works in a similar way and is often best taken as a daily preventative to respiratory tract problems. Cat's claw is one of the strongest immuno-modulatory herbs and really helps pick up your energy when you are feeling low from respiratory tract infections, whilst sage is one of the oldest and most effective cough and cold herbals that has been used to strengthen the body.

Remember that often you need to treat the underlying causes of respiratory tract problems. This can often be elusive and takes a good examination of the precursors and possible triggers. The fastest way to heal a cough, cold or other respiratory problem is not always the most obvious. Look for clues by taking the time to remember all activities and foods eaten in the last week or two before the problem occurred.

Upper respiratory tract wellness is important

A congested head cavity, if left unaddressed, can become an infected head cavity. This will cause you more down-time in the long run than if you had nipped it in the bud right away. There can be post nasal drip, followed by a sore throat that spreads mysteriously to the lungs which can create all manner of respiratory tract illnesses. This congested system can be naturally and very quickly helped using respiratory tract herbals. Often people use sinus and hayfever clearing herbal extracts; one good time-proven formula is fenugreek, mixed with olive leaf extract. You should have results within about 20 minutes of taking the first therapeutic dose. Take this with warm water which has the benefit of helping herbs absorb quickly into your system. Ensure you drink lemon juice, with honey and water, two to three times a day as a preventative.

Make a note of any plants, foods and cleaners, etc. that may be contributing to the problem. This formula and the lemon juice can be given to people of all ages. Even small children respond to this combination and feel better fairly swiftly. If you notice that it takes longer to see results, then you may be more congested than you think. Often it can take up to six months of progressive improvement, taking the herbs daily, before you get a completely clear result. Eat garlic and ginger daily. Garlic is delicious when added to cooking, whereas garlic extract has a nasty taste and is very strong.

If you ignore an upper respiratory tract infection, such as in the sinus, hayfever or rhinitis, then you are prone to stagnation of the mucous and further infection which can be debilitating. There can be a constant and sharp pain above one or both of your eyes in the forehead. The best things you can do if you are in this position, is to take antibiotics and some probiotics and start your herbs ASAP. If you have a particularly bad strain which is antibiotic resistant, then you may need the following aged garlic extract, it is an excellent remedy but needs to be taken in strong doses to get results. The other time to use this extract is topically, if you have a skin infection. You may never need to use this recipe, but it's better to have the information if you want to try it out.

Homemade garlic antibiotic

Take ten bulbs (not cloves but the full bulb) of garlic and peel off the skin. Roughly chop the garlic and place in a jar. Add to this 500 ml of 40% vodka. Leave for three months sitting in a sealed container in your cupboard. Strain off the liquid, and press the garlic to get trapped liquid. Use by the teaspoonful, as necessary.

This will last for three years in the fridge and there are some styles of medicine that suggest aged garlic is better the older it gets. You will need about 30 to 60 ml per day to get rid of a heady respiratory infection, taken for three to seven days. This needs to be combined with complete cleansing except for hot vegetable soups and fresh vegetable juices such as carrot and lemon juice. You won't want to eat as this formula has a way of making you feel even sicker than you should. It has the worst taste. You will get better, but you'll be suffering every step of the way. You may need to take other herbs with the garlic extract, and remember to seek the assistance of your Health Care Professional to get the best healing regime possible for these infections.

The garlic remedy sounds terrible doesn't it? But it's a sure-fire way to decongest your system. In fact, you'll be feeling marvellous after you have recovered, with beautiful strong clear blood running through your body due to the complete clearing the garlic has given you. You will smell, so take parsley in juice constantly throughout the process as chlorophyll always combats the stench of garlic on your breath. But body odour is another issue all together. You will smell like a garlic bulb instead of a rose for days! Chlorophyll needs to be taken as fresh and close to the pick as possible. Add some wheatgrass juice to your diet for a week or so and you'll be bouncing with energy.

Never ignore a sore throat

When you get a sore throat you need to look after it and ease the pain and minimalise your chances of infection as quickly as possible. Many ear infection, sinus and lung infections can be avoided if you address the problem at its cause by healing the sore throat in the first place.

Wrap up in warm clothes, keep your feet and head warm and your chest well covered. Layers of clothing are good. You may need to make an onion poultice, place it in a scarf and wrap around your neck as soon as possible after the sore throat has started. You need to take olive leaf extract, turmeric extract, fenugreek extract and liquorice extract. Drink lemon juice and hot water. Talk as little as possible and rest as much as you can until you are better again. With a sore throat, it's easy to stop taking your herbs and looking after yourself as soon as the symptoms subside. This is a mistake as you need to continue taking the herbs for at least three days after the symptoms have gone. This is because you can easily have a relapse. Sipping honey off the spoon and taking throat lozenges can also be beneficial. Just remember that it's a lot easier to heal a sore throat than to heal a deeper infection.

Recipe for onion poultice

To make an onion poultice, thinly slice a raw onion and wrap inside a scarf that you wrap around your neck.

The fumes from the onion will enter your nostrils as you breathe and help clear up any type of throat, sinus or lung infection. You need to change the onion every 12 hours and replace with freshly chopped raw onion.

Within half an hour of placing the poultice around your neck you will decrease coughing frequency and severity, have less pain in your throat and also have a stinging sensation in your eyes. The stinging of the onion fumes in your eyes will subside quickly. Just close your eyes and rest for a while, as once your eyes are closed they will not feel the onion sting.

You will find that you get used to the smell rather quickly, as the benefits of this poultice far outweigh the smell. If ever you want to get rid of an acute cold or flu quickly, make this poultice and wear to bed each night and remove the following day when you need to get on with your work. This poultice is also good for earache and if you are concerned about getting infections in the head, throat or lungs.

The five best herbs to avoid the flu

Each winter is a rotten season for flu. It's difficult to avoid exposure to the seasonal ills and chills when we have central heating systems, air conditioning and environments where a lot of people gather for celebrations, work and education. The only defence you have is to strengthen your immunity and boost your resistance against these savage intruders.

We are faced with a world where new and more complicated viruses and bacterium enter each year. There are always going to be new bugs about, no matter where you live, and the same challenges to protect your system against the sudden onset of flu-like symptoms. Just do your best and make sure you keep you and your family in the best of health as far as is environmentally possible.

There are antibiotic-resistant strains emerging and these herbs can help you avoid these, or if you fall prey to one of these antibiotic-resistant strains of bacteria then herbs they may be your healing solution. You need to stay off pharmaceutical antibiotics as much as possible. This way if you are ever exposed to a bacteria that needs antibiotics, when you do take this medicine your body is more likely to respond with a better chance of healing.

Stay away from commercial foods that contain antibiotics, such as some chicken and meat. These will alter your body chemistry and make you less susceptible to the healing powers of antibiotics. The best thing you can do for your immunity is to take some preventative herbs and hope that you can avoid any bacteria floating around in hospitals, schools, your work place and anywhere else you go during the winter months.

Astragalus

Remember that prevention is better than cure.

Flu fighting qualities

Astragalus is your number one herb to take daily from the onset of flu season until the end of spring. This herb has been shown through research to help boost T-cell and B-cell production enabling your defence system to be strong and robust through exposure. Research has shown that the antiviral activity of astragalus is most likely the result of positive effects on immune function from enhanced interferon production. The bitter principles are the main actives in astragalus and it also has a relatively high content of zinc and silicon, which may also attribute to the strong anti-flu qualities of this herb. Astragalus combines beautifully with most other herbal formulations, however you need to take this herb as a preventative or a recovery herb. Do not take astragalus when you are in the throes of the flu or an acute cold, wait until the symptoms have subsided.

How to use it

Take 5 ml of liquid herbal extract twice a day for two weeks, and then decrease dose to 5 ml daily for the duration of the flu season. If you are exposed to any viruses or feel the flu coming on, then simply increase the dose to the original dose for the next week. If you are taking capsules, simply have 5 grams a day for one week and then decrease to 2 grams a day for prevention.

Garlic

Throughout time, immortal man has used garlic as the best herb to prevent the onset of many an illness.

Flu fighting qualities

Garlic contains allicin, which contributes to its antimicrobial, antifungal, expectorant and immune stimulant qualities. Research has shown that garlic is an effective immune stimulant, and when you exercise aerobically and consume garlic in your diet you may increase the quality, quantity and killing power of natural killer cells tenfold! This certainly is reason enough to take garlic from the beginning to the end of the flu season. Garlic produces a wide spectrum antimicrobial effect on intestinal bacteria, fungus and some parasites, which helps keep you in tip-top health.

How to use it

There's an old saying about garlic, 'fresh is best'; however, the odour may have your lover fleeing the bed later in the night. So, to avoid the nasty odours, simply eat green parsley or chlorophyll with your garlic. Add raw garlic to your salads and vegetables. Freeze either a clove of garlic or some garlic capsules for 15 minutes before eating and they will pass through to your small intestine intact, which may help you avoid some of the odour. The liquid extract of garlic is very effective and very smelly. It is best taken in acute situations where you want the medicinal benefits of garlic to work very fast and efficiently, especially when you have caught the flu and wish for a speedy recovery. There are contraindications to garlic and you must check with your health professional if you are taking any medications.

White horehound

'Oh no … I feel the flu coming on' … a dose of white horehound may stop it in its tracks.

Flu fighting qualities

When you have the first signs of the flu, the best herb to take is white horehound. This herb seems to stop the flu in its tracks. Take a good dose and take it within a few hours of the first signs of the flu such as weakness, cold symptoms, and personal indicators that you know are signs a flu is coming. White horehound has expectorant, spasmolytic and bitter principles. This is a traditional favourite for warding off the impending cold or flu.

How to use it

White horehound liquid extract is invaluable. Take 5 ml at the onset of the flu and then another 5 ml one hour later. You will need to take about 25 ml over a 12 hour period for effective avoidance of the flu onset.

Take one tablespoon of fresh leaves, add to one cup of boiling water and seep for ten minutes, strain and drink. Have five or six cups of this tea over the next 12 hours. If you don't manage to avoid the flu completely, be assured that you have worked preventatively and will likely have fewer symptoms and the duration will be shorter.

Olive leaf

The super antioxidant and antimicrobial properties of olive leaf work like a coat of armour for your immune system.

Flu fighting qualities

Oleuropein was shown to potentate a macrophage response, resulting in higher nitric oxide production, which is believed to be beneficial for cellular protection. Oleuropein is an antioxidant. The hydroxytyrosol in olive leaf has shown broad antimicrobial activity against bacteria known to cause intestinal and respiratory tract infections. Patients often comment on the increased health and vitality they feel after a course of olive leaf extract. It works wonderfully and gently on people of all ages. So, you can use this herb on babies, children and the elderly.

How to use it

Olive leaf capsules are best taken in the morning regularly from the onset of the flu season until it is well over. Take 2 grams of olive leaf each day for each 30 kilos of body weight. This should offer you effective immunity strengthening and avoidance of the flu. The liquid extract is very popular. Like other flu preventing herbs it offers a wide array of health benefits, making olive leaf a definite herb to take for flu prevention.

Andrographis

This herb has been traditionally used in Chinese, Thai and Ayurvedic medicines for it's wonderful repairing abilities.

Andrographis and isolated andrographolide stimulate both antigen specific and non-specific immunity. Research has shown that andrographis demonstrates an immunostimulant action, especially on macrophages. This is good news for avoiding and curing the flu. Imagine all those killer cells in there gobbling up the toxins and flu invaders!

Andrographis is a good herb to take when you want to avoid the flu, and if you happen to be flu bound then take a good dose of andrographis until you are better. Research has also shown that andrographis extract given to children over flu season has significantly decreased their chances of catching the flu. Andrographis has traditionally been used by Western Health Care Practitioners for any bacterial or viral respiratory tract infections, and the prevention of common colds and enteric infections.

How to use it

Take 5 ml of herbal extract daily for two weeks as a preventative, and decrease the dose to 2 ml a day for the duration of the flu season. If you find yourself down with the flu then increase dose to 10 to 20 ml a day for the duration of the flu until you are feeling well again. I do not know of any contraindications of andrographis. However, as with all herbals, it's best to seek the advice of your Professional Health Carer before adding herbals to your routine if you are on medications or suffer any illnesses.

What to do when you get the flu

Rest as much as possible. Go to bed and keep warm, if possible. If you get home from a busy day and feel the flu coming on, then take white horehound straight away. This will help arrest the onset of the flu. Take a good relaxing hot bath or shower, the heat will help sweat out the flu and allow your body to begin the elimination process. If you have some echinacea root or white horehound take these herbs throughout the first 12 hours to continue the process of avoidance. If you are planning to relax the next day then you need to allow the healing crisis to run its course. At the beginning of any flu it's a good idea to take vitamin C powder in juice or water, 5 grams every four hours for four doses. This helps loosen the digestive tract, allowing you to eliminate the toxins from your body efficiently, whilst allowing you to gain the antioxidant benefits that vitamin C offers.

The flu foods

Less is best. When you have the flu the last thing you feel like doing is cooking gourmet foods. Mono flu foods such as soups and casseroles are good when you feel on the edge of the flu. Just make a big pot of that food and place the leftovers in the fridge for instant heating as required.

With flu foods, if you are in a position where you must cook for children or other adults, you can add extras such as rice, pasta, tofu and meat to feed the non-flu-affected members of your household. Simply take your portion and place it aside and add the extras as required. However, there is an old saying related to cooking and energy: if you have bad or sick energy and you cook, then the food will also taste that way (i.e. bad or sick), and it's true. So, try to get someone else to cook whilst you are sick and rest yourself. However, if you must cook, then keep it light and stress-free as possible. The flu foods are simple, vegetarian and light. You can have soups, salads, steam fries and juices. Herbal teas and basic yet light drinks to soothe hunger and aid cleansing which is always required when healing from the acute flu.

Soups

Carrots, cabbage, onions, garlic, broccoli, tomatoes, pumpkin and any other vegetables you have handy. Simply make up a vegetable soup with these ingredients and place it in the fridge. When you feel hungry heat some up, you will have the satisfied feeling of fullness yet still be eliminating toxins and allowing your body the digestive rest required for efficient flu recovery. Add garlic to the soup and sprinkle some brewer's yeast flakes or kelp flakes over the soup each time you eat some. Depending on your taste you can also add some fresh chilli, mint, parsley, or other chopped herbs to the soup.

Steam fries

Steam fries are when you take your wok, turn it up really high and add water instead of oil to steam the vegetables you wish to eat. For a flu, steam fry, combine green curry paste, lemon juice, fresh ginger, mint and vegetables. Usually the vegetable base is your traditional flu base of carrots, cabbage, onions, garlic, celery, broccoli and pumpkin with a little tomato added at the end. A steam fry is most convenient as you can prepare the food quickly without much ado and eat what you want instantly. Then you can take the leftovers, place them in the fridge and reheat the next time you are hungry. Once again you can add extras such as chilli, brewer's yeast, kelp, tamari, soy sauce or sea salt for flavouring as desired. You can even add some sesame seeds, flax seeds, sunflower seeds or pumpkin seeds for extra nutrition and taste.

Salads

When you have the flu, eating a fresh salad has a wonderfully refreshing energy that flows through your body instantly from the first bite of crunchy vegetables with the delicious tang of good vinegar and zest of garlic running through your taste buds.

To make a salad when you have the flu, just use lots of vegetables. Either loads of carrot with cabbage and onion and garlic and add some ginger and yummy broccoli. Don't make any more than you wish to eat as it doesn't keep so well in the fridge. Use whatever fresh vegetables you have at hand. The dressing needs to be vinegar based and light.

Traditional dressing

Mix together one tablespoon of apple cider vinegar, one tablespoon of good cold-pressed oil (such as olive or apricot), a teaspoon of French mustard and a little honey and sea salt.

You can use lemon juice instead of apple cider vinegar and you can also add some chilli if you want the heat. This will be cleansing on your liver and gall bladder as well as soothing on your digestive tract. The apple cider vinegar is very healing in many ways and always a good addition to any flu meal. The flu salad is cooling and a delicious change from hot flu soups and steam fries.

Juices

Regularly mix up carrot juice with lemon juice and garlic and drink it over the day at two hour intervals when you're down with the flu. The juicer doesn't need to be washed between each drink (as who wants to juice and wash up when you're sick?). Just throw a clean tea towel over the juicer between juice sessions and ignore it until the end of the day. This juice combination of carrot, lemon and garlic is so good; it clears the liver, reduces mucous and adds the healthfulness of garlic which is easily assimilated and keeps hunger at bay. This is your ultimate flu food as it promotes a really good recovery. You can go for a few days on this juice as your mono food if you are particularly unwell and lose a few kilos to boot!

Other juices are beneficial too. Depending on what you feel like, you can rest assured that most juices will be beneficial for you when suffering from the symptoms of common cold or flu. These keep your fluids up in a nutritious and cleansing way.

Other drinks

Herb teas are great and ones that taste refreshing are a delicious change from standard flu foods. Liquorice root, thyme, peppermint, ginger, melissa and asparagus are all good flu teas. The asparagus cleanses your kidneys, allowing you to flush out more toxins from your body faster.

Fenugreek seed tea

Simply boil the kettle and pour a cup of water over two tablespoons of fenugreek seed and allow this to sit overnight or through the day (about eight hours). Then each time you need a drink of fenugreek tea, take a teaspoon of the seeds and about a tablespoon of the water from the original mix, pour fresh boiling water over this and drink it as it cools down.

This is the best flu tea as it will help detoxify your system and eliminate the flu symptoms. You will sweat a bit, and it may smell like curry but the benefits far outweigh the taste. And when you're flu ridden you will appreciate the effects of the mucous drying up and being removed from your system.

A fishermen's cure from coromandel

Here's one to get your body in a healing fizz. The fishermen make this mixture up and take it out with them at night in the winter to keep the flu at bay and help them through the night on the fishing boats. They mix a teaspoon to a tablespoon of this formula with each cup of coffee they drink through the night to keep cold and flu at bay. These fishermen even add milk and sugar to the instant coffee and then add this flu recovery blend to the cup! It's a good cure for those determined to keep up the coffee whilst sick.

Instead of coffee you could have a herbal tea such as lemon and ginger but you'll be lucky to taste the herb tea as this brew is very strong with capsicum.

> Take a bulb of garlic and peel the skin away, chop it up and mix it with 3 inches of chopped ginger and two tablespoons of chopped capsicum pepper or ten hot chillies. Mix it all together (or blend it) with a cup vinegar and place in a jar with a lid.

Keep this mix in the fridge and whenever you want a drink simply add between a teaspoon and a tablespoon of the brew to your drink. It's very hot, very yucky and very effective.

Herbs to help

Good herbs for respiratory tract recovery include white horehound, thyme, fenugreek, wild cherry bark, sage, ground ivy, liquorice root, olive leaf, andrographis, cat's claw, fenugreek, elderberry, and nettles. There are no hard and fast rules when it comes to what herbs will help you when you are struck down with the common cold or flu. Rest is essential and often it's best to relax, not eat much, fill up on good old-fashioned chicken and vegetable soup and take regular warm baths to help soothe tired bones and muscles. You often need to let these situations run their course.

But, when it comes to other respiratory tract problems, if you act fast you can often avert illness. Infrared saunas or normal steam saunas are good to help you sweat out the flu. However, don't think you can just get on with work and fill up on suppressive pills containing pseudoephedrine to keep you going. These are okay to have occasionally, but when you rely on them to cure the flu you are setting yourself up for a congested system in the future.

In many ways the flu is a sign that your body needs to stop, eliminate toxins and allow rest and room for you to just relax and get better. If you fill up on suppressive medications and try to avoid the problem at hand, you may even end up sicker than you thought. Herbs and natural alternative solutions are often the best course of action on the road to recovery. You need patience and you need to accept that for your Wellness Zone, you need to take the time to listen to your body and slow down a pace or two.

Herbal cough medicine is easy to make at home

Herbal cough medicines are natural and are often able to heal the coughing problem as well as stopping or helping you to recover from deeper respiratory illnesses such as pneumonia, pleurisy, bronchitis and other lung diseases. If you have a persistent cough, especially through the night, then your immunity becomes more compromised and you will be tired and weak which opens you up to secondary infections. This can also decrease your recovery time.

Herbs that help alleviate coughing are tea tree, olive leaf, sage, thyme, nettle, liquorice root, elecampane, lime flowers, wild cherry, marshmallow, schisandra and chamomile. If you are able to have some of these herbs at home, either as a powder or in herbal extract form, you can easily make up a cough formula when you need one. Or make up a big bottle and refrigerate for when needed.

Herbal cough formulas made with concentrated herbs can be mixed down with honey and warm water and taken as required. A good herbal cough formula is a combination of liquorice root extract with thyme, which is often given for deep coughing such as whooping cough or the persistent night cough that almost makes you sick. Add to that some nettle, which is very good at stopping lung infections developing and olive leaf or tea tree for the extra antimicrobial properties.

All of the herbs mentioned here are good to stop a cough in its tracks and heal the illnesses that can develop. Using the onion poultice around your neck is very good as it relieves the throat and the onion essences go into your lungs through each breath which can retard bad night coughing when worn to bed at night.

Lemon juice and honey drink is also a must-have when you have a bad cough. Even babies can benefit from this drink mixed with chamomile tea instead of water, as chamomile tea is your number one tea when it comes to cough relief. Chamomile cough medicine can be made as required and will help as long as you keep taking it through the day or night.

Easy chamomile cough medicine

Take four chamomile tea bags and soak them in 200 ml of boiling water until it cools down. Add one tablespoon each of runny honey and apple cider vinegar. For an instant cough medicine, sip this for relief each time you cough.

Nettle tea for cough relief

Drink nettle tea when you have a long-term daily coughing problem. This tea has been used traditionally to help heal all manner of lung diseases, including tuberculosis and whooping cough. You will need to drink the tea three to four times a day for good results. It will not stop a coughing fit once it has started but it will help to decrease the frequency between coughs and help decrease the bouts of coughing by shortening them in severity and duration.

Tea tree and olive leaf tea

Mix one tablespoon of olive leaf extract with 2 ml of tea tree oil and one teaspoon of honey or a few drops of stevia extract. Boil an onion in one cup of water and reduce the water until there is only a very little left in the pot. Separate the onion from the water and mix the liquid with the olive leaf extract, tea tree oil and honey.

Herbal extract cough medicine

Herbal extracts can be made to taste more like cough medicine and less unappealing by adding warm water and runny honey to your dose of herbs. Take 15 to 30 ml of liquid extract, add an equal amount of warm water with 2 to 5 ml of runny honey. Mix well and sip as required. Also, if you use 50% liquorice extract in any cough medicine mixture, this will make the herbs taste deliciously like liquorice, which also sticks to the throat and helps the other herbs to be absorbed.

Other tricks to help make your respiratory herbs taste better, is to add soy milk to blends that contains liquorice root or mix the herbs into your hot lemon and honey drink.

Ready-made, instant cough syrup

Take 50 ml of liquorice root, 50 ml of other herbs, one tablespoon of raw honey, and 100 ml of boiling water and mix together. Keep it stored in the fridge. If you can get the pure extracts and water them down with your own flavourings, you will be saving money in the long term by having the concentrated product and adding your own water and flavourings as required.

CHAPTER FIVE

Nerves

Your nervous system should be a high priority for maintaining your Wellness Zone. Once you know that you are absorbing nutrients well and breathing clean oxygen to ensure clean cells, then you need to repair any damage or exhaustion to this system. You need to have a balanced and level nervous system that is operating optimally.

There is the somatic nervous system which is in your control and then there is the autonomic nervous system that is out of your control. This is the part that helps control smooth unconscious muscle contractions such as digestion and bowel movements, also nervous system responses to assimilating food, breathing, heart beat and other automatic processes.

The reason why your nervous system is so important in your Wellness Zone is that your brain is the master controller of this system and nerves affect the functioning of every system in your body. Your nerves are the electrical wiring system, and if they aren't functioning well you are in trouble everywhere! It's interesting to note that when you have a healthy nervous system, as a whole, then you will be able to handle all aspects of your life well, everything else seems a little better than it would if your nervous system was stressed!

Nervous system illnesses certainly put your life on hold and these are to be avoided as much as possible. The best way to avoid them is to have a healthy diet and also to use herbs regularly as a buffer against stresses. Stress is the biggest problem for your nervous system, this can be physical oxidative stress, such as toxins from your body add stress to the nervous system, or it can be emotionally or mentally triggered.

Foot baths are an ageless remedy for stress relief

At the end of a busy day, why not relax and have a warm foot bath to help you unwind. Foot baths increase circulation to the peripheral parts of your body, they help relax your whole body and you can add specific herbs or essential oils to the bath to help you enjoy the experience even more.

Foot bath

You will need a wide bucket that is deep enough to add hot water, herbs and both of your feet. Place a towel under the bath and soak your feet in your favourite blend of essential oils, herbs and other moisturising oils. This is an ageless remedy that works well with everyone. Children just love this treatment, followed by a gentle foot massage.

Herbs and foods for a healthy nervous system

Often, when the nervous system is stressed, you will not be hungry and run the risk of under-nourishment if the problem persists for a long time. Many people either eat too little food when they are stressed, or they go the other way and eat too much of the nurturing emotional foods that are often low in nutrition. As you can imagine, you will either become thin or fat. It's a difficult juggling act to live in constant stress and stay healthy. So your constant attention is required if you plan to be stressed and healthy.

Pay attention to your diet daily, and even if you feel overwhelmed with cravings for the wrong foods, or if you feel as though you couldn't eat a thing, make sure you do eat, and make sure you take the appropriate herbs and nutritional support to balance your body.

The best herbs for your nervous system are, undoubtedly: oats, chamomile, valerian, passionflower, hypericum, melissa, fennel, peppermint, geranium and any herb that acts as a buffer between the nerves. The herbs for the nervous system are often not the nervines themselves, but the herbs that are softening, nurturing foods for the nervous system. You need to watch your foods when you want to add extra support to the nervous system. Eat soft fruits, such as apples, pears, guavas, paw paws, apricots and strawberries. Keep away from hot chilli and really stimulating herbs. Turmeric and fennel are digestive aids. Peppermint tea is a good beverage mixed with a bit of honey and chamomile flowers. The chamomile is very nurturing whilst the peppermint is just stimulating enough to add positiveness to the nerves. When you are nurturing and supporting your nervous system you would do well to have regular small meals containing first class complete protein such as eggs, tofu, fish, lean red and white meats and lentils. Take B group vitamins in combination with protein as you require these co-factors and co-enzymes to help the amino acids do their job and magically join together to make those beautiful healthy cells. Your brain loves L-glu-tamine, the amino acid, so does your liver and nervous system. So, this can be taken in times of nervous tension and when you need nervous support.

Keep away from ice, cold drinks or plain water when you are on a nervous system support diet. Keep your drinks warm and a little sweet and sip regularly through the day. Soups and broths are good as are room-temperature vegetable juices.

Don't attempt to cleanse your body until you have a strong nervous system, as your body may not cope well as the toxins are thrown up into your blood stream, which can bring the focus to your problems and weaknesses more than ever. Make sure you get iron, zinc and magnesium every day when you are repairing your nervous system. Magnesium can be taken at up to 5 grams of amino acid chelate per day, the worst scenario is that you will have looser bowels but the magnesium will do you the world of good, supporting your muscles, nerves, adrenals and mental capacities.

Don't go on a special protein or other diet when your nervous sys-tem is stressed. Be rational and have a good general diet that takes into account your favourite foods, emotionally nurturing foods and all the essential nutrients you require to balance the defects in your nervous system. These can show up as: a vulnerability to respond excessively or inappropriately to a given situation, the potential to under or over react to circumstances and the possibility that your body clock just won't turn off into sleep mode, relaxation mode or any mode that isn't hypersensitive. Imagine the damage you can do to your body when you live constantly in this manner.

Until you have your nervous system in good working order you will find that you are mentally less focused, emotionally less balanced and physically compromised. No matter what the illness, no matter what the problem, work from the top down. This means that you are concentrating on getting your brain in good condition and the nerves are a direct reflection of the brains' health.

Take herbals that have shown pituitary gland support, such as astragalus, which really helps with all aspects of the body. But when you work on the brain and nervous system you cannot go past the adaptogenic herbs as an added support to help bring everything into balance. Therefore brahmi, gotu kola and liquorice are also very helpful herbs. Withania is wonderful if nervous exhaustion is the main issue. Combine herbals that are offering anti-depressant, nervine, adaptogenic and replenishing qualities.

Don't eat unless you are hungry, however, saying this, you need to eat small amounts of nutritious food regularly throughout the day no matter what your hunger mechanisms tell you. This is because nervous system dysfunction is deceiving and as mentioned earlier you may tend to eat too little or too much depending on your personality and circumstances.

Make each meal count nutritionally when you are repairing the nervous system. If the person is recovering from an addiction then focus on nervous system repair in conjunction with your detox therapies; however, make the detox as slow and easy as possible until you feel sure the nervous system can handle the added pressure of detoxification.

If you are recovering from an addiction, get hold of some passionflower and take a therapeutic dose at regular intervals through the day. This is a good herb for any withdrawal as it tends to mimic the feeling of satisfaction on a nervous level.

Nervines

Nervines are nectar to your nervous system. They have a calming effect on your central nervous system and can't be overlooked as the first approach to any situation where you need nervous system support.

Herbal nervines are non-addictive and gentle, they do not create a sensory perception of loss or state of narcosis like some sedatives and tranquilisers. Some nervines have the benefit of becoming sedative in larger doses. This can be a good thing or a bad thing depending upon your situation. Always consult with your Health Care Practitioner about how much herbal nervine to take for your constitution, body size and circumstances.

Nervines are delicious to the nervous system and they can help restore depleted energy as well as help overcome debility and depression. Taken at night some nervines become hypnotics and induce sleep. These are good herbals for anyone suffering from insomnia. Nervines taken in herbal extract form, last thing at night, with equal parts herb to rather warm water helps induce sleep. This helps the simple diffusion of the herbs and allows the nervine and sedative effects to kick in quickly, inducing a good night's sleep.

The active constituents in nervines are the alkaloids and essential oils

Small fat soluble molecules of photochemical alkaloids and volatile oils cross your blood-brain barrier. Nervines can interact with neurotransmitters and chemicals released at synaptic junctions between your neurones. Neuro-transmitters include; dopamine, serotonin, y-aminobutryic acid, (GABA), melatonin, histamine, autonomic nervous system hormones, noradrenaline and acetylcholine.

Nervines can assist with any condition where you think you need nervous system support. This includes anxiety and depression, nervous debility, nervous tension, stress, insomnia, headaches, neuralgia, shingles, convulsions, epilepsy, hyperactivity or any attention focusing deficits. Therapeutic doses of nervines help children who are having difficulty focusing at school. The nervines can take the edge off their worries and they are able to relax enough to absorb the information given, instead of spending their day in a state of frustration and panic. Anyone who is having difficulty with any mental task would do well to add a small dose of nervines to their breakfast each day and see for yourself whether you feel calmer throughout the morning.

Take chamomile tea or other nervous system supporting teas such as oats, hops, passionflower, hypericum, melissa or valerian instead of coffee when you are under a lot of nervous system stress. Coffee is not a good substance for anyone under stress. It tends to put your nerves on edge and make you lose mental clarity and focus. Coffee might be good to keep you awake when you are working long hours, but it does nothing to help keep you on task and relaxed. Take bacopa or ginkgo biloba for concentration during stressful times. These herbs are good for the over-worked business person who just can't stop at the end of the day.

Nervines can have the synergistic added qualities of sedatives, spasmolytic, hypnotic relaxants, anodynes, tranquillisers and act as a tonic. If you want the best results get a Health Care Practitioner to make you extracts especially to suit your requirements. Try a one week supply of these herbals to test the waters and see what results you are getting. Often you need to adapt the formula as the nervous system becomes more steady and healthy. Also doses can be adjusted, depending upon the acute situation.

The herb hypericum is useful as a pain reliever as well as a nervous system balancing herbal. Hypericum is good for anyone who needs to pick up their spirits and calm their nervous system. It can be used topically as a cream and is excellent for arthritis and muscle pain. Remember that hypericum tablets were given to the British soldiers during the great war to take if they were shot by a bullet. This aspect of hypericum has been dwarfed by its popularity as an anti-depressant. So many people who have any pain can benefit from the addition of this nervine, pain reliever in their health care regime.

Some good nervous system herbs are: melissa, valerian, skullcap, hops, hypericum, chamomile, passionflower, kava kava and motherwort. Melissa is a good herb to give someone who is already on prescription anti-depressants and needs some solid nervous system support. Perhaps many people would be able to avoid these pharmaceutical anti-depressants in many cases if they were able to balance their nervous systems and have a good nutritional profile. Consider this information before you take yourself off to your Health Care Practitioner for synthetic support for depression and anxiety.

Sometimes older people need this pharmaceutical support following years of nervous system wear and tear. They have a crisis in life and need to subscribe to medicines because the body responds with chronic depression, nerve shakes or anxiety and excess worry that is almost impossible to shake off. There are times when these pharmaceuticals have their place in health care and you need to use wisdom to decide what a good medicine for your condition is and what can be prevented with herbs and nutritional support. Visit your Health Care Practitioner and discuss the options. If your practitioner is open minded, then they will also be practical and help you find the right solution for your nervous system dysfunctions. However, always do your best personally to keep your nerves in good order, this is one way to prevent future severe responses to the events of life.

Migraine headaches

Any inflammation in your brain needs to be addressed quickly so that it doesn't develop into a migraine headache. These can be caused by many triggers, including hormonal imbalances and stress. Remember that your brain is in charge of your entire nervous system and that if there is a mental problem this will be reflected in all nervous system activities.

Feverfew has been used successfully as pain relief for migraine sufferers in cases where orthodox treatments had failed to be effective. Some people had a distinct improvement within days of regular use of feverfew, others taking a little longer. Patients taking feverfew for migraines have found added benefits and relief from menopausal symptoms, indicating that feverfew can also help with hormonal headaches.

Feverfew has been shown in research to inhibit prostaglandin synthesis, decrease the rate of blood clotting, inhibit histamine and enzyme release from immune cells and have a mild sedative effect. The active constituents are sesquiterpene lactones, which are bitter compounds that have a variety of physiological effects substantiating the traditional uses of feverfew for migraines. The main active has been found to be parthenolide which has an anti-inflammatory, prostaglandin antagonising, antithrombotic and serotonin inhibiting action.

Feverfew is very similar to common aspirin in action; there are few side effects except the occasional allergic response from respiratory allergy sufferers and stomach upsets from eating the fresh raw, bitter leaves. Consult your Health Care Practitioner if you are on conventional medications and avoid feverfew without Health Care Practitioner consent during pregnancy. Take 2 grams of dried herb capsules or 2 ml of herbal extract daily as a preventative. Initially take 5 ml of the extract or 5 grams of dried herb daily for a week to help the herb absorb into your system, then cut back to the daily preventative dose.

Often a migraine headache will come suddenly and unexpectedly and last for days on end. This is the classic case of stress and imbalance of the nervous system. Magnesium is a good supplement here as it will help bring this system into balance. You can try many nervine herbals; however, often strong pain relief is necessary. If you take this pain relief stay in touch with your Health Care Practitioner and talk about the results and the time frames for response. You may require assistance to bring the skeletal system in balance as this can often be the cause of a migraine. You may also like to have acupuncture to help relieve the pain and have head massages. Loosen those muscles and just rest. Look out for exposure to toxins and an overload of poisons in your body as a trigger for a migraine.

Strong ginger tea increases circulation and also helps relieve all headaches, from hormonal cyclic headaches to migraines.

Strong ginger tea for migraines

Take a full knob of ginger about 4 inches long and at least 1 inch across. Grate the ginger and place in a pot. Cover with 400 ml of boiling water. Leave to infuse for ten minutes and pour a small amount into a cup. Sip throughout the day until you have drunk the whole brew.

Often with migraines you will feel nauseous and not want to eat or drink anything. Vomiting is common. Taking tiny amounts of this tea will help relieve the feelings of nausea as well as help ease the migraine.

Relaxing eye bag for headache relief

Are you a person who gets headaches and migraines regularly? If so, you need to make a relaxing eye bag that you place over your eyes when you want to lie down and relax whilst recovering from the pain.

Eye bag

Sew a small sack, about 10 by 15 cm, out of some cotton or natural fabric. Fill it loosely (so that it sits comfortably over your eyes) with a mixture of equal parts of dried lavender flowers, raw wheat grain and dried feverfew herb. Next, make up a small bottle containing 10 ml each of; chamomile essential oil, lavender essential oil, peppermint leaf oil and rose oil (if available).

When you get a headache simply heat the bag in the microwave for one minute until warm and then add a few drops of your essential oil blend to the warm bag (not the side that you place next to your eyes, but the far side that does not contact with your body) and place over eyes. Now lie down, place the eye bag over your closed eyes and relax. These oils and the weight of the bag are relaxing and can often be the comfortable nurturing factor as you wait for other medicines to help relieve your headache. This eye bag can become an integral part of your first aid kit, you can use it any time that someone needs to lie down and close their eyes and relax as part of the healing process.

Memory

Bacopa is an adaptogenic herb, which helps to bring all aspects of your body into balance. Research has shown that the active nitric oxide in bacopa has an extremely positive effect on learning and memory recall. Antioxidants and B-sitosterol, a powerful fatty acid, are found in bacopa which may be why it is revered so highly as the intellectual and brain rejuvenating tonic. Bacopa is an excellent herb for students, stressed business people and those who wish to improve memory capacity. Research with patients has found consistently that people who take bacopa daily have better short-term memory than before they started taking this herb.

Bacopa is a herb you need to take regularly. Expect some benefits within a week of taking 3 to 4 grams of herbal capsules daily, the benefits will last as long as the herb is taken. Bacopa helps with Alzheimer's and other conditions such as Meniere's disease; it is a herb best taken long term and preferably before you note any memory loss. Other good herbs for memory are panax and Siberian ginseng, lessor periwinkle, ginkgo biloba and gotu kola.

Improve your mental focus and vision

Omega-3 DHA fatty acid, specifically helps central nervous system function and visual system structure. Omega-3 helps improve and strengthen your eyes and balance your nervous system. This essential fatty acid is great for children who have learning difficulties and those who have trouble concentrating or staying focused on task. Research has also shown that supplementation of omega-3 can help decrease mental depression.

Some essential oils help increase your focus and concentration

Burning essential oils or even smelling their aroma in a cup of herbal tea can help increase your focus and memory for the short term. Have an oil burner in the room and add some fresh rosemary twigs, or the oil of rosemary and some water. Heat the burner and you will notice increased concentration as time goes on. You can also use sandalwood, grapefruit or other sharp oils for the same purpose. Experiment and see for yourself what oils increase your focus. Sage is another traditional favourite herb for memory, take as an infusion, extract or essential oil. Make sure you have a rest from concentrated mental tasks every 40 minutes or so, to help you stay focused and do your best job.

Smooth muscle restoratives

There are herbs called spasmolytics that relieve spasms and cramps in smooth muscle. Smooth muscle is part of your autonomic nervous system, and also the part that is out of your conscious control. Their effect may work throughout the body or on specific organs or systems. Most nervines are secondary spasmodics.

Alkaloids, flavonoids, saponins, essential oils and polysaccharides are the actives you need for these autonomic nervous system relievers to be effective. They work on neurotransmitters which operate at the nerve ganglia (wiring system). Sometimes these also have an effect on your central nervous system. They are effective for muscle cramps, dysmenorrhoea, cholelithiasis and cholecystitis, urinary calculi and renal colic. Use them in combination with carminatives or nervines if you need relaxing and restful healing herbs.

Often just a dash of one of these herbs in a potion will make the difference between a relaxed and functioning digestive tract in times of utter stress and a just functioning system. The gustatory nerve runs through your digestive tract and this nerve often plays havoc with stressed people who find themselves with loose bowels, pains in the stomach and other symptoms of digestive unease. These problems can be solved simply by adding some restful herbs to your meals and learning to avoid food when you are stressed.

Include all nervines in this category to help ease the spasmodic responses. But specific herbs are wild yam, cramp bark, and pasque flower.

Visionary

Your eyes are so closely related to your nervous system that often they are affected when you suffer from stress. Often the more chronic the stress becomes, the more problems you have with vision and seeing clearly. Make sure you look after your eyes when you are under stress.

Bilberries can improve night vision and strengthen your eyes. Studies have also shown that bilberry extract can arrest the progression of cataracts and diabetes-related eye damage.

Anthocyanidins are bitter compounds that inhibit collagen destruction, scavenger free radicals, reduce capillary permeability and increase blood circulation to peripheral blood vessels in the brain. Bilberry is also known to relieve muscle spasms. Anthocyanidins are known to regenerate 'visual purple' in your eyes, which is a protein that breaks down in sunlight and can dim your vision.

Bilberry is a good herb, used regularly to prevent eye damage for people who spend hours in front of computer screens, as well as night drivers and airline pilots. Blueberries and other dark red pigmented berries such as mulberries work in a similar way to bilberry and can be taken as a substitute. You will need to eat about two tablespoons of fresh or canned blueberries a day for good visual results.

Bilberry extract can be taken daily for good eye health, 2 ml of extract a day, or a single 2 gram tablet should help. Bilberry combines well with lutein and selenium, as these have been shown to increase the density of the macular pigment in the eye; also, the herb eyebright is good mixed with bilberry.

There is an interesting connection between loss of vision and blood sugar imbalances. Often people will have cravings for sugar and have signs of 'Type 2' diabetes at the same time they notice that their vision is deteriorating. The herb bilberry leaf also has chromium picolinate in it which helps increase the uptake of insulin in the blood stream and balance blood sugar levels after meals. Bilberry as mentioned is also excellent for vision.

It is indeed interesting with bilberry that Mother Nature has provided us with this one herb that takes care of two jobs, in the arena of middle age degenerative health care.

Any type of vision degeneration can be improved with a combination of antioxidants, bilberry, eyebright, vitamin C and vitamin A. If you have a vision problem you need to do eye exercises and you need to address all factors of your health. If your vision starts to weaken you need to ask why? Then act on this information.

Learn to say 'no' to stress

Stress is inevitable. However, there is good stress and bad stress, the stress we need and stress we don't need. You need to sort this out for yourself and decide what stress is acceptable to you and what stress is to be reduced, eliminated or altered. It's your life, it's your stress and only you can do something about it. Even if you are unable to change the stressful situation, then at least you can take your B group vitamins and listen to some relaxing music. You can make stress easier to cope with, and you can even make stress work for your body so that you are not so physically depleted from the experiences. Learn to say 'no' when you know you don't really want to take on a task which will cause you unwanted stress. The nervous system herbs help and you need to try to stay within your Wellness Zone most of the time. Over work and not enough time for family, friends and a social life can add pressure to your nervous system. Take time each day for some silence and allow yourself time to just reflect on life.

Sometimes we say *yes* to people when they infringe on us their own desires, without considering the impact of their actions on other people. This can result in unnecessary conflict and stress that you would rather avoid. Say *no* when someone wants to compromise your lifestyle or your plans to suit their own agenda. This is not bad manners, and it certainly is healthier for all concerned in the long run. If others become offended because their plans don't fit your needs, then it is good to talk about this and get it out in the open at the earliest convenience. This way you can avoid excessive and unnecessary stress. Also, don't be offended and try to understand when someone says *no* to you. Life is a two way street and respect needs to be shown in all relationships in order to avoid or minimalise stresses. The skill of listening and communicating clearly certainly helps when you want to avoid stress.

Alcohol adds to the stress load

Alcohol is one of the worst tools you can use to de-stress; however, it is the number one stress recovery tool used by many people. You have a few drinks with the intention of unwinding but what you are actually doing is loading your nerves with tension and your body with more toxic waste to get rid of, which adds to the stress load on your eliminative organs.

After a busy day you have a drink. This first drink is excellent, very relaxing and that's when you should stop. One drink can do wonders to allow you to forget your stress, but then you have another couple of drinks. You don't eat properly, and you don't rest as you should. When you finally get to bed you wake up in the middle of the night and worry about all the things you shouldn't worry about. This is typical but it is something that you should avoid when you are stressed. You actually need silence, rest, herbs, nutritional food and some more of those water-soluble B group vitamins. Keep off alcohol and caffeine and try to support yourself as much as possible. Rest, take memory herbs and nervous system support herbs along with a good clean diet and your antioxidants and you will be doing the best you can.

If you do have a drink of alcohol to unwind then make sure you have water to help stop dehydration. Also make the effort to have a meal which is nutritious and delicious to help you unwind. It may be tempting to have two, three or four drinks but draining the whisky bottle is not the path to wellness. Furthermore, the next day you will not be thinking clearly and will be adding even more stress to your nervous system. You would do well to go for a long walk or run after a stressful day and limit your alcohol.

Do you get depressed?

Everyone gets depressed from time to time. This is a feeling when, no matter what you do, you are feeling down and out. You are in the pit and wanting to get out, but unable to do so easily. All too often people turn to anti-depressant drugs too soon before they have tried natural solutions.

One natural solution is the herb hypericum, a natural, non-addictive anti-depressant that works fairly quickly in mild to moderate times of depression. You can also support your nervous system with B group vitamins and a magnesium supplement to help lift your spirits. When you are depressed, nothing can help you when you are not prepared to help yourself. You need to take responsibility for your depression and eliminate the problem before it becomes chronic and you find that depression is normal to you.

Often women become depressed after having babies, or through other hormonal problems. Men can become depressed when they become too stressed in work and feel that they are not coping. Anyone can get depressed when finances are tough, when hormones are out of balance and when ideas are not flowing freely, allowing you the freedom of feeling successful. Often depression comes about after a trauma or accident. In fact depression can become cyclic throughout the day.

People can be depressed at a certain time each day, each week or even each month, it is very individual.

The good thing about herbal anti-depressants is that they work quickly and help lift your morale without side effects; however, if you have a chemical imbalance or some deeper depression, make sure you see your Health Care Practitioner for a correct diagnosis and appropriate care. Herbal and vitamin anti-depressants are here to help balance you and in many incidences they are all you may require. However, if you are not getting results from your herbs and vitamins, then please seek further assistance. Your Health Care Practitioner can often make you up a stronger herbal formula, or other vitamins may be added to your regime.

Herbs to consider are: hypericum, melissa, chamomile, calendula, passionflower, kava kava, astragalus, valerian and maca. Some herbs are contraindicative to other medicines and each instance needs to be addressed individually.

Remember that children get depressed too and the herbal solutions are often gentle solutions. Simply give the child a chamomile tea before bed and some hypericum extract before school. Essential fatty acids and B group vitamins are important additions for any child who is depressed or feeling out of whack emotionally. The herbs for focus and concentration such as bacopa and gotu kola plus ginkgo biloba can also help with depression. The amino acid L-tryptophan, taken daily in combination with the herbs helps reduce depression.

There are some simple foods you can eat to help relieve depression

Hot rolled oats are a good food to nurture your nervous system and help relieve depression on a daily level. If you are depressed, eat old-fashioned hot rolled oats for breakfast. You can also add oats to cakes and other meals as they are nurturing to the nervous system. If you feel depressed regularly eat warm and nourishing foods in small amounts. Don't eat too much food as obesity certainly will add to your depression. If you are obese and depressed then lose some weight and you may find that your mood lifts as the weight goes down. Depression responds well to exercise. So get those endorphins going with a good daily walk where you can talk with a friend or to yourself for half an hour or longer. The more depressed you are the longer you should walk each day. For example, if you feel really depressed and are determined to make yourself feel better, time yourself to walk for one hour in one direction and then one hour home again. Walk at a gentle pace and stay safely on the footpath or way off the edge of the road. Do this for four to seven days a week and you will soon start to feel uplifted. You will become fit and toned and your mind will soon find other things to occupy itself with instead of feeling down and out. Other ways to deal with depression are to watch funny or light-hearted movies, talk with friends about good times and help someone else out on their rainy day.

Lighten up—it's the best choice

Depression can often be genetic or environmentally induced. If this is the case you need to realise that you are capable of helping yourself become stronger and removing yourself from your mental dilemmas. Seek professional assistance when you are depressed and also seek happy people with a positive attitude to life. Make the most of your day and take pleasure in the small things. This may be difficult at first, but persistence does bring rewards. Especially when you find that you are recovering from your depression and feeling joyful in your life again. Never give up on yourself or your loved ones when they are depressed. Always remember that cliché, there is light at the end of the tunnel where there is hope, love and eternal happiness. Isn't that a better picture than depression?

Chronic Fatigue Syndrome (CFS)

Chronic fatigue is often triggered by a burnt-out nervous system created by too much stress for too long. Have you ever felt so exhausted that you could sleep for a month? What about having an endless flu? Or perhaps you've suffered from a virus, started to recover only to crash again into total illness accompanied by an ever-growing depression? Any of these scenarios could be an indication that you are suffering from myalgic encephalomyelitis (ME) also known as chronic fatigue syndrome.

Until recently, those suffering this condition were medically ignored, considered hypochondriacs or classified as suffering from 'Yuppies flu', the result of high-flying lifestyles and late night parties. Now, thankfully ME/CFS is taking its place as a legitimate illness that deserves medical support, research and respect.

Amongst natural Health Care Practitioners, ME can be acknowledged and managed with some simple therapies and practices that will eventually help you back to health, back to a lifestyle where you are recovering and re-energising. Even if you don't get back to your previous fitness levels, you can still heal and lead an active life after ME/CFS.

CFS and ME, often interchanged, are the names for this debilitating set of symptoms that leave you incapable of functioning properly for a period of time, anywhere from six months to several years. There is no set time frame. The onset can be sudden, following an illness or it can be slow with no particularly astonishing event to justify the sheer exhaustion.

Symptoms can be so severe that you can take to your bed for months on end and have no energy for any activities. The results are often frightening, with broken health, broken careers and broken families.

What is this condition? Who is likely to get it? And what are some natural solutions to help manage recovery back to good health?

Spot the symptoms

It is generally agreed that if you have the following chronic symptoms lasting for six months or more you may well be suffering from ME/CFS:

1. Profound exhaustion exacerbated by minor exercise
2. Memory and concentration impairment
3. Intense flu-like feeling
4. Muscle pain
5. Sleep disturbance
6. Headaches
7. Disturbed balance
8. Depression or anxiety

Other less common symptoms include sore throat, painful lymph nodes, depression, nausea, mild fever or chills, etc.

According to research, women are more likely than men to get ME/CFS. There is no specific test for diagnosis, and it is often only diagnosed after eliminating other conditions. It can be more tiring and very frustrating for those suffering ME to undergo a whole swag of tests, which may result in an inconclusive diagnosis. So currently all you can do is to look at your history and symptoms and accept that you may be suffering from a condition that, although it has been recorded since the 1700s, there is as yet, no definitive procedure of medical confirmation.

What causes chronic fatigue?

The cause of ME/CFS is unknown, the symptoms may be caused by a continuing immune response, due either to a persisting infection or to the failure of the immune system to 'turn off' after an initial infection. Disturbances in brain chemistry may contribute to the symptoms, and some are examining alterations in cellular metabolism which could also be of significance.

In many cases, ME/CFS begins with a viral infection. The onset is sudden, with typical 'viral-like' symptoms. ME/CFS can begin with a bacterial or parasitic infection, a vaccination, or exposure to a toxic chemical or allergen, some sort of challenge to your immunity. Other contributors, such as strenuous physical activity or psychological stress can exacerbate the situation. In other cases, the onset of ME/CFS is gradual, with no recognisable precipitating event.

Many people experience 'viral' infections under similar circumstances, but what distinguishes ME/CFS is that the symptoms remain for a minimum of six months and frequently for many years. For this reason, researchers are examining whether people with ME/CFS have a genetic predisposition to developing the illness, and whether certain viruses which can evade the immune system are present in people with ME/CFS. For example, a history of glandular fever, Epstein Barr virus, Ross River fever or Lyme's disease are examples of precursors to ME.

Cytokines are the chemical messengers of the immune system. They play an important role in the communication between different immune system cells and the destruction of some organisms which invade the body. Some cytokines, such as interferon and interleukin, are used to treat diseases such as cancer and hepatitis B. When these cytokines are administered to patients, they develop symptoms very similar to CFS. Possibly continual production of cytokines by the immune system is the cause of many of the symptoms of CFS

Anyone can have ME/CFS, the old adage that you needed to be a yuppie has long gone. If affects mostly people between the ages of 18 and 45, these people can come from any socio-economic environment. You could have had a virus, or you could have no evident precursors to ME. It is such an unknown condition that we can only take it case by case and accumulate information on what therapies are working and how each person responds to different treatments.

Recovery and revitalisation

There is no better Health Care Practitioner than Mother Nature. With ME you need to take each specific indication and treat it synergistically with every other symptom. You also need to take into account the precursors and incorporate therapies to eliminate any residues from your system. This will involve cleansing the body, balancing the nervous system, ensuring that sleep patterns are normalised, treating depression appropriately, relieving pain and learning to pace yourself; mentally, emotionally and physically.

Try to be accepting, relax and recover gently with trust in your body's ability to let Mother Nature cure you with a little help from the many natural therapies available. It's not easy. Often you will be dealing with financial and emotional stresses that were unplanned. You will become frustrated because just as you are starting to feel energised, down you go again in another bout of sheer exhaustion.

It's very easy to overdo it with ME/CFS. Often people can go for a few weeks where they feel on the road to recovery, only to wake up one morning feeling worse than ever before!

In orthodox medicine it is stated that there is no specific treatment for ME/CFS; that there is only a management plan to help with recovery. Anti-depressants, painkillers and anti-inflammatories are often prescribed. You will need to decide whether any of these can help you. If so, then talk with your Health Care Practitioner. You can combine these orthodox prescription medications with natural remedies providing there are no interactions that may affect your health. Make sure you talk with your Health Care Practitioner about any medications or herbs you are taking. The last thing you need when suffering from ME is negative setbacks from herb/drug interactions.

Just take each day one at a time and remain positive with the firm belief that you will recover. Have an open mind and let the results from any therapies you try speak for themselves. If any form of therapy offers relief, that is wonderful and keep it up! Don't forget that time is an effective healer too, so if you make sure you look after yourself on all levels, there is light at the end of the tunnel.

Physical activity

Take it easy, with the gradual introduction of an enjoyable exercise plan. It's true that yoga, Tai Chi, walking and water exercises are often beneficial to the treatment of ME.

Try not to get depressed if you can hardly walk to the kitchen today. Just remember that you are suffering a debilitating condition that needs your full cooperation. This cooperation includes the acceptance that energy is low, and you now need to rest. When you feel ready, start your exercise regime with some gentle stretching in bed and then progress from there to the floor where you may be able to practice some yoga to tone your digestive tract, energise your organs and get some flexibility in your legs, back and arms. This may seem like a big call to begin with, but as you take on a regular daily routine, you may soon start to feel alive again. Tai Chi offers some very easy movements that tone your body too.

Rest when you need to rest, but try to stay out of bed as much as you can during the day to avoid sleep disturbances at night. Try to get a small amount of mobility going as often as possible. Gradually increase your exercise regime in graded steps. For example, you may only be able to do ten minutes of yoga a day this week, but next week increase it to 15 minutes, if you can, and keep it at that level for a few weeks before you step up again. Then you can add another form of exercise such as a short walk through the garden. Remember that you can crash back into exhaustion at any time, it's important to take the exercise plan gradually making sure you don't get too over-enthusiastic. Don't plan two big days in a row. If you need to go into work one day, make sure you have the next day at home to recuperate, the same for social activities.

Eat simply

When we consider that ME/CFS could be a post-viral condition, it seems fairly obvious that the lymph nodes and eliminative organs may be due for a cleanse. This is because your system will be sluggish and often symptoms such as irritable bowel syndrome and digestive congestion can be present.

Keep your diet light, fresh and delicious. Don't go clogging up your digestive tract with heavy meats and starchy breads. Instead opt for steamed vegetables, fresh salads, seasonal fruit and some quality protein in the form of eggs, lentils, fish and skinless chicken. Try to keep your fat intake fairly low as this will help to keep the load off your body in more ways than one. Take a supplement of essential fatty acids if required.

Make sure you get your essential minerals and vitamins. Eat regularly and in small amounts. This can also help speed up your metabolism, which could be running slowly at the moment. If you are preparing your own food, just remember that the less processed it is the better. Go for a couple of bananas and a glass of juice for lunch instead of processed commercial options that may add extra stresses to your eliminative organs.

It's easy to whip up a drink in the blender combining some protein powder with fresh fruit, or combine some herbs and supplements with soy milk and fruit for a super-healthy meal! Juices are always cleansing and they can be of great benefit for you when you are recovering from ME/CFS.

Natural supplements can help

Herbs can be slow to work, but you can have some good results if you look at some adaptogens such as: ginseng, astragalus, schisandra, withania, gotu kola and ganoderma. Perhaps the antimicrobial herbs of Chinese wormwood, olive leaf, cat's claw, black walnut and garlic will help eliminate any invaders. Antioxidants are also required: grape seed extract, maritime pine and vitamin C powder can all help. Liver herbs such as milk thistle and dandelion can help boost your system. Nervines are also very helpful when you feel stressed and sick.

Talk with your therapist and decide what's best for you. Each of us is individual and therefore all aspects need to be taken into account to come up with the best plan.

Severe flu-like symptoms can be treated like any other case of the flu with garlic, sage, thyme, andrographis, echinacea, fenugreek and bowls of warm vegetable soup! Just remember this, flu is dragging on a bit longer than usual, so you'll probably be completely sick of these remedies by the time you're feeling better! Muscle pain can be assisted with hot baths, steaming showers, massage, body work, magnesium, hypericum and some mental affirmations. White willow bark could also be of assistance.

Sleep disturbances can be tackled with valerian, a cup of chamomile tea before bed or some melatonin. Try to keep a regular sleep pattern going, sleeping during the night and staying awake during the day. This is not always easy; however, if you can get some good books and movies and have others to communicate with, you will be better off.

For unsteadiness or feeling off-balance, ginkgo biloba and feverfew may be of assistance, and you should also incorporate some balancing exercises into your daily regime.

Irritable bowel syndrome needs good fibre and fresh fruit and vegetables. Oat bran and rice bran can be good, Try to stay off the laxatives on a regular basis. Eat some rhubarb, drink some prune juice and plenty of water; also, try to keep your nervous system in balance as the autonomic nervous system has a direct impact on your digestive tract. If you are suffering from IBS then you may well have other digestive disturbances. In this case consider some aloe vera juice, acidophilus and slippery elm powder as part of your diet.

Headaches need rest, meditation, good bowel movements, an aligned spinal cord and some feverfew. Perhaps even the simple act of drinking a glass of water can help relieve your headache. This is one area with ME/CFS where orthodox medications are used regularly by many sufferers. If you do need to take painkillers make sure you balance it out by cleansing your body afterwards with some juices and herbs. Ginger tea daily helps.

Natural anti-depressants can be Sam-E, hypericum, chamomile and other nervines. B group vitamins are also important in keeping your nervous system in good condition.

Depression can be overcome with your own free will. Write affirmations, get out of the house and do some activities that you enjoy, as often as you can. Stay positive, stay focused on your healing and you will overcome ME/CFS.

Look at your options

Traditional cultural practices such as Chinese acupuncture and Indian Ayurvedic medicines have approaches to ME/CFS that can help revitalise your chi/prana. Look at techniques such as reiki, holistic pulsing, energy healings and crystals. Perhaps some flower essences are just what are needed to help lift your spirits, or the beautiful scent of pure rose essential oil. Keep your ears and eyes open for new information and therapies that can help.

Multiple Sclerosis (MS)

Multiple sclerosis is a nervous-system-triggered auto-immune disease that needs serious help! With an ever increasing patient list each year, it is estimated that up to 5% of Australian women will have this condition during their adult lives. Much research has been carried out over the years about MS, it has been prevalent in developed countries only, placing itself in the category of 'developed country diseases'. Now patterns are forming that suggest people who suffer from MS have had viruses in the past such as retrovirus and Epstein Barr virus. Could MS be another manifestation of post-viral syndrome fatigue that specifically targets the nervous system? There are natural solutions for MS sufferers to help ease the stress and lengthen the time span between relapses of this cyclic condition. These include dietary, herbal and lifestyle solutions.

What is MS?

MS is an auto-immune disease where the nervous system is damaged gradually over time. The pattern creating more severe symptoms and disabling the person's physical abilities to the point where the sufferer may be incapacitated for long periods of time. This is often followed by periods where you are able to move more freely and capable of having an active life, only to be followed by another period of debilitation. There may be some cells in your body that are programmed in your own unique genetic structure to turn off or die off at a certain point in time.

However, there are steps you can take to help retard this cell degeneration that occurs with MS. What you need to take is dependent upon your own situation. If you want to help yourself with MS, the first place to start is to repair the nerve sheaths that may be programmed for this auto-death situation. Use nutritional and herbal medicines to help this nervous system as your priority.

To be more specific, your nervous system is like an electrical wiring system circulating around the body. With MS the myelin sheaths in the central nervous system are destroyed gradually. They are reduced to hardened and non-functioning sheaths called scleroses. The loss of the myelin, which is due to an immune attack on myelin basic protein, results in short-circuiting and shunting of the current which ensures the successive nodes are excited more and more slowly, until eventually the impulse conduction completely stops. The interesting part of this action is that the nerve axons are not actually damaged. This results in growing numbers of sodium channels that appear automatically in the demyelinated fibres. This may explain why there are periods of relapse and periods of wellness.

How does MS affect you?

MS is most often diagnosed in young people between the ages of 20 and 40. It is predominately a developed country disease which suggests that lifestyle and exposure to environmental toxins may be a trigger. Women can get MS after the birth of a child or, as research is showing, MS can be a post-viral disease. A common symptom is visual disturbance including blindness. One early diagnostic sign of MS is looking at the eye using an ophthalmoscope and observing the demyelination where the optic nerve enters the back of the eye.

The symptoms are not always consistent and it may take time before an accurate diagnosis can be made. Because MS is a progressive disease of the nervous system, there may be a disturbance in the sensory nerves, especially in the peripheral parts of the body such as feet and hands. There can be a feeling of walking on air and the sufferer may start to stumble more than usual. There may be a disturbance of the nerves controlling movement followed by the dragging of the legs and walking stiffly with a slowdown in the response to any given situation. This can include many muscles in your body, including the jaw, arms, and legs.

Eventually MS affects the intestinal muscles and the bladder sphincter which may be put out of action. As the disease progresses the mouth and vocal cords can be affected. MS is a fairly painless disease, pain is rarely present and when it is, it is not unbearable.

The patient is easily depressed, often puts on weight and can suffer from low self-esteem through the constant stress with MS. There can be added financial strains on the family and emotional stresses as you experience the 'bad' parts of the cycle.

Studies conducted by Wagner et al. Viral Immunol 2000 showed that 100% of MS sufferers in their research were Epstein Barr virus (EBV) seropositive, with a lack of evidence of a current EBV infection, suggesting its role as a persistent latent virus. Other tests have been conducted since then, which strongly support this finding.

Endogenous retroviruses have also been identified with MS plasma samples, but not in controlled research. Elevated antibodies to these retroviruses have been found in MS sufferers. It has been suggested that the presence of both the Epstein Barr virus and retrovirus is a trigger for MS. However, the presence of retrovirus may be endogenous and it is activated by the EBV infection.

Relapses

Infections and weakened immunity tend to trigger another relapse in sufferers of MS. You can do well whilst taking immunity boosting herbs, a good diet, and some excellent antioxidants only to relapse when you stop this regime even for a short period of time and pick up another flu or bug doing the rounds. Even exposure to the cold or getting caught in the rain can trigger a relapse if the immunity is not strong and boosted.

Studies in England have shown that many MS sufferers are also chronic sinusitis sufferers. MS sufferers are generally sensitive and allergic to many environmental triggers. Stress tends to be another trigger for a relapse. Often if there is an emotional argument, financial stress, a death in the family or any shock a relapse will occur.

Relapses can be regular or they can occur randomly depending upon the events, support and health of the patient. The best active practice in helping a MS patient is to boost their immunity, strengthen the nervous system and delay the time frame between each relapse as much as possible.

How can you cure MS?

Injections of beta interferon have been successful with orthodox medicine in reducing the frequency of the attacks, but do not eliminate the symptoms whilst the attack is acute. Bovine myelin has been used in research trials and it is suggested that this therapy provokes the production of suppresser cells that inhibit the immune attack against myelin basic protein.

Is there a cure? Not yet. However we can ease MS naturally, by living a healthy lifestyle with good dietary practices and using alternative health care approaches to enhance the good times and delay the relapse into bad times.

Keep your diet healthy

The diet needs to be specifically tailored so that you are not eating foods you are allergic to. Therefore keep low on dairy and gluten if they affect you. Also, stay away from environmental triggers such as pollution, cigarette smoke, chemicals, insecticides, pesticides, artificial fertilisers and fragrances that may trigger an allergic response. Petrochemical products can also trigger allergies along with paints and synthetic fabrics.

Use alternative approaches

Floatation tanks, rebirthing and Neural Linguistic Programming (NLP) are all options to alter the way you perceive a situation. With MS it's important to look at the alternative realities and the choices you have when faced with your darkest days. These alternative therapies, including counselling, can really help boost your confidence and make you see the world in a lighter way.

Regular massage

There are many types and styles of massage that can help MS. When you are in a relapse make sure you get regular gentle massages that will keep the circulation going and also keep your body toned as much as possible. This will help you in the long run as the relapse ends and you find yourself feeling more comfortable. When you are experiencing good health, massage is important to help keep your body in that state, it can also make a difference to the time frame between relapses and it is certainly a pleasant way to extend the MS good health period!

Herbs can help

- The immune modulator herbs, such as Chinese wormwood, astragalus, echinacea, cat's claw and olive leaf, can all help with boosting the immunity.
- Antiviral herbs, such as hypericum, play a double role as hypericum is also a favourite anti-depressant herb and certainly helps MS.
- Anti-inflammatory herbs, such as celery seed, turmeric, ginger, hops and gotu kola, help relieve inflammation and reduce excess fluid retention.

- Adaptogenic herbs, such as withania, ginseng and bacopa, are excellent to strengthen the system and act as a good tonic.
- Cleansing herbs, such as dandelion and milk thistle, are good taken regularly for MS as they will help keep your body cleansed of toxins on a regular basis.
- Allergies need to be addressed herbally with fenugreek and other specific herbs depending upon the situation.

Make sure you address all the other side effects that have started to creep into your body since the onset of MS. These include arthritis, weight gain, depression, multiple allergies, and bad habits, such as smoking or drinking alcohol in excess. Once you have a complete picture of all your personal problems, then you can specifically tailor a lifestyle, medicinal and exercise plan to have maximum healing potential?

What to do if you're worried about a child's attention, behaviour and nerves

Too many children are on medications these days for various nervous system based health conditions. Too many parents allow their children to be placed on these medications thinking they are doing the right thing to help decrease conditions such as behavioural and attention disorders. Often these medications can be avoided when the parents look at natural alternatives that nurture and balance the child's nervous system and help increase their ability to focus and concentrate. Giving your children a good nutritional profile and eliminating toxins from their diet and environment goes a long way towards helping your child take responsibility for their own actions and decisions about appropriate behaviour. As parents we need to lead our children by example and treat them with the utmost of respect and mentoring to help them develop into self-responsible and self-monitoring people. The nervine herbs, B group vitamins, natural unprocessed foods, and love are all part of this process.

If you have trouble with your child's behaviour, the first course of action after eliminating the rubbish from their diet and toxins from the environment is to give them B group vitamins, essential fatty acids in the form of omega-3 and some herbs such as chamomile, valerian, hypericum and oats. Children do well on hops and valerian to help them sleep at night.

Help your children create silence in their day and routine as this helps stabilise and balance the nervous system. All behavioural problems can be relieved with therapeutic doses of nutritional and herbal medicines. With the help of your Health Care Practitioner your child can be healthy and develop naturally.

Many people worry that their child may have some type of attention deficit syndrome. Look at old-fashioned solutions such as spending time with the child and treating them with respect. Once again the nutritional profile and dietary habits are paramount.

The basic regime for these children is simple

- In the morning they need one good quality B group vitamin tablet with zinc. They need the herbs ginkgo biloba, hypericum, astragalus and bacopa mixed together in a therapeutic dose for the child's body weight.
- They need omega-3 fatty acids in a therapeutic dose to their body size.
- A good breakfast containing some protein such as egg with whole grain toast and some fruit juice.
- Send small nourishing and healthy snacks for a day at school.
- When they arrive home from school they need some magnesium powder mixed in a drink with some L-glutamine the amino acid.
- Dinner needs to be early with protein and vegetables.
- They need rest, relaxation and no television in the evening. Teach them to read, draw or write.
- Before bed they need nervine herbs such as valerian and chamomile.
- Early to bed and early to rise. Lots of positive energy and support.

If the child isn't responding to this regime, then look at the parents' attitude and lifestyle and encourage them to follow a similar regime. This usually produces results as the whole family becomes balanced again, together! Often children are canaries to the environment at home, if there is a lot of stress or worry in the home then these can be reflected directly and unconsciously in the child's behaviour. In the world today, too many parents are working and life gets harder for younger people as they have to juggle school with after school care, homework, stressed parents, financial difficulties, relationship conflicts, personal development, play and a myriad of other problems that adults can often overlook as they get on with their own lives. This can all contribute to the nervous system balance being tipped in the wrong direction and children responding in inappropriate ways to situations.

It's all a learning process and to balance children's focus, behaviour and nerves it often takes a whole family. Remember the saying, 'It takes a whole village to raise one child', and your child deserves the love, contribution, mentoring, time and appreciation of the whole village too. So, as a parent, make time for your children and don't overlook their problems. The worst thing a parent can do for their child is to place them in a category and leave them there. The best thing a parent can do is to overlook the labelling and help the child develop, with research, love and safe nutritional healing solutions.

CHAPTER SIX

Cardiovascular

You need to know as much about your genetics as possible in this area of your Wellness Zone. If your father, mother or grandparents had any problems with their circulatory system or heart, then you cannot afford to sit in ignorance and think that you are safe from one of the biggest killer illnesses in our world today. Yes, for your Wellness Zone you need information, and you need to learn about specific conditions that may be genetically passed to you and your children. For example, if there is a history of cardiac arrest in the family, and you know that your father and grandfather had this condition at a certain age (usually in their 40s or 50s), then you may well be predisposed to exactly the same rerun in your life. The risk is even greater if you smoke or handle stress in ways that make a situation worse.

Women are not excused from this position either. Up until menopause, women's hormones act as a protection against many forms of cardiovascular disease. However after menopause women are at risk in much the same way as men. So, protect your heart and circulatory system as a priority in your life. Varicose veins and stagnant pooling of blood in the pericardium of the heart are all too common symptoms of women's cardiovascular disease.

Keep your blood flowing freely with the assistance of white willow bark, ginkgo biloba and bilberry. Keep your cholesterol under management with natural techniques. Make sure your arteriosclerosis is under control and do all within your power to keep your cardiovascular health in good condition. Make sure you keep your vision good with eyebright and bilberry. If your feet and peripheral circulation become cold or numb, make sure you are aware of this and that you take ginkgo biloba, bacopa, ginseng, hawthorn berry and other herbals and natural solutions to help keep your body functioning optimally. Remember that if your cardiovascular health is poor, then the chances are that your memory is not functioning efficiently either. 'Use it or lose it' is very relevant when it comes to cardiovascular health. Get fit, get thinking, get busy and don't stop. Cardiovascular health is the key to long life and good health.

High blood pressure means that your arteries and veins could be heavy and solid, like plastic; this is an indication that they may also be constricted and blocked with arteriosclerosis. All of these indicate that you need to soften these vessels with apple cider vinegar and lemon juice. You need to take antioxidants and you need to take protective measures against genetic and other cardiovascular problems that may lead to your instant death.

The lowdown on cholesterol and arteriosclerosis

The relationship of high cholesterol to arteriosclerosis is developed in a series of events that are often brought about by diets high in saturated fatty acids leading to an overload of LDLs in the body which carry the cholesterol through the system to deposit in arteries causing the end product of arteriosclerosis.

Cholesterol is a waxy substance that occurs naturally in your body. It's produced by the liver to build cell walls and make certain hormones. You can't function without a certain amount of cholesterol but the body makes all that it needs; 80% of cholesterol is synthesised in your liver and only 20% actually comes from dietary animal products we eat. It is common for many of us to have an unhealthy accumulation of cholesterol.

Triggered by damage to the tunica intima caused by blood borne chemicals, viruses or physical factors, such as a blow or hypertension, injured endothelial cells release chemotactic agents and mitosis inducing factors, which begin to transport and modify greater amounts of lipids picked up from the blood, in particular LDL's.

LDL's are the type of lipoprotein that delivers cholesterol to tissue cells in the bloodstream. When the sequestered LDL becomes oxidised it damages neighbouring cells and acts as a chemotactic agent to attract monocytes to the area. The monocytes then cling to altered endothelial cells and migrate beneath the tunica intima where they become macrophages. These macrophages then gorge on oxidised LDL's and become transformed into lipid-laden foam cells and lose their scavenging ability.

Soon, these macrophages are joined by smooth muscle cells migrating from tunica media and they also take up lipids and become foam cells. These accumulating foam cells initiate the fatty streak stage.

The smooth muscle cells also deposit collagen and elastin fibres, thickening the intima and producing fibrous lesions with a core of dead and dying foam cells called arteriosclerotic plaques. These fatty moulds of muscle and fibrous tissue begin to protrude into the vessel lumen which is the condition arteriosclerosis.

Some people have the added disadvantage of lipoprotein (a) which is involved in delivering cholesterol to sites where tissue repair is occurring. Lipoprotein (a) is a special LDL that is presumed to assist in wound healing, but it backfires when present in excess. Lipoprotein (a) binds to the subendothelial tissues more avidly then other LDL's. It is thought to promote the mitosis of cells in vessel walls. Because it resembles plasminogen, it can call upon it at sites where clots have formed. However it lacks plasminogens clot-dissolving ability, so it competes successfully with that clot buster and may prevent the disposal of undesirable clots.

Arteriosclerosis is the end stage of the disease. Enlarged plagues hinder the diffusion of nutrients from the blood to deeper tissues of the artery wall. Smooth muscle cells in tunica media die, elastic fibres deteriorate and are replaced by non-elastic scar tissue, and calcium is deposited in the lesions. These events cause arterial walls to fray and ulcerate, encouraging platelet adhesion and thrombosis formation.

The increased rigidity of the walls leads to hypertension which increases the risk of myocardial infarcts, strokes and aneurisms. Too much cholesterol in the blood is a major contributing cause of heart and blood vessel disease. Cholesterol forms clots and plaques that clog the arteries causing arteriosclerosis that can choke off the supply of blood to your heart (causing heart attacks) and to your brain (leading to stroke).

By lowering your cholesterol level you take personal responsibility and may be able to stop plaques from developing in your arteries, and shrink clots that have already formed. This is true preventative medicine where you actively contribute to your Wellness Zone.

If you have already had a heart attack or bypass surgery, your Health Care Practitioner can check your cholesterol level regularly. Keeping the level low is your best insurance against blocked arteries. Understanding your cholesterol level is an important key for anyone who wants to ensure good health in later years and also for anyone who eats dietary fats regularly or who has a family history of coronary heart disease or strokes.

The high-density lipoprotein (HDL) cholesterol is referred to as the 'good' cholesterol, because of its ability to cleanse the arteries and act as a carrier to remove the slower accumulating low-density lipoprotein (LDL) cholesterol, or the 'bad' cholesterol, which builds up and clogs the arteries. Technically, we want to increase our levels of HDL and lower our levels of LDL cholesterol in the blood. The higher the HDL level, the lower your chance of having a heart attack or stroke.

If you don't know your cholesterol readings, call your Health Care Practitioner for testing. The cholesterol test is best done after a 12 hour fast. The blood test will also measure blood components such as triglycerides. Like cholesterol, triglycerides are a type of fat that is found in foods, including meat, cheese, fish and nuts, and is also manufactured by the body. There is a relationship between high triglyceride levels and heart disease. Cholesterol and triglyceride testing will help you determine how likely you are to develop heart disease.

How to lower your cholesterol level

Getting regular exercise, maintaining a healthy weight, and limiting the amount of alcohol, carbohydrates and saturated fat in your diet will help lower your cholesterol and triglyceride levels. Globe artichoke assists in lowering cholesterol levels, helping the gall bladder remove the cholesterol efficiently through the small intestine and eliminate it thoroughly. Sugar cane waxes are proving popular especially when taken in a therapeutic dose each day. The phytostanols have been attracting quite a bit of attention as they are have effective results in comparison to statin drugs. They get the blood flow moving and clear low-density cholesterol; they shake up the arteriosclerosis with some good old-fashioned garlic, turmeric, ginger and capsicum, which are good to remove the plaque. Also adding selenium to the diet and Coenzyme Q10 are good for anyone who is at risk of having high cholesterol.

Avoid high-fat and cholesterol-rich foods such as French fries and other fast foods: tortillas, sausage, bacon, hot dogs, cake, cookies and other desserts. Do not fry your food. Common sense prevails here; it's fairly obvious that if you eat more fatty foods then you have more chance of absorbing them into your blood stream. The phytostanols work as cholesterol blockers, and they act as a barrier between your small intestine so the cholesterol laden fatty cells do not get diffused through into your blood stream. Essential fatty acids are good fats and these can be eaten freely by anyone, including people with high cholesterol levels.

However, saturated fats increase blood cholesterol levels. There is often hidden cholesterol in commercial foods, so check the labels, or better still, avoid them altogether.

There is no daily recommendation for total fat intake. Just look at the obesity in the world and you will see that your body has an amazingly huge appetite for foods that create fat in your cells. So avoid the temptation and try to restrict fat calories to 20% or less of your total calories each day, and fewer than 5% of these fat calories should come from saturated fats.

How to reduce saturated fat in your diet

Eliminate fatty animal products from your diet, such as hamburgers, bacon, sausage, and processed meats. Cut the visible fat from meat and remove the skin from poultry. Read labels carefully and avoid foods that contain hydrogenated vegetable oils, cocoa butter, beef fat and lard. Be kind to your body, only have these foods if there is absolutely no alternative (which shouldn't be often).

Use skim or low-fat milk and milk products. Enjoy fat-free snacks, including pretzels, air-popped popcorn and fruit. Avoid lollies and desserts, especially those containing butterscotch and caramel (this is extreme for most of us, so do your best to cut down your sweet tooth).

Are you overweight? If so, losing weight will help you lower your cholesterol level. It's best to lose only a half to 1 kilo per week; exercise will also help you lose weight and lower your cholesterol.

Phytosterols—natures new cholesterol cutter

One key for optimal health is to keep your cholesterol levels low. Have you ever wondered about cholesterol levels and how you can keep them in a healthy balance? Research is showing that phytosterols are the new cholesterol cutters, so use herbs and plants as a preventative measure.

How do I keep my cholesterol levels in balance?

The key to a healthy cholesterol balance is to keep the blood serum levels of cholesterol low and eliminate any cholesterol that is not needed for immediate hormonal use. Now if you have a diet that is high in plant sterols, then you will produce less LDL and you will have a better chance of taking the LDL safety out of your body.

The aim when balancing cholesterol levels is to lower the total levels, inhibit its production by the liver, lower triglyceride levels, increase HDL levels whilst decreasing the LDL levels, inhibit the oxidation of LDL's and help prevent blood clotting and platelet stickiness.

What is a phytosterol?

Plant sterols and plant stanols are collectively known as phytosterols. Plant sterols are plant hormones with chemical structures similar to that of cholesterol. Especially high sterol levels are found in rice bran, wheatgerm, corn oils and soybeans. In a more concentrated form, these substances are called plant stanols. Structurally these compounds are chemically similar to cholesterol. However, unlike cholesterol derived from animal sources which absorb easily and raise the body's own cholesterol levels, phytosterols are present only at very low levels in the body because they are difficult to absorb.

Interestingly, phytosterols so closely resemble cholesterol that they can actually block food-based cholesterol from being absorbed into the bloodstream. The result is that both phytosterols and dietary cholesterol end up excreted in waste matter.

Food manufacturers have begun to incorporate plant sterols and stanols into margarines. Nutritional supplement manufacturers also offer phytosterols in tablet form for those individuals who don't want the extra calories of cholesterol-lowering margarine. However you don't need to take margarine to get phytosterols. Many common and nutritious foods contain these essential sterols which you can add to your daily menu.

How do phytosterols work?

Put simply, phytosterols block your body's ability to absorb cholesterol. They work by fooling the body into thinking they are its own cholesterol, so instead of making more, the liver makes less. Also, they are carried about harmlessly attaching themselves to other cholesterol in the system. It's a real win–win situation for your body and certainly is worth trying if you are suffering from the effects of high cholesterol.

Sitosterol (a phytosterol) is a white waxy substance, made by plants and is contained in many plant oils, especially corn oil and avocado oil. It has the effective action of blocking cholesterol from being absorbed through the villi of the small intestine, whilst being quite safe and not blocking the assimilation of other nutrients.

It's quite an amazing product as it doesn't matter how much cholesterol is contained in foods in the gastrointestinal tract, sitosterol will prevent it from getting into the blood stream. With adequate amounts of sitosterol taken in oil or tablet form you can eat your favourite rich foods with less worry about the cholesterol.

Foods high in phytosterols

Avocados are a number one source of phytosterols; remember that as phytosterols are plant hormones, most plants will have them in trace amounts. However, because they are suspended in fatty acids, the oilier the plant the more phytosterols will be in the food.

For example, flaxseed oil is high in phytosterols, as are the vegetable oils derived from many plants including soybeans, olives, coconuts and seed oils including sunflower and sesame. Sunflower seeds, nuts and grains of all types contain phytosterols. Phytostanols are concentrated forms of plant hormones and found in the oils of plants such as pine trees and sugar cane. These oils are readily available commercially and are often esterified for access to the active stanols such as polycosinal.

Because phytosterols are not easily absorbed into our system and they work by picking up random cholesterol and carrying it out of the body, you can add them to your diet easily and naturally incorporating the benefits into almost any meal!

The best herbs to lower cholesterol

Some herbs have proved themselves through time to help reduce cholesterol problems. Simply add these to your diet high in phytosterols and you are well on the way to good cholesterol levels.

Chilli

Hot chilli is the herb of choice to help eliminate cholesterol problems with patients who do not suffer complications. Capsicum is known to help break down arteriosclerosis and help remove it from the body. It also acts as a stimulant and helps with circulation.

Take 400 mg capsule of chilli daily with food. Or add a teaspoon of honey to half a teaspoon of capsicum powder four times a week. A few drops of the extract can be added to food or drink daily.

Globe artichoke

Globe artichokes are known to help eliminate cholesterol from your body faster by acting as a choleretic and by increasing the contractive power of the bile duct which improves the flow of bile from the liver to the gallbladder. The mode of action is considered the indirect inhibition of an enzyme as part of cholesterol biosynthesis.

Globe artichoke also helps increase liver tissue regeneration, increases liver circulation, increases the RNA content in liver cells and stimulates cell division. All adds to cholesterol cutting.

Take 5 ml herbal extract with juice or water as a preventative measure, preferably before meals mixed with a teaspoon of apple cider vinegar and a teaspoon of flaxseed oil to help block the cholesterol uptake.

Garlic

Garlic has been used to lower total serum cholesterol and prevent clotting of blood in traditional Western herbalism. Research has shown garlic to lower serum cholesterol levels and inhibit the oxidation of LDL cholesterol. Use fresh garlic in your cooking.

Garlic potion

Juice fresh garlic bulbs (leave the skin on) and refrigerate to age. Use a teaspoon in salad dressings and on top of vegetables.

Ginkgo biloba

Ginkgo biloba is one herb you hear a lot about. Everyone knows its popular benefit of increasing blood circulation and nutrition to the brain. It increases your short-term memory and because of its flavonoidal actions ginkgo is a very good general tonic and an excellent antioxidant. An antioxidant is a substance that mops up free radicals in your system and assists them to flush out harmlessly. Too many free radicals create disharmony and can lead to gradual deterioration of your body. This can manifest as ageing, cancers, illness and general lowered vitality and strength.

The combination of ginkgo biloba with hawthorn is now widely used by Health Care Practitioners for conditions such as high blood pressure and circulatory problems. This combination is particularly good because it combines the benefits of ginkgo with hawthorn's action of dissolving deposits in thick and sclerotic arteries. It also improves circulation to the heart, providing it with rich oxygenated blood and helps reduce; blood pressure, prophylactic stroke and heart attack. Ginkgo and hawthorn work synergistically together with excellent results, therefore offering a natural remedy as an alternate to prescription drugs.

Cardiovascular tonics

These either work directly on the heart, in which case they are called left cardio tonics, or they work on the venous system entering the heart, in which case they are called right cardio tonics. Most that work on the left heart are scheduled agents that work by strengthening the heart muscle and regulating coronary output. Actives involved are flavonoids, procyanidins, cardiac glycosides, alkaloids and amines. Omega fatty acids DHA and EPA are excellent to help reduce your chances of cardiovascular disease.

Most herbal remedies are based on constituents like tannins and flavonoids rather than potentially toxic cardiac glycosides and alkaloids. The most widely used cardiotonic is hawthorn. Hawthorn also contains procyanidins and flavonoids, which have potent antioxidant effects on blood vessels, helping prevent atherosclerosis, heart disease, high cholesterol and arteriosclerosis. Cardiovascular tonics are used for congestive heart disease, hypertension, as a preventative for heart disease, peripheral vascular disease and arrhythmias.

You can use the following herbs for preventative cardiovascular tonics: hawthorn, ginkgo biloba, bilberry, grape seed and myrrh. Combine these herbs together for a delicious little heart tonic, circulatory tonic—strengthening the vascular system—or memory enhancing potion which also assists vision. The antioxidant actions of these herbs make them an almost must-have combination for anyone who runs the risk of heart disease. This is actually just about everyone today in our over-stressed and overfed world! The cardiovascular system is certainly affected by bad dietary choices and exposure to pollutants and environmental toxins which brings about the need for super strong antioxidants.

Everyone who smokes should have antioxidants and cardiovascular tonics daily. Everyone who is exposed to stress, bad diet, pollution and has a genetic predisposition to any vascular conditions would do well to adopt these herbs.

Horse chestnut cream

Mix together the herbs horse chestnut, in a cream with bilberry for topical application. This can help varicose veins and also helps shrink the little capillaries on the surface of the legs. Apply this cream blend if you are standing on your feet all day, especially on cement, or standing still more than you are moving.

Do shoulder stands for five minutes at least three times a week in the evenings. This gets the circulation going the opposite way and can greatly assist oedema and the pooling of blood that occurs with some cardiovascular disorders. If you are unable to do shoulder stands then lie on the floor with your feet up against the wall. This is effective too!

Just lie there and watch the news each night. You will find that toxins find their way down into your peripherals and also the blood will move up towards the body and you will enjoy less stresses on your legs the next day. This can assist in decreasing varicose veins and stop them worsening. Shoulder stands, and opposite positions are also good to help improve your memory as the blood rushes to your brain.

Keep your veins and arteries soft and flexible. This is where the herb bilberry can assist, as it helps strengthen the walls. You also need collagen, vitamin C and apple cider vinegar in your diet regularly to help keep your venous system flexible and soft. Smoking is the fastest way to make this system stiff and constricting and of course the build-up of plaque on the inside walls of veins and arteries can block them which is a very hazardous situation.

Hot chilli and garlic in combination helps remove this plaque. It is well known amongst Health Care Practitioners that these two herbs work well to break the plaque away from the internal walls and help to carry it out of the venous system, excreted via the kidneys. Drink plenty of water, as even though your kidneys are part of another system, they are also intrinsically related to the venous system and they help monitor your blood pressure as well as discriminate between what will be staying in your blood stream and what will be eliminated.

Look after your kidneys by flushing them regularly with lots of fresh clean water. This is another preventative for your cardiovascular system that is often overlooked as people consume sweet soft drinks and stimulating coffee instead of clean water. Make your Wellness Zone a clean cardiovascular zone!

Cardiovascular disease

Many aspects of cardiovascular disease can be improved with an increased consumption of omega-3, such as decreasing systolic and diastolic blood pressure levels, which is helpful in hypertension. Omega-3 has antiarrhythmic properties and research has shown supplementation prevented fatal ventricular fibrillation, tachycardia and ventricular premature beats. Omega-3 also lowers LDL and VLDL cholesterol levels and triglycerides in the blood and helps raise the HDL good cholesterol assisting in the management of cholesterol and arteriosclerosis.

Anybody who has suffered any problems with their heart or cardiovascular system needs to ensure that they keep their body weight within a good healthy range. So, if you are even slightly overweight you are adding load to this system of the body and putting yourself at risk. Don't smoke, look after your heart health as though your life depended upon it, literally. You see, if you have one kidney fail, the other will take over, if your digestion is not operating well, you may get very sick through lack of absorption of nutrients, if you have a lung collapse, there is another one there operating, if you have almost any illness there is time. But, with cardiovascular attacks, time is not on your side. If a blocked piece of arteriosclerosis breaks away and gets stuck in your heart, then you may die instantly. If your heart stops functioning for any reason, well, that could result in instant death. So, don't take this for granted.

If your heart still beats, you are very lucky to have got a second chance once you have already had a coronary bypass or other such operation. However, don't risk it and pretend everything is OK. With some good health practices you can recover, come off all medicines and have a very healthy life. You can also become very sluggish, develop multiple illnesses and grow more depressed and obese after such operations and life experiences. A lot of the results are your choice. It's your Wellness Zone, make your choice and make the effort to get the results. You don't get fit and healthy by being a lounge lizard, and you don't get healthy on a fatty and overfed diet!

Keep your blood thin and your veins strong

Keeping your blood thin and running freely through the venous system is your best preventative method for strokes and other cardiovascular blockages in the venous system or heart. The herbs ginkgo biloba, capsicum pepper and white willow bark are specifically targeted to this end. You would do well to eat garlic in your diet daily and also have beetroot regularly as this is a premium blood cleanser and strengthener.

Other herbs to keep your blood clean and strong are: garlic, sarsaparilla, rehmannia, nettle, onion and bilberry. Bilberry also works on keeping the veins and arteries elastic and strong, helping eliminate your chances of high cholesterol. Apple cider vinegar is good to keep your venous system soft and elastic as you want to avoid the possibility of your system becoming plastic and hard which is a precursor to many cardiovascular diseases. Keep triglyceride levels down with omega-3 fatty acids. These fatty acids also assist with keeping your veins and arteries strong and functioning optimally.

Varicose veins

Horse Chestnut has shown itself to be the herb of choice if you wish to minimalise varicose veins and prevent future ones. The active compound aescin helps to seal weak capillaries and veins, reducing the swelling and relieving pain in existing varicose veins.

Research has shown that horse chestnut effectively reduced leg pain from chronic venous insufficiency. Horse chestnut will not reverse the deep veins protruding from your limbs; however, it will help arrest the situation and relieve the strain on your venous system by helping to eliminate some of the smaller less offensive veins.

Horse chestnut is a must-have herb for those who are on their feet all day and for anyone with a genetic tendency towards varicose veins who doesn't want them to get worse. Take horse chestnut regularly for a month or longer to notice a difference. The benefits will only last as long as you are taking the herb and veins will start coming back within a couple of weeks of ceasing the treatment. Topical creams are effective for decreasing varicose veins.

Keep your blood pressure down naturally

There are natural solutions to keeping your blood pressure down, even after years of Western living you can take measures to help yourself naturally reduce blood pressure. Magnesium is one mineral which is gaining a reputation for helping to balance your blood pressure levels. You also need to keep your kidneys in optimal condition as they are regulators of blood pressure. To do this make sure your adrenal glands are in good health with herbs and good fluid intake. Also keep your system as non-acidic as possible as this will help your kidneys function optimally, which in turn helps your blood pressure.

The amino acid taurine helps cleanse the liver and regulate blood pressure. Keeping your liver clean and detoxification pathways operating optimally is key to keeping your blood pressure down. Once you develop a beer belly or fat around your abdomen then you are certainly in the running for increased blood pressure. This fat is a clear indicator that your health is on a downhill slide towards degenerative illness.

Stay trim, fit and healthy and you have a better chance of keeping your blood pressure lower. Keep as stress-free as possible and also ensure that your cholesterol levels are in check. High cholesterol can lead to arteriosclerosis, a sure-fire way of blocking veins and arteries with plaque that can lead to high blood pressure as these passages narrow.

Keep your veins and arteries soft and healthy with bilberry extract and apple cider vinegar, this will help your blood pressure stay normal due to the flexibility in the veins and arteries. If you do find that your blood pressure is creeping up, then simply take a detox, lose the excess weight, drop the stress load, reduce the cholesterol, repair the kidney or liver dysfunction and you will find yourself back on the road to health.

Talk with your Health Care Practitioner about any other nutritional herbs and supplements to help reduce the blood pressure problem such as co-enzymes and co-factors to amino acid synthesis. You may be surprised at how simple it is to make the change to good health again, once you see some results from simple lifestyle changes.

Hot chilli cardiovascular protecting formula

Take 100 grams of hot capsicum and cayenne pepper powder. Mix with 100 grams of fresh runny honey, 100 ml of boiling hot water and 100 ml of apple cider vinegar in a glass jar. Stir mixture well and place in fridge.

Each time you need to use the formula shake the jar first. Take one teaspoon and add to meals or drink with water four or five times a week. This will help break down arteriosclerosis and also increase peripheral circulation.

CHAPTER SEVEN

Immunity

If, as babies, we are fed our mother's breast milk, we will acquire her immunity for the period of time that we are breastfed. This is an awesome protection against the environment. Once we become independent, we need to acquire our own immunity (protection) against the world. This is when our parents often take us along for artificially acquired immunity in the form of immunisation vaccinations. This is good when there is potential for certain diseases to come into our sphere of contact. But you need to ask yourself, is it so good when you are not likely to be exposed to these foreign pathogens?

Immunity is a loaded subject. Science is finding out more and more about the artificially acquired immunity programmes and their benefits and downfalls every year. You need to make your own personal call when it comes to this artificially acquired immunity. However, remember that every time you are exposed to anything pathogenic, your body recalls it in its immunity. This immunity gets stronger and stronger as we get older and acquire for ourselves, naturally through exposure, many defences against future attacks to our internal environment. When your immunity is good, you are generally strong, healthy and vibrant. This is where you want to be for your Wellness Zone.

You want a good immunity. To do this, get plenty of rest, keep your body as toxin free as possible, exercise well and live today knowing that what you do with your energy levels has consequences on your immunity tomorrow. Too much stress, work or play and not enough nutrition, sleep and positive experience in your life can all cut through your immunity and leave you weak and lifeless. Once this happens, you can open yourself to any passing disease which may lodge itself in your system, hence illness which can start as an acute attack can become chronic fatigue in a few month time. Keeping your immunity strong is really a cornerstone in your Wellness Zone.

If your immunity is weak, then you will be weak in every respect. You will be compromised environmentally both externally and internally. Your immunity is your body's armour. It's your defence against pathogens, disease, virus and bacterium vulnerability. Your skin acts as a physical barrier to the rest of the world, your mind acts as a mental barrier and protection for your body. Your lungs, your digestive tract, your eyes and your blood are all vulnerable to many invaders who want to take you alive and spit you out in their bid for life. These are the places where your immunity needs to act.

When you cut yourself, your white blood cells, hence immunity, kick in and try to stop the bleeding and control the invasion of infections. Your digestive tract and lungs make mucous as a protection against any invaders as they cause allergies. Allergic responses are your body's way of trying to protect your Wellness Zone, this is good, your immunity is good. You need to enhance and protect your immunity as much as possible at regular and constant intervals for you to achieve your optimal Wellness Zone.

Herbs to help immunity are the immuno-modulatory herbs: echinacea root, cat's claw, astragalus and of course the old olive leaf extracts. This combination is beautiful. Add some rosehip extract and of course the reishi mushroom has its place in immuno-modulatory herbal blends. Elderberry is excellent against viruses and to boost immunity.

There are many herbs that can be taken to improve your immunity; for example, if immunity is compromised with your throat and lungs, then blend liquorice with some thyme and olive. But if your digestive tract is compromised, then bring in pau d'Arco with its active lapachol that tends to starve the pathogens outright.

Use pre- and probiotics to bring the good floras back into play. Garlic is awesome to help heal any immune compromises in the digestive tract. If your blood is compromised, nettle and smilax combined with cat's claw are good weapons for health. Pau d'Arco and cranberry are good if you are concerned about urinary tract infections.

Any compromised immunity gets B group vitamins, L-glutamine— the amino acid and a good diet along with a blend of herbals that will act as an adaptogenic as well as an immunity modulator. Don't be afraid to move sideways on these herbs and get specific to the illness if the situation calls for it. Don't double up on the job, use one immuno-modulatory herb to help, blend with some adaptogenic alternatives and specifics for the condition. It's all individual. Each of us needs our immunity strengthened in different ways and we need to decide what is causing the problem in our immunity.

Is it emotional? Was it triggered by something that is worrying us? In this case you can't go past adding hypericum or melissa to the herbs as we need to strengthen our resolve as much as our body!

Have we overdone it and neglected our health? In this case we need some vitamin C, zinc and herbs that will build cellular integrity and help with energy production. Were we exposed to something environmentally? Then we need to add some herbal cleansers to boost the immunity.

It's amazing how your thoughts, beliefs and emotions can have a huge impact on your immunity. Lighten up, be kind to yourself and you will notice an improvement in your health. Every time your immunity is compromised it is the result of some previous action or exposure you have experienced. Lowered immunity is your bodies signal to give it some attention and to rest, recover and get back in your Wellness Zone.

How do you know when your immunity is down?

You need to be aware of when your immunity is compromised as early as possible and mitigate the possible problems that may follow many illnesses. If you start to get a sore throat then that is one sure sign that an allergen is trying to compromise your immunity. Another sure sign is inflammation anywhere in your body. If you feel a little more tired than usual, more stressed, or are not able to eat quality foods for a time, then look out for lowered immunity. This can occur after we have had a late night, been exposed to cold, wet weather or even when we have been exposed to an allergen and not even noticed that it is having an effect on our body. Make sure that you protect yourself when you are around others who are sick, as air borne illnesses are common.

Adaptogenic herbs

Bring yourself back into harmony when your defences are down

Increase your ability to adjust to changes within your environment. An adaptogenic is a herbal blend that helps the whole system come back into balance. Adaptogenic herbals are non-specific in their action, but very specific in their ability to heal just about everything. They really increase your resistance and your immunity faster than other herbals. They bring your body energy levels up into a more energetic plateau and help you get through some tiring or stressful situations. These herbals help to normalise your system and the good news is that they are silent workers. They work without interrupting the rest of your body or the way it operates.

When you need to boost your immunity and bring your body back into your optimal Wellness Zone make sure you take some zinc, magnesium and B group vitamins as well as the herbals specifically targeted to the immunity. Maca helps make your body stronger faster. Also a good shot of fresh barley, wheatgrass or seaweed juice can help boost you in your worst moments!

Adaptogens are your herbal armour, they reinforce the non-specific power of resistance against any stressors and increase your ability to deal with any sickness or pathogens, they guard against disease. In fact adaptogens are harmony remedies, many are oriental in origin and are used widely in Chinese healing. These herbs promote vitality and disease resistance.

Stress, depression and anxiety are all relieved with adaptogenic herbs, also impotence, infertility and chronic illness. Everyone needs adaptogens in their life, the adaptogenic herbs are: panax ginseng, liquorice, Siberian ginseng, bacopa, schisandra, *Sambucas nigras*, gotu kola, withania, reishi, astragalus and maca extracts. These herbs need to be used in synergy for best results, sometimes single herbs are too strong and can take your body out of balance instead of helping the immunity problem.

If you have a chronic illness, there will be an adaptogenic herbal that you can add to your daily regime to help your recovery. Adaptogenic herbs can make the difference between a smooth and a stressed healing process. Many people are able to avoid conditions that can make sickness worse, such as depression and complete exhaustion, because they have added adaptogenic herbs to their morning vitamin and herb intake.

These herbs are also beneficial for anyone who is withdrawing from an addiction. They bring the body back into balance rather nicely and often are not contraindicated to other medications you may be taking. However, as with all herbs you need to check for specific interactions and contraindications before mixing herbs and drugs together.

Immune protection

Omega-3 helps your body repair itself easier and faster, this helps to protect you from invading toxins. Omega-3 helps retard progression of many types of cancer including breast and prostate.

A combination of the herbs astragalus, cat's claw, olive leaf and ginger extract at 1:2 extract equal parts of each is a good immunity boosting and protecting blend. You can take a small amount of this preventative blend daily and then if you are exposed to a new environment, such as travelling overseas or when you are surrounded by sick people, you are protecting your own health.

Antimicrobial herbals

Antimicrobials assist the body to destroy or resist pathogenic invaders. Some chemical constituents directly inhibit the survival or reproduction of specific organisms. Antimicrobials are used for bacterial, viral and fungal infections, intestinal parasites, complimentary therapy for carcinoma and conditions of lowered immunity. The actions can be antibiotic, immunostimulant, antiseptic, antibacterial and antifungal or vulnerary.

Antimicrobial herbs include Chinese wormwood, black walnut, calendula, garlic, sage, pau d'Arco, wild indigo, rosehips, thyme, tea tree, myrrh, cat's claw, grapefruit seed, echinacea root, papaya, turmeric, ginger and olive leaf. It's good to get a few of these herbs and add them to your first aid kit at home. Then when anyone in your home becomes exposed, you can give them these herbs and hopefully avoid any pending illnesses.

Infectious diseases

Don't ever think that you are safe from infectious diseases. Tuberculosis (TB) was a major killer until the advent of antibiotics to kill the infection. It is still prevalent in many parts of the world. We live in a transient world with people travelling to and fro with no real checks in place to determine how far and how fast TB is travelling through communities. The incubation time can be from a week to 100 years. If you had a relative who had tuberculosis as a child, or if you have been exposed to people with this disease in your travels, then it may very well be incubating in your body waiting to rear its ugly head when your immunity is sufficiently low.

Tuberculosis can appear in any part of your body; it is not limited to the lungs. This is why you need to be diagnosed as soon as you suspect this condition to stop it spreading, through your own body, let alone the community. A persistent and bad cough is one sign of TB, a hacking cough that just goes on for months on end. Another sign is ulcers that may appear on your neck. The first ulcer needs to be tested as, if you do have TB and the ulcer is ignored, it becomes weeping and then other ulcers will appear, until eventually there is a rosary of ulcers around your neck. This will also indicate the disease is far advanced and you may be close to death.

Scarring on the lungs is a typical sign of TB, if you have the bad cough and have lung x-rays you will find that the scarring shows up, this is an indicator that you have been exposed to TB and are a carrier. You may find there are none of the problems mentioned as the incubation period is one week to 100 years. However if you do have scarring on the lungs then you are prone to develop full blown TB at some stage when your immunity is low. Coughing blood is another indicator of TB and must never be ignored.

There is a lot of negative stigma that is associated with TB and people mistakenly think that it's a condition developed where living standards are poor and where hygiene is lacking. This is untrue. There are no social, racial nor hygienic barriers with TB, it is one infectious disease that is sitting, waiting to rear its ugly head in the Western world once more. You need to remember that TB is still a serious problem in many countries. There are other infectious diseases controlled by antibiotics at this point in time. Just be aware that the world is an infectious disease waiting to happen if we are ever in the situation that antibiotics and immunity are compromised to breaking point.

If you are diagnosed with TB and you do take the series of antibiotics that are very strong and the only solution to the problem, you can also take some liver supporting herbs such as milk thistle and dandelion. These will help your liver to cope with the onslaught of medicine. Nettle is good to heal lungs and you may want to take astragalus, cat's claw and olive leaf extracts to help boost your own immunity and give you maximum healing potential. Don't be frightened of infectious disease, just be aware. They can certainly be a problem and, if you travel, you are more prone to these conditions which, although silent in their approach, can have deadly consequences.

HIV/Aids is another huge world problem which can be helped with herbal medicine. HIV is a deadly disease which has, as yet, no definitive cure. If you have HIV/Aids or cancer, the herb sutherlandia, also known as cancer bush, is being used successfully in Africa to help alleviate the symptoms and strengthen the body. Bitter melon has also shown success in some research. There are many stages of this disease and you will need to work with your Health Care Practitioner to develop a good immune boosting plan to extend your life and health status.

There are some infectious diseases that are able to cross species and cause disease through eating the meat, milk or other products from the animals concerned. Make sure that you eat quality meats and animal products that are produced to a high hygienic standard. Also, if you work around animals beware that there are some infectious diseases that do pass across to humans and you would do well to keep you immunity strong and address any problems as soon as you become aware of them.

Cancer

Cancer is too common in the world today. Surely, the environment must be influencing the cells in our bodies so that they are unable to consistently reproduce appropriately. There are many kinds of common cancers that you should take every measure to prevent for your Wellness Zone.

Many common products are suspected and best avoided, for example using aluminium deodorants under your arms right next to the lymph nodes is not good for your body. Talcum powder to eliminate sweaty underarms, breasts, legs and genitals is another toxic option as this may lead to cervical cancer and other cancers located near the areas where you use this substance.

Eating poisonous foods, petrochemicals in all their forms, smoking and breathing in toxins are other ways that you may be exposed to enough poisons to set your body into a cancer programme.

We are able to get cancer and to heal ourselves from cancer unconsciously many times in our lives without even being aware of this fact. Yes, you too may have suffered from cancer. This is because your body was able to cope with the mutation of cells and your immunity was strong enough to fight the cancer alone. Cancer becomes a problem when it gets out of control and your body is not able to kill off the cells either naturally or with some extra, outside help.

Breast cancer risk can be reduced when you take turmeric extract regularly to help the detoxification pathways in the liver to detox excess oestrogen, which can lead to some types of breast cancer. Prostate cancer can be reduced with broccoli and antioxidants such as grape seed extract and apricot seed extract. You can help yourself avoid digestive tract cancers and colon cancer with fibre, beetroot and parasite cleanses. Lymphatic cancers can be averted with fenugreek and lemon juice. Liver cancer can be delayed or avoided with carrot juice, and regular cleansing with seaweeds. Many cancers can be delayed or avoided with juice cleanses.

You must be aware of your emotions and responses to life, as often the cause of cancer is not environment, it is actually triggered by other events such as emotional trauma. If you want to avoid cancer then you are in for an uphill climb, there is far too much of it in the world and we all need to address every aspect of our lifestyle and take positive preventative steps if we are to effectively protect ourselves. You need to keep your body as strong as you can and your environment as clean as possible. You don't know that what you do today isn't going to show up in your body as cancer in 20 years' time.

You can make up a lovely cancer preventative formula using herbs listed here. If you do have cancer in any part of the body, then you need to make sure you have an excellent support network of people and medicines that can ensure you have a good nutritional profile. Also, the appropriate herbs and medicines to kill off the tumours, cancers and compromised cells and allow your body to grow back perfectly as nature intended.

The herbs that are often referred to for cancer treatment in various cultures are: sutherlandia, Chinese wormwood, cat's claw, astragalus, black walnut, turmeric, maca, pau d'Arco, paw paw, grapefruit seed, apricot seed, sheep sorrel, plantain, olive leaf and nettle. Taking a herbal blend of black walnut and Chinese wormwood not only alleviates parasites from the body, but it also helps prevent and protect you from cancer.

Much money and research has gone into the modern-day dilemma of cancer. Quite simply our world is not a natural world anymore and cancer will become more common as the world becomes more crowded and people lean more toward the artificial and less towards Mother Nature.

It is sad that people think of natural products as being primitive, or wholefoods as being less attractive than the processed versions. It is also sad that we use so many chemicals in our lives which can lead to disease and illness, especially cancer. Many people in their fight against cancer have gone back to nature and won the battle back to good health.

There are many cancer diets and detox programmes available. You need to look at the alternatives and decide for yourself. The use of raw calves liver juices followed by the herb Chinese wormwood 12 hours later is a good anti-tumour method that has been used in clinics. Basically, you need to recognise that tumour cells love iron. So the idea is that you feed the cells iron and then 12 hours later move in with the Chinese wormwood and blast the cells open as this herb has active constituents that break the cells open, effectively killing off the tumours. Many advocates of herbal medicine use Chinese wormwood and also black walnut for killing toxic cells in the body.

Some advocates of cancer therapy say that you need to have a good dose of folic acid to help prevent the side effects of radiation and chemotherapies. Apparently the side effects of these treatments are minimalised whilst the benefits are still present when you take folic acid before each treatment in therapeutic doses.

Everyone gets a bit scared when we start talking about cancer. It's a hard healing path when you are faced with the myriad of options. There are herbs and nutrients you can take to make each day a little more comfortable and to give your body a greater potential to healing with cancer.

Coffee enemas are a popular treatment. They help the liver flush toxins and help you eliminate poisons from the body. Some cancer treatments advocate regular coffee enemas through the day in combination with organic juices, especially green juices, each day. There are cancer therapies that advocate one month or longer on pure juice cleanses, oxygen therapies and large doses of nutrients such as Coenzyme Q10 in combination with the herbs.

Protein plays an important role in some cancer treatments; however, it has been found that a high protein and low carbohydrate diet tends to make you sicker when on radiation and chemotherapies. You need to eat nurturing and cleansing foods while on these programmes. Make sure you have adequate protein but don't eat anything that places the body in ketosis for long periods of time on an anti-cancer diet, as this will also weaken you and may not help your health. Green vegetables tend to be the mainstay of most natural cancer healing regimes.

Detoxing has a part to play but only you can decide how to approach this arena of health care. The process of fasting is known to heal the body of many illnesses. With cancer, this is the principle behind the juice cleanses and also the protein ketosis diets that many people choose to undertake. These place the body into gluconeogenesis where the body eats its poisons and toxins first before body fat, followed swiftly by muscle tissue. If you are going to do this style of dieting, please remember that you also deserve some enjoyment in life and that the occasional rest from strict diet plans is healthy and beneficial.

Drinking raw paw paw leaf juice daily and also fresh red grapes in a mono juice are also advocated in some natural methods of cancer treatment. All juice cleanses are incorporated in many preventative and healthy diets for many illnesses, not just cancer.

When there is a genetic disposition in your family towards a certain type of cancer, you must not ignore this. Take whatever measures are reasonable and accessible to ensure that you can delay or hopefully circumvent this disease in your own body. Genetics are not always inevitable and with cancer sometimes the lifestyle or diet of past family members has had an impact on their health status. Make sure that if this is the case that you do not make the same mistakes.

Taking a daily tonic can help prevent the onset of cancer. Once you have assessed your genetic risk for cancer then find out what herbs are the best to help reduce your risk and make yourself a daily preventative tonic. Prevention is better than cure and often cancer can be stopped in its tracks by simple measures such as raw juices, green foods and nutritional support.

Daily cancer preventative tonic

Take the juice of paw paw leaves at therapeutic doses depending on your personal situation. Make sure you eat well and take the preventative and beneficial herbs to bring you back to wellness.

Just remember green organic foods are your best friends and fresh raw cleansing foods are excellent. There are techniques to help break up tumours and kill off cancers that your Health Care Practitioner can talk to you about.

CHAPTER EIGHT

Stimulants

In this ever increasing busy world, often our bodies feel sluggish and low on energy. Most adults today drink coffee. However it's a habit that you would do better without. Because coffee is a stimulant and too much stimulation in your body can lead to exhaustion and chronic fatigue, which is certainly a common state of exhaustion today. When you consider stimulants for your Wellness Zone, remember that there are times when the body requires this class of herb to help bring it back into balance. Just be moderate, as stimulants increase metabolic activity and increase physiological functions. They arouse latent lifeforce and vitality. They act predominantly on circulation and the nervous system but their influence pervades throughout your whole body.

There are two classes of stimulants. The circulatory stimulants that are hot and spicy and the agents which act directly on your sympathetic and central nervous system. The term stimulant is applied in a more general sense increasing certain activities, diuretics stimulate urinary output whilst bitter agents stimulate bile production in your liver and aid digestion. The true stimulants through their circulatory effects can synergistically potentate the effects of other medicines and are often added to herbal formulas because they work faster. This is especially important when someone has no energy and a very sluggish and over-worked system.

You will want results from the herbs to get in on a cellular level and start making balancing changes as soon as possible. So, add a dash of stimulant to the blend taken in a therapeutic dose for your weight, height and formula, and you will be healing and energised sooner than if the stimulant was left out of the formula. This is very good when you want to get up and go.

For example, you can take a combination of green tea extract and ginger before you exercise. This takes about 20 minutes or so to kick in and helps you have more energy and a stronger threshold for the activity than you would have otherwise had. However, if you take caffeine you will get the same kick, if not more and sooner with a faster flat-out rate, which means that you will fade faster. The green tea and ginger blend is healthier and certainly keeps you going as well, if not as initially fast as the caffeine. Ginger is a good stimulant to add to many herbal formulas as it will help to boost the working rate of the other herbs.

Don't overuse stimulants—there are alternatives

Overuse and misuse of stimulants can lead to exhaustion when you have little vitality. Have you had too much coffee and feel completely washed out in the early afternoon? With only the next coffee to keep you going? If this is the case you could take a herbal adrenal support formula and get your adrenals back into good health.

Too much stimulation can aggravate inflammatory conditions and should be used with caution in disorders of excess heat. Stimulants are often used for congestive respiratory disorders, especially where breathing is obstructed. Stimulants are fast acting agents but their effect is short-lived and can become addictive as you will need the next coffee after the first has worn off. Ginger and capsicum are safer stimulants and don't have the same mental implications as our favourite, coffee. If you find yourself in the position where you are constantly under stress and constantly drinking coffee through the day, then take adrenal supporting herbs such as liquorice root and ginseng regularly to help balance and take the strain off your adrenal glands. Coffee can also be dehydrating, so drink extra water.

The active constituents in stimulants are olea resins, essential oils and alkaloids

Stimulants increase vasomotor activity and arterial blood flow. They create warmness throughout your body. Circulatory stimulants increase the blood flow to every part of the body; they also assist to reduce blood cholesterol and lipids and decrease platelet aggregation. This is a bonus for those eating rich fatty foods who may wish to combine the stimulants in their meals to help decrease the risks of cardiovascular problems. Capsicum pepper is especially popular for this job. They can also act as appetite stimulants and carminatives. In large doses they can be strong irritants to your stomach lining which can exacerbate digestive tract problems.

So, in many ways stimulants are better taken when you are in optimal health, anyone else who takes them is only masking the energy depletion problem and uses the stimulant as a band aid which can come off very quickly leaving you with less energy than ever. Unless you are using them as a cardiovascular protection, in this case you would do well to eat hot chilli meals and incorporate the stimulant in your diet.

You can use stimulants for circulatory insufficiency, cold extremities, acute infection characterised by cold and chill, congestion of respiratory organs, chronic bronchitis, asthma and many digestive disorders. Added to formulas they will assist transport of other herbal medicines as the stimulants will help to speed the process of the formula.

The main stimulants available that you would use are; capsicum, ginger, prickly ash bark, horseradish, guarana, green tea leaf and ephedra.

CHAPTER NINE

Skin care

Keep your skin healthy and beautiful

Skin is the biggest organ in your body. It can be clear and beautiful if all systems are working in harmony and balance. However there are times in our lives when skin becomes congested and reflects an inner imbalance or reflection of the toxins we have exposed ourselves to.

We all want to have radiant, clear and healthy skin. Often with the excesses of stress, busy lifestyle, inconsistent diet and general exhaustion, our skin becomes dull and we develop a sallow look instead of the desired glowing complexion. When our body goes into overdrive, it affects all systems, and the basic pathways of daily functions are slowed down or compromised. This can lead to your skin taking over many elimination processes that would normally be carried out by your kidneys, lymphatics, liver and large intestine, that are our regular eliminative organs. If your skin is exposed to environmental toxins or allergens the result could be one of many skin conditions that are unsightly and uncomfortable. Also at different stages of our lives hormones can create havoc with our appearance.

Hormonal skin problems occur when there is an imbalance of oestrogen and progesterone or the male androgen hormones. This is often common in teenagers, women who are pregnant or breastfeeding and also in women going through peri-menopause or menopause. Men fall prey to hormonal fluctuations at any age and this can easily be reflected as skin blemishes, rashes and irritations.

If you are experiencing hormonal skin problems it's often good to keep soap away from the skin and use a gentle skin wash. Witch hazel and rose water are both good for hormonal skins. Washing the skin with apple cider vinegar diluted with water will help restore the pH levels and cleanse the surface dirt from your skin.

Herbs need to be assessed individually, often women do well with the herb vitex; however, if you are taking the contraceptive pill then vitex is contraindicated as it could decrease the effectiveness of the pill. Another herb to use to help clear hormonal skin conditions is red clover which is an alternative herb and works well to adjust your skin. This herb is especially successful for teenage boys and men with hormonal blemishes and acne.

Allergic skin conditions are many and varied. Eczema and psoriasis are two common conditions. You will need to address diet and environmental toxins that you have been exposed to. Often you will need to complete a programme of dietary elimination to find the cause and also address all allergens. In the process you can only relieve the condition with skin nutrients and quality pure plant-based skin creams and lotions. Dark circles under the eyes are a common symptom of food allergies. Sometimes a juice cleanse will help temporarily eliminate these allergic responses. Turmeric and dandelion mixed together in a topical cream, can help relieve the symptoms of psoriasis.

Psoriasis is a particularly difficult condition to treat. When you apply topical creams, it only seems to stop the immediate problem. A new irritation is just under the surface, bursting out from under your skin to create a bigger problem and to spread further as time goes on. Many people suffer from this condition for years with no luck in treatments. Psoriasis is an auto-immune condition—your body will have triggered itself into a mode of psoriasis which is difficult to reverse. You need to cleanse your liver, boost your immunity and have excellent stores of essential fatty acids to even start to heal psoriasis. Any topical application is often a temporary treatment and you may need to change the treatments regularly as each one loses its healing benefits over time. Often you can try one cream and it is successful for a few months and then suddenly it has no benefit to the condition. Turmeric, dandelion, chickweed, comfrey and calendula are the herbs that have some healing effect. Alternate these between a beeswax base and a cream base over time and you may be able to keep your itchiness down and the rash under control.

Excessive perspiration can be eliminated if you attend to the health of your kidneys, colon and lymphatic system. Sage tea along with good kidney tonics, such as dandelion and burdock, melissa and ginger, are all recommended to help bring your skins eliminative functions back into balance. Using a natural deodorant is good, they are safer than the aluminium-based deodorants which can contribute to adding toxins to your body. Sea salt deodorants are also good; however, make sure you don't get the salt deodorants that contain aluminium salts.

You can try essential oil blends such as tea tree oil mixed with pure corn powder. The herb panax ginseng is known to help eliminate excessive perspiration over time; however, you will need to take the herb on a daily basis to get results. Often you will perspire excessively at a certain time of the year, or when your body has reached a certain threshold of toxicity. When you do find that you perspire excessively then eat lots of fresh fruit and place yourself on a detox for a week or so and see whether that helps relieve the symptoms. Decrease your intake of alcohol, coffee and other dehydrating beverages and increase your intake of water, peppermint tea and melissa tea. Add some essential oils to your hair and clothes to help mask the smells of the excessive perspiration and make sure you wear clean clothes at least twice a day to help you feel and smell fresher.

Rosacea (excessive redness) is caused by congestion of the capillaries. This condition can worsen and cause a chronic irritation on your face that worsens with stress, hot weather and environmental exposure to irritants. Wild lettuce boiled gently to make a decoction with purified water makes a soothing face wash. Do not use soap on your skin, instead use finely ground oatmeal.

It is best to avoid all types of heat with this condition. Once again you can use the recommended nutrients for skin, attend to any hormonal imbalances and make sure you cleanse your liver, kidneys and digestive tract. Make yourself a hydrating refresh spray using the wild lettuce decoction and pure water. Horse chestnut is another herb that can be added to your refresh spray to help eliminate surface capillaries. Often a red face can be caused through liver conditions, gout or other medical problems. You will need to address the underlying cause with medical diagnosis and ensure that you cleanse your body properly and care for your skin in the process so that you do not end up with chronic skin conditions arising from medications and prescribed creams.

Does your skin bruise easily?

Then consider strengthening your venous system. Take vitamin C and bioflavonoids. A herbal formula of rosehips, chickweed, fenugreek and golden seal can help you resist vulnerability to unsightly regular bruising. Keep your B group vitamins up and also make sure you eat protein with most meals to help minimalise bruising. Placing one raw beaten egg in a poultice with slippery elm bark and placing this over the hurt area is also a way to draw the stagnant blood to the surface, helping to eliminate the bruise more quickly. Arnica cream is another remedy to help stop bruises from surfacing.

Cold sores are very common. Herpes simplex can be relieved by regular supplements of L-lysine—the amino acid. Also, consider keeping your immunity high with cat's claw, complete multi-vitamin B group and astragalus. Tea tree oil can be dabbed onto the lips at the first sign of a cold sore. Keep applying regularly until symptoms are relieved. If you get a cold sore, then you know that your immunity is down and you need to rest more and rejuvenate your body. Often cold sores go hand in hand with late nights, too much stress at work or just sheer exhaustion. It is difficult to stop a cold sore from developing once it has started; you can try 100% pure tea tree oil, placed on the cold sore every hour or so. Cold sores are determined to run their course. Take some olive leaf extract internally at a therapeutic dose for two or three days to help prevent other immunity compromised conditions from surfacing. Always view a cold sore as a basic warning that you have done too much and it's time to rest and start looking after yourself again.

Thinning skin can be found in ill and older people who are not absorbing nutrients properly. The best solution is to take protein powder regularly in your diet as this will give you easily absorbed quality protein in a drink form. Just add a couple of tablespoons of quality concentrate protein powder to a cup of fresh juice and blend. Take this daily as a nutritional supplement along with the other skin nutrients. Thinning skin needs to be addressed by clearing up the villi in the small intestine which is the entrance point for nutrients to be absorbed across into the blood stream. You will need to clear any excess mucous from this area, which can be done with fenugreek extract, a gluten-free diet and balanced digestive enzymes including bile secretions. This is a complete process and can take many months. However, once the digestive pathways are open again, you will find that nutrients are absorbed into the body and the skin condition will improve along with all other aspects of health.

Wrinkles are inevitable; however, the rate of their appearance is not so predictable. You need to eat skin foods and nutrients. Also, use quality botanical skin care that is not contaminated with chemicals. We should be able to eat what we put on our skin. Avoid the sun as much as possible. Keep your body clean internally and externally. Keep your skin well hydrated and remember to laugh and smile a lot. What a sad thing to have wrinkles shaped in a frown and a grumpy face. When you do develop wrinkles, make them happy ones.

Once again, protein and essential fatty acids are good to keep skin healthy. Vitamin C keeps skin elastic and regular face massage helps keep your skin relaxed and flexible. Good circulation is important to keep the blood flowing to your skin, and exercise is the best way to keep your circulation strong. You will not have good skin if you don't look after your whole body from the inside out. It's not good enough to mask your skin with makeup and chemicals. The chemicals found in makeup can contribute to unhealthy skin. Keep your skin well hydrated naturally and you will have less chance of developing faster wrinkles than necessary.

Herbs to help with skin conditions

Aloe vera

The gel contains glucomannan, a polysaccharide. Aloe has antibiotic, biogenic stimulators, wound healing hormones and minerals. Internally, aloe will help cleanse the digestive and urinary tracts, it will also assist in liver detoxification. Externally, to help with sunburn, blistering from burns, and cleansing cuts. It will help clear skin blemishes, acne and rashes.

Burdock

Burdock is used internally for blood purifying. A diaphoretic which promotes sweating and perspiration, it can also be applied externally to assist with psoriasis.

Calendula

One of the most common herbs used for skin care is calendula. This herb is used internally as an antimicrobial, antifungal, antiviral and haemolytic; it has immune boosting properties. Calendula is used for internal inflammations, liver and digestive tract imbalances, thrombophlebitis and varicosis.

Externally, calendula is beneficial for inflamed skin of all degrees, and it assists with wound healing, burns, varicosis and is generally soothing and comforting to irritated skin. Calendula has been used to clean new wounds and to assist in healing skin lesions.

Kelp

Kelp is rich in many minerals and is a blood purifier. When taken internally, kelp will help ensure that you are getting many of the necessary minerals for skin care including zinc, vitamin A, and silicon.

Kelp makes a healing detoxifying body wrap. Mix one cup of kelp powder with three cups of hot water, add 30 ml of vodka and mix thoroughly. Rub over body and wrap yourself in some fabric, then lie in the sun for 20 minutes (mid-afternoon/morning is best as the sun is not too hot and you can enjoy the warmth without burning). Afterwards, shower off and massage your body with a good oil blend.

Chickweed

Used externally, this will help solubilise toxins in the abscesses and rashes. Chickweed will increase the effectiveness of bactericides by increasing the permeability of bacterial cell walls. This is great for cleansing skin with blemishes. Mix some freshly ground chickweed with aloe vera juice or gel for a soothing and cooling experience. Ideal for people of all ages from babies to older folk who have sensitive or irritated skin.

Red clover

Taken internally, red clover is beneficial for all hormonal and inflammatory skin conditions; it is an alterative herb and also works as a reproductive tonic for both males and females. Young men and women with acne, benefit well from the addition of this herb to their routine as do those who are older and suffering from menopausal hormonal skin problems.

Peppermint

Taken as an infusion, this can help with many skin conditions that evolve from inner toxicity. Dandelion is another herb that works well as an internal cleanser to help eliminate conditions such as rosacea, blemishes and rashes caused through a sluggish metabolism and ineffective elimination.

Olive leaf

Olive leaf is good to help fade sun spots

Chamomile

Combined with hypericum, chamomile should be your first herb of choice for any burns to the skin.

Other nutrients to keep your skin in top health

Zinc

Try some extra zinc in your diet if you are suffering from eczema or skin rashes; it may just be the key to clearing up some stubborn skin conditions.

Zinc is an essential mineral, which assists in the DNA replication, detoxification of chemicals, hormonal production, and synthesis of carbohydrates, proteins and lipids. Zinc contributes to the growth and health of all body systems including skin tissue. If you are having skin problems such as rashes and eczema, white spots on your nails or conditions such as poor vision, immune deficiency or possibly cardiovascular problems or even mental disorders, then you may be lacking in zinc.

Seafood, such as oysters, are the highest source of zinc with each oyster containing about 2 mg zinc. Salmon, beef and lamb are also good sources with about 4–5 mg per 100 grams of meat eaten. Cashews, sunflower seeds and oats are good plant sources containing over 6 mg per cup.

Vitamin C

Vitamin C works as an antioxidant, protecting your skin when taken internally. It can also help promote healing if applied externally as an exfoliate rub.

Vitamin C rub

Simply mix one teaspoon of calcium ascorbate powder with one tablespoon of runny honey. Place contents in a small jar and keep in the shower or bathroom for skin care. To use, simply wet your face with warm water and dip your fingers into the mixture, rub gently onto the skin in circular movements for a couple of minutes then leave on for another few minutes. Rinse and feel the softness of your skin.

Alternately you can take a natural cream base and add one teaspoon of vitamin C calcium ascorbate powder to 50 ml of base cream. This will add the protective and antioxidant properties of vitamin C to your creams and can be used all over the body.

Essential fatty acids are necessary for the metabolism of all cells. Each cell membrane contains essential fatty acids. So, technically your skin is loaded with these nutrients. Often people with chronic skin conditions have improved with the daily intake of omega-3 and omega-6 fatty acids. These improvements have been for conditions such as eczema, psoriasis, rosacea and hormonal skin conditions for all stages of life. Even dry, scaly skin has improved with a daily dose of essential fatty acids.

Sulphur is found in collagen (the protein in connective tissue) and keratin (the protein in hair, skin and nails). Sulphur will give your tissues shape and firmness, so if your skin is lacking in elasticity, then you may wish to add some extra protein to your diet. Eggs, milk products, nuts and seafood all contain sulphur.

Face mask for dry and ageing skin

Beat one egg and then mix together with one teaspoon of ground almonds. Place a small amount on your dry face and leave on for 15 minutes then rinse off. This mask is recommended for dry, ageing skin about once a week. You can even use it on hands and feet for a deliciously moisturising and toning treat. Keep the remaining mixture in the fridge (or better still share the experience with a friend).

Silica

Wonderful to detoxify skin tissue, it also works as a skin toner. Horsetail taken externally as a skin wash in extract form can help with many skin conditions.

Horsetail skin tonic

Simply take 25 ml of herbal extract and add 75 ml pure water. Rinse your skin with a small amount of this mixture when needed.

Vitamin E

Vitamin E is often used as a sunscreen as it protects the skin against sunburn. Many gardeners use a mixture of vitamin E oil and fresh aloe vera or cucumber to protect their skin from the harmful rays.

> Prick a vitamin E capsule open with a pin and mix with either 50 grams of fresh aloe vera or 50 grams of fresh cucumber which has been blended or ground with a mortar and pestle. Place this on the exposed areas of skin and go gardening.

Clean water and fresh air are two of the most important components to ensure that you have a healthy and vibrant skin. Add some good regular exercise to relieve stress and get your heart pumping, then your skin will be in the best condition possible for your age and lifestyle.

Complex carbohydrates and complete protein

Keep your diet high in unprocessed foods. Eat complete proteins and complex carbohydrates regularly. If you have a good digestive system and eat wholesome organic foods, chances are you will not suffer from many of the ills that plague our society.

If your body is good on the inside then that will be reflected in your skin. However, there are certain environmental conditions and hormonal stages of life that will test even the best skins. All you can do is to ensure you address each problem as it arises and research any possible underlying causes for your skin problems.

CHAPTER TEN

Women's cycles

A s a woman you will know that hormones can rule how you think and feel in a cyclic pattern that can almost control your life if they are unbalanced and out of hand.

There are some aspects of hormonal health care that you need to understand and avoid. The first one is that if you crave sweet, wheat-based and sugary foods you will need to address your oestrogen levels. Make sure that you are eliminating oestrogen from your liver through the optimal functioning of the specific detoxification pathways in the liver that eliminate oestrogens. This is not the only sign of too much oestrogen in your body, but it is a warning call.

There are many types of oestrogen and not all of these are good for your health. Often, if you have an excess of oestrogen, then you will be stressed and too busy in your life. This needs addressing. If you find that you have this problem then please look at your adrenal glands and your thyroid hormones to see whether these are functioning optimally.

You may be caught in the stress cascade of adrenal burnout where the thyroid hormones take over and the stress continues, leading to thyroid problems such as hypothyroidism. You then pump a lot of oestrogen to compensate for the adrenal burnout and the hypothyroidism, which leads to peripheral obesity. Then, when you hit menopause you will just become fatter and fatter as there is no functioning system in your body to control the energy of metabolism which can lead to insulin insufficiencies and syndrome X. This is often followed by cardiovascular disease and all the associated problems.

It is too common to see women overwork in their 20s and 30s only to put on stubborn fat in their 40s and onwards. There are solutions, including exercise and diet. But what you really need to do is look after yourself and take preventative measures when you are younger to help avoid this cycle.

There are two types of fat, the worst kind is abdominal fat around your belly caused simply by working too hard and not taking preventative measures to stop it from happening. The second type of fat, around the peripheral thighs and bum is healthier, but this still indicates that you may not be hormonally balanced and maybe your body is not as balanced as it could be. If you are overweight, address the problem now and also address the issues associated with too much stress.

Many women will do well taking a good, high grade magnesium amino acid chelate powder. Take 3 grams every night before bed combined with L glutamine and taurine. This will help to balance the muscular skeletal system and also repair adrenal stress. You would do well to take a high grade B group vitamin complex with zinc every day as this will support your nervous system.

Taking a herbal blend of turmeric, vitex, kelp, nettle, hypericum and liquorice root will help balance your thyroid hormones and adrenal glands and assist with oestrogen detoxification whilst helping you maintain energy whilst under stress. Women under stress with the daily grind of family, work and other commitments need to future-proof themselves against all the modern Western diseases that can creep up on us as we age.

Too thin is too dangerous

Keep your bones strong and avoid being too thin. Often when women diet and keep a very slim figure they are compromising good health in the equation. As the years pass, often the women with the strongest bones and the least incidence of osteoporosis are the ones who maintain a good body weight to their height and bone structure. Don't be foolish and create any form of unnatural eating disorder or diet regime whereby you are missing out on essential nutrients to help build your body optimally. If you are too thin then you will become weaker and possibly have more problems with your health.

Do not allow yourself to go under the Body Mass Index (BMI) for your height and bone structure. Make sure you are well-nourished and then you will have less hormonal and other health problems as you age. If you weigh 20% under the recommended body weight, you may stop getting your period. You may also stop storing calcium in your bones and be in the same position as women who have completed menopause. This means that you will age faster and look older than your friends who are not so underweight. If you really want to be thin, then the healthiest path is to have a strong muscle mass which is achieved through exercise and good nutritional profile. If you are thin with a poor muscle mass then you are at risk of many illnesses.

Hormonal balancing

Often women find it difficult to balance lifestyle with hormones. Successful women try to juggle a career, family and social life with their monthly menstrual cycle, or lack of it. Hormonal fluctuations can cause many symptoms from severe pain, frayed tempers, hot flushes, bursts of anger, crying, headaches, suicidal tendencies and lethargy through to conditions such as osteoporosis, endometriosis, infertility, amenorrhoea, breast lumps, cervical cancers and hysterectomy. Other women are lucky and seem to breeze through each month and have a balanced cycle without complications.

Wherever you are in this treadmill of womanhood, you will need to ensure preventative health care to keep reproductive cycles in harmony and to prepare for each phase. From monthly regulation, contraception, childbirth, peri-menopause and menopause, right through to the post-menopausal stage and the implications that hold for health.

The monthly cycle—women's hormones for reproduction

The hormones are initially stimulated by a lowered concentration of oestrogen, which causes the lower anterior lobe of the pituitary gland to release follicle stimulating hormone (FSH) and luteinising hormone (LH). FSH is secreted in its greatest amounts in the first half of the menstrual cycle and LH has its peak secretions mid-cycle. FSH and LH cause ripening of the follicle and ovulation; they also stimulate cells of the follicle wall to secrete oestrogen into the blood stream. The ripened follicle ruptures, discharging an ovum from the surface of the ovary to make its way to the fallopian tube. This is ovulation.

Once the ovum has been expelled, the follicle is transformed into a solid granular mass (the corpus luteum). LH begins to produce proges-terone and more oestrogen. The high levels of progesterone depress the secretion of LH. With decreased LH levels the corpus luteum ceases to function and shrivels. This causes the concentration of oestrogen and progesterone to drop rapidly causing the endometrium to begin to shed in menstrual flow. The low oestrogen at menstruation causes the FSH to rise and start the cycle again. During pregnancy, the corpus luteum remains active.

There are four phases to the menstrual cycle

The first stage is the proliferative phase where oestrogen in the bloodstream stimulates preparation of the endometrium for possible pregnancy. The endometrium progressively thickens over two weeks as uterine glands and blood vessels within the lining proliferate. This stage is terminated by the rupture of the follicle and liberation of the ovum about 14 days before the next menstrual cycle begins.

The second luteal phase is when the endometrium increases in thickness. The corpus luteum in an ovary is developing and secreting progesterone. This phase lasts 10 to 14 days. During this time, the ovum travels through the oviduct to the uterus.

The third premenstrual/ischaemic phase occurs one or two days before menstruation when the endometrium becomes anaemic and shrinks. The corpus luteum begins involution. The phase ends with breaking off of small patches of endometrium and the beginning of menstrual flow.

If the ovum is not fertilised when passing through the tube, it disintegrates soon after reaching the uterus and circulating levels of oestrogen and progesterone fall off sharply. If the ovum is fertilised, it takes about seven days to pass to the uterus and become implanted. The implanted ovum secretes gonadotrophic hormone which stops the secretion of FSH. Finally menstruation uterine bleeding accompanied by shedding of the endometrium, lasting an average of 4–6 days. Before the flow ceases the endometrium begins to repair itself through the growth of new cells. Within the ovaries a new ovum ripens and the cycle begins again.

In the following pages are three hormonal situations that many of you are familiar with. There are also some herbal and natural medicine ideas to help ease the associated stress on your body.

If you are taking any medications, please check with your Health Care Practitioner before mixing herbal medicines with pharmaceuticals as this can lead to dangerous health implications if the wrong combinations are mixed. Also inform your Health Care Practitioner what herbal supplements you are taking before going on any medication. It is best to be safe when taking any form of medicine, whether herbal or otherwise.

Premenstrual Tension (PMT)

PMT is a condition where you feel a distinct change in your body, any time from day 14 of your cycle to the first day of your period. The symptoms are anything and everything that you can think of; in fact, there is no defined set of symptoms for this condition. It can be pain, emotional stress, mental fatigue, tiredness, headaches, swollen ankles, depression or forgetfulness. The only way that you can determine whether you are suffering from premenstrual tension is to keep a diary of three consecutive cycles from day 14 until your period. If you find a recurring symptom at the same stage of every cycle, then you can assume it may be PMT.

The symptoms are nearly always related to hormonal imbalances, most commonly an excess of oestrogen and a deficiency of progesterone during the second half of the cycle. It is possible that hormonal secretions from the ovaries reach a peak in the blood at ovulation, at the same time toxins are withdrawn from other areas such as lymph glands, liver and soft tissue, placing a strain on the liver and kidneys, leading to fatigue and fluid retention. Diet can affect this cycle too; however, the main cause is hormones.

Herbally, vitex is the most important requirement as it improves progesterone secretions and can balance or reduce oestrogen levels. Mix the vitex with hypericum for emotional support and the other balancing benefits that this combination offers. Vitamin B6 (pyridoxine) is given to reduce tension, aggression and irritability. If you suffer from cramping, a good calcium/magnesium supplement can be taken for ten days before your period. Turmeric helps to balance your oestrogen levels because this herb helps detoxify excess oestrogen in the liver.

Celery seed and juniper or dandelion are beneficial for fluid retention. Also, omega-6 gammalinolenic acid as found in evening primrose and spirulina can assist symptoms. The omega-3 fatty acids in linseed and fish oils can also reduce symptoms. If you know you need a change in diet and are overweight, then address this issue as you may find a decrease in symptoms as your weight becomes natural and appropriate.

Women suffering from PMT would do well to have a good vegetarian cleansing diet whilst they are enduring the symptoms. This includes regular juices of carrot and celery to cleanse the toxins from the liver and also to help eliminate excess fluids. Also, consider spirulina as a regular part of your diet. Eat small meals that are easily digested to help reduce the overall stress on your body at this time. If you want to use aromatherapy oils, consider camomile, jasmine and melissa which all have a balancing effect.

Peri-menopause health care

Lucky you, if you have made it to your mid-30s and not suffered from any of the afore-mentioned premenstrual symptoms, you will be amongst only 10% of women in the Western world. However, whatever the past has offered in hormonal reproductive cycles, now is the time to prepare for the future and make your journey through menopause as comfortable as possible.

Some people are just plain unlucky, they get every reproductive condition imaginable and nothing they do helps. Others are a bit luckier in the genetic stakes and tell stories of mothers and grandmothers who didn't experience symptoms of peri-menopause or menopause.

Unfortunately for us, we don't have the clean environment and wholesome organic foods that were eaten in the past. So, unless we consciously create a clean environment in our body and in our outside world, then we can fall prey to many toxic conditions. Peri-menopause is one of these telling times, when the condition of your body has as much to do with how you feel, as your hormonal fluctuations do.

Peri-menopause is about keeping your cycle as regular as possible

Give your body a thorough cleanse and health check. Make sure you address the whole picture: alcohol, smoking, junk food, weight management, nutritional intake and exercise. Look at your reproductive cycle and see where you need help. Take the amino acid L-glutamine to clear out the toxins in your brain and the liver-cleansing herbs milk thistle and dandelion to get any excess fats and toxins out of your liver. Visit your Health Care Practitioner and get tested to see whether your hormonal levels have decreased.

It is a good idea in your mid-30s to get blood and saliva tests done to see what your hormonal levels are as you may require these readings in the future if you consider hormonal replacement therapy during menopause. Make sure you eat sufficient calcium in your diet as blood bone calcium levels should be at their peak during these years, thereby reducing the risk of osteoporosis in later life.

If you are feeling the brunt of peri-menopause, then consider the addition of the following herbs. Dong quai has a tonic action, it is a relaxant and a nervine and is extremely useful for reproductive problems. False unicorn root contains steroidal saponins and glycosides; this has an oestrogenic action and improves the cyclical function of the ovaries. It is very good taken in the first half of the cycle for problems related to dysfunction of the follicles and insufficient oestrogen secretions. Also good during menstruation if you have pain, cramping or heavy bleeding, ovarian cysts or other ovarian pathergies.

A vitex and hypericum combination can be very good during the second half of the cycle. Also, consider black cohosh as it has an oestrogenic effect and depresses luteinising hormone secretion. LH secretion occurs in pulses in some peri-menopausal and menopausal women coinciding with hot flushes. This herb has been found to be useful in decreasing hot flushes, as has sage.

Keeping your body healthy and taking regular cleanses ensures that all organs are functioning well and that you are not creating unnecessary stress due to an unbalanced system. Look at the whole picture and not just the symptoms. Therefore a little prevention and awareness goes a long way in health care.

Menopause

We are offered so many options to alleviate the symptoms of menopause that it can be difficult to choose. There are many herbs packaged in different ways and marketed with famous faces on the packs. Do they really work? What about hormone replacement therapy (HRT) in the form of patches and oral pills that create relief and extra tension at the same time?

Many women make it to menopause untainted by the perils of excess weight gain, mood swings and depression only to find themselves raving lunatics and feeling fatter than ever before after a bout of HRT. Others flow through the HRT programmes without a mishap, they take the pills for years and feel fabulous, not an extra ounce of weight, not one hot flush and certainly no bad tempers. HRT certainly has its place in health care and can have many benefits. Discuss your options with your Health Care Practitioner; this is not the right choice for everyone and you must personally weigh up your options considering all aspects of your health regime and history.

Herbally, many women want to try the natural way and avoid HRT. Your Health Care Practitioner can help develop an individual programme incorporating herbs, diet and other relevant factors. Many women choose to go it alone and they try every packet of expensive pills on the pharmacy shelf only to be left with an empty purse and no relief. Others scout the shelves and finally hit the right product that offers some, if not full, relief from hot flushes, pain, frayed emotions and other problems.

There is no 'cure-all' for everyone. Often herbal extracts work well because they are concentrated and you can get a good therapeutic dose tailored individually. You can only read as much information as is offered and try whatever you think you need to get relief. Just remember that you are not alone in this menopausal pursuit of peace and sanity, there are many women out there feeling just like you.

You can try some of the herbs mentioned in this section to see if they work for you, but also consider diet, lifestyle, genetic factors and attitude. There are a variety of hormonal wild yam creams which are known to work well in combination with oestrogen replacement.

Herbally you would consider hormonal balancers and oestrogenic herbs such as black cohosh, red clover, wild yam, false unicorn root, dong quai, and vitex for symptoms similar to premenstrual tension. Maca extract is a good general hormone balancing herb and has a good reputation for relieving hot flushes. Other herbs specific to hot flushes are black cohosh, sage and hypericum. Perhaps a few anti-depressant herbs are also needed, in the form of hypericum, lavender and rosemary.

Nervines are good to help with anxiety and mental symptoms, these are herbs such as pulsatilla, passionflower, verbena, dong quai, withania, oats and scutellaria.

The adaptogenic herbs of astragalus and liquorice root are always good to mix with other herbs as they help balance the whole body. You may also feel the need for some vaso dilators and memory enhancers like ginkgo biloba and bacopa to add mental harmony, concentration and focus.

Foods rich in oestrogens are worth considering, including soy beans, alfalfa, barley, carrots, cherries, sunflower seeds, beans, peas, rice, sage, wheat and yeast. You will also need to be very conscious of your calcium and magnesium levels, as once you pass menopause your body is vulnerable to osteoporosis. Make sure you have a bone density test and act accordingly. The best sources of calcium are almonds, comfrey, kale, sardines and other fish with edible bones and some fresh dairy foods.

Good luck. Menopause is certainly a trying time for some women. However you need to look at the big picture and stay as calm, positive and healthy as possible. There are many women who experience menopause with no symptoms. Even one generation ago, women were not suffering in the ways we do today. This is where we have to consider our lifestyles and the impact it has on our bodies. There is one fact you can rely on: menopause is a temporary condition and will pass. The reproductive cycle is very simple; however, there are many conditions and complications that arise. If you detect any unusual pains, lumps, sores or symptoms that are disconcerting, visit your Health Care Practitioner and discuss the details. There are very accurate tests these days and it's better to be safe than sorry.

To maintain good health, we need to take the best of the orthodox medical world and the best of the alternative medical world to create our own unique blend of personal healing and health care.

CHAPTER ELEVEN

Fertility

This has become a big social issue as many couples are unable to conceive. The infertility rate in men has increased over 50% in the last half century. Women are having babies later in life and of course other factors such as environmental stresses, toxicity and illness can all have an impact on your fertility. With a little planning help, you will hopefully conceive and have a healthy bouncing baby!

Research has shown that 25% of infertility cases are unexplained with no medical condition involved. These couples often have the most success using herbal support. Even if there is a medical reason why you are having difficulty, herbs can help you prepare for conception in the best way possible. From detoxification, to increasing sperm count and helping hormonal levels and ovulation, we are having increasing success helping patients become pregnant using modern science and good old herbal medicines!

Find the problem with fertility

If you have been trying to fall pregnant for six months or longer unsuccessfully then you should visit your Health Care Practitioner for all the tests that modern science can offer, as there may be a problem with either partner's ability to conceive. Or possibly the situation will be unexplained medically.

Whatever the outcome of your tests, herbal medicine can help increase your chances of becoming pregnant. If you decide to take fertility drugs, there are herbs that can also be taken, in a complimentary way, thereby helping your potential to conceive. You need to check for any contraindications with fertility herbs and drugs in each instance throughout the process.

Don't self-prescribe herbs for fertility as you really need support and the right herbs for the right phase of your cycle. Your Health Care

Practitioner can create the best complimentary regime possible for your situation. This is different in each case depending upon the problems you are facing. Keep your hopes up and do everything you can to help enhance your fertility.

Plan for a healthy pregnancy

Often a detoxification and pregnancy preparation plan is designed for both partners before they plan to conceive. This is one of the healthiest and most loving things you can do for each other and your future children. The plan consists of full internal cleansing, energy boosting and of course hormonal balancing for both partners. If you have had trouble conceiving in the past then this could be your next step to success. Sperm takes four months to mature, which is a good time frame for preconception care. Your hormones may need some balancing and one of you may need to gain or lose body weight. Remember, if you are lucky enough to conceive and carry the pregnancy through full term, then the baby will be taking all of its nutrients from your body. If you have a clean, well-nourished and healthy body, the chances of a healthy future for your baby are a lot better.

Preconception herbal care

Milk thistle is the premium liver detox herb. Before you even think about conception, have a good look at your lifestyle choices and exposure to toxins. Both partners can take milk thistle for up to three months before conception. Black walnut taken in small amounts daily helps get in and detox your whole body, this herb also helps eliminate parasites and other foreign pathogens hiding in your organs.

Adaptogenic herbs will help balance your adrenal glands as well as bring your whole body into balance again. These include liquorice, Siberian ginseng, astragalus, maca, asparagus and withania. Coenzyme Q10, which is found in avocados, is a must-have nutrient when you are planning to conceive, as it assists in adenosine triphosphate production (ATP) production and boosts mitochondrial energy.

Multi B vitamins, depending upon the problem, can be used specifically and as a complementary approach to traditional infertility solutions. Good doses of B group vitamins taken at meals with quality protein are recommended for all couples planning to conceive. The B's are so important as enzymes for the synthesis of all new cells in our body and combined with protein, you are ensuring that the amino acids are getting the support they need to make healthy new cells.

Essential fatty acids and the minerals zinc and magnesium are added to the menu of anyone planning to conceive. Along with good antioxidant herbs such as grape seed extract and antimicrobials such as olive leaf to really prepare your body in the best way!

Female infertility

Women's infertility can be caused by a number of factors. Weight problems can contribute, as both under and overweight women tend not to ovulate, possibly because of the over-production of androgens and oestrogens, suppressing ovulation. Research has shown that women who are overweight and lose only 10% of their body fat have a better chance of conceiving. If you are over the age of 35, your chances of conception diminish with each passing year. So, you will need to bring your hormones back into play again.

Other factors could be stress, toxicity and specific hormonal imbalances such as insulin resistance, luteal phase defect, excessive or insufficient oestrogen or thyroid disturbances such as hypothyroidism and hyperthyroidism. Or you could even have sperm antibodies or cervical mucous problems, endometriosis or polycystic ovarian syndrome causing infertility.

Reproductive health

Omega-3 fatty acids are necessary for optimal prenatal and pregnancy health. Labour is affected by prostaglandins made during pregnancy, the metabolism of EPA is important for the production of these prostaglandins and many others in your body, as well as for the proper and optimal development of your baby. Babies who are not breastfed need to be supplemented with omega-3 to ensure optimal brain and body development.

Fertility herbs for women

Tribulus specifically helps follicular maturation and the menstrual cycle by helping facilitate conception. Tribulus also elevates the FSH and can be contraindicated if you are already producing enough of this hormone.

Vitex can be used to help increase progesterone and reduce prolactin; it has the ability to balance female hormones. Depending upon your hormonal imbalance, your Health Care Practitioner can mix you specific herbs which could also include; dong quai, black cohosh, sage and peony.

Panax, Siberian ginseng, coleus and noni are good for women with thyroid dysfunction contributing to infertility. Green tea and ginger are amongst the more beneficial herbs available to help reduce your weight and bring your fat index into healthy range.

Male infertility

Stress is a major cause of male infertility and low sperm count. Research has shown that men who are exposed to heavy metals and shift workers and who are under a lot of external stress tend to have lower sperm counts then their more relaxed buddies! Other causes of male infertility are poor sperm morphology (which is the form of the sperm) which can be caused by toxin and oxidant damage. Poor sperm motility (the ability of the sperm to swim) is another common male fertility problem. Prostate problems can also attribute to male infertility.

Therefore, any man who is having trouble with fertility needs to relax, detox and get healthy. Male fertility needs time. So plan on conceiving four months after you have completed your detox and are in good health, having addressed your nutritional status and taken preparatory herbals to assist with sperm health.

Fertility herbs for men

Tribulus helps to regulate the luteinising hormone levels, which increases testosterone mobility, this increases sperm count. Glutathione can increase the excretion of mercury toxicity and alter the antioxidant effect on the body.

Folic acid and zinc are two minerals that have been shown to increase the numbers of normal sperm. Maca has been used traditionally to alleviate impotence, and improve male fertility and sexual function.

Panax ginseng specifically helps regulate the effects of stress. Hypericum is an excellent herb for men to take when planning conception as it helps balance the autonomic and the somatic nervous system. Often men have a high stress threshold and thrive on excess stress. Hypericum and other nervine herbs, chamomile, passionflower and melissa, will relax the whole body.

Grape seed extract and green tea help reduce free radical damage along with selenium and vitamins E and C. Carnitine has been shown to help increase mitochondrial energy and contribute directly to sperm motility and levels. Sperm has a lot of mitochondria in each cell and this need to be enlivened with Coenzyme Q10, often taken with ginkgo biloba to help maximise potential.

Damiana, saw palmetto and small leaf willow are traditional male herbs reputed to help increase a male's fertility when given in therapeutic doses for specific conditions.

Your best plan for conception

Once you have all the information required about the physical problems that may be preventing you from conceiving, then try to stay positive. Visit your Health Care Practitioner and work with them to maximise your chances, but bear in mind it is not always possible to conceive. There are, however, herbs that can help to self-empower you and your partner, allowing you to make decisions and have some control of the outcome, whilst increasing your health and maximising your potential to have healthy babies!

CHAPTER TWELVE

Kidneys and urinary tract

If you have any problems with your kidneys or urinary tract then you need to have a diet based on fresh fruit and vegetables. The wholesome vegetarian cleansing detox is the perfect diet for kidney health.

Protein in many ways is the enemy of your kidneys. Protein is harsh on kidneys; the little nephrons that act as filters in your kidneys are destroyed by a high protein diet, and this is one reason why these diets are not sustainable for a long period of time. When your body is in ketosis, you are at risk of kidney damage. It is okay to be on low carb diet, where you eat a lot of fresh fruit and vegetables, but to be on a high protein diet is not good for your kidney's health. Keep your kidneys in tip-top order with lots of fluids, especially cleansing waters and foods that are high in chlorophyll.

The most common urinary problems are bacterial infections. These need to be noted and measures taken as quickly as possible to get rid of the infection quickly. Garlic extract, aloe vera and cranberry juice are all good to help eliminate this problem. Also, you need to remember that flushing your kidneys with clean water is the fastest path to cleansing infections, often these have developed because not enough liquids are included in the diet.

Secondary infections occur in the kidneys after another infection in another part of your body has been eliminated and the residue of that infection is caught in the kidneys. If you are on any antibiotic herbals or medications for an infection, make sure that you finish the course as prescribed. This will help to eliminate the residues of the infection from your body via your kidneys and you will have less chance of kidney infection.

Look after your kidneys and bladder as you age

Nephrons in the kidneys are naturally lost through age and you will be unable to concentrate your urine as effectively if these are damaged. Therefore, you will have more toxins running freely in your blood in older age than when you were younger. The best way to help yourself is to eat fewer toxins and make sure you have a lower protein intake in older age. Keep alcohol and acid-forming foods to a minimum. Smoking and taking other drugs and medications can also add strain to your kidney's main job of filtering toxins and unwanted wastes from the blood stream.

As you age your bladder capacity and strength can also decrease. Doing pelvic floor exercises and keeping your body in good tone and fitness can help eliminate bladder problems such as incontinence. Many women suffer from this problem after childbirth.

Ensure that you keep your core strong and do exercises to stop incontinence occurring as you age. This is an avoidable situation but unfortunately many people don't even think about their bladder, let alone trying to prevent incontinence in the future! Your Wellness Zone when you are older depends upon you taking small measures in this area throughout your life.

Keep your prostate healthy

Prostate disease is an increasing problem in men over the age of 50, and even younger men are suffering, which must be a reflection of lifestyle and environment. Prostate disease starts with the prostate gland swelling and it's difficult for urine to pass, blocking off the urethra. This stops you from urinating in large amounts, a common symptom is frequent nocturnal urination and cancer can develop if the situation worsens.

Broccoli is rich in antioxidants and is known as a good healing botanical for prostate problems. You also need to take zinc, vitamin C, antioxidants in the form of grape seed extract and lycopenes from tomatoes. Bilberry and other cardiovascular herbs can also be of benefit. The main prostate herbs are: saw palmetto, small leaf willow, nettle, damiana, olive leaf and tribulus. These herbs are often blended in combination depending upon the exact problem.

Often men find that if they make the effort to become more physically fit, lose any excess body weight and adhere to a good prostate healthy diet containing lots of fresh fruit and vegetables along with some good cleansing regimes, then the prostate swelling will ease and the PSA levels will decrease again, or at least stay low after an operation.

Prostate health really starts when you are young and the best prevention is to take plenty of anti-inflammatory and antioxidant foods in the diet. Taking hormonal herbals such as turmeric, tribulus and red clover also help ease this problem.

Once again you need to avoid the beer belly as this truly is an indicator that your body is ready to receive degenerative diseases. Prostate disease can often be avoided entirely by having a fit healthy body and a good regular exercise regime in place. You also need an optimal clean diet, regular detox therapy and you can take herbs to help prevent the problems occurring.

Once you start to feel that there is a problem with your prostate, ensure you are diagnosed correctly and that the possibility of cancer is eliminated.

Broccoli—one of nature's miracle foods

Brassica oleracea var botrytis.

Learn to love broccoli

The active health properties in broccoli are its mega antioxidant content, in particular indole-3-carbinol. Some research links indole-3-carbinol to a reduced risk of breast, prostate and other hormone-dependant cancers. Isothiocyanates found in broccoli, may suppress tumour growth and hormone production. Flavonoids also demonstrate protection against cancer.

Sulforaphane, produced by the body from broccoli, has shown to trigger the production of phase II enzymes, these can detoxify cancer-causing chemicals and are among the most potent anti-cancer compounds known to man. Broccoli is also a great source of folic acid, magnesium, vitamin C, beta-carotene, calcium and potassium.

But … be careful how you cook your broccoli—a recent study published in the *Journal of the Science of Food and Agriculture* found that boiled broccoli loses two-thirds of its flavonoid content, compared with a mind-blowing 97% loss induced by microwave cooking. So use your wok, stir-fry, steam or eat the young sprouts for best results.

Broccoli sprouts fight cancer

Researchers at Johns Hopkins University School of Medicine have discovered that three-day-old sprouts have very high amounts of the natural cancer-fighting compounds isothiocyanate and sulforaphane, which help support antioxidants such as vitamin C and vitamin E. The researchers found that when testing young shoots of broccoli at this three-day stage, the shoots contained 20 to 50 times more of these cancer-fighting actives in concentrated form, than was found in mature broccoli.

There are many reasons to eat sprouts. In addition to providing very high levels of vitamins, minerals, proteins and enzymes, sprouts deliver them in a form which is easily assimilated and digested. In fact, sprouts improve the efficiency of digestion.

Prevent heart disease and protect your lungs with broccoli

Other studies have shown that the consumption of broccoli is strongly associated with a reduced risk of coronary heart disease death in post-menopausal women. This is because the health benefits of broccoli are able to help delay the degeneration of cells in the body, slowing down the ageing process, delaying inflammation and thereby altering their risk of heart disease.

It was found that chemicals present in broccoli, cabbage, bok choy and other cruciferous vegetables may protect against lung cancer. Researchers studied more than 18,000 men, and they recorded 259 cases of lung cancer during the study's follow-up period. The researchers found that the men with detectable amounts of a substance known as 'isothiocyanate' in their bodies had a 36% lower risk of developing lung cancer over a ten year period.

How does broccoli help with prostate disease?

For years we have been recommending broccoli treatments in natural clinics for men who have prostate disease. It has been shown consistently that when you have broccoli, steamed, in juices, or as sprouts added to your daily diet, the prostate heals faster and returns to normal function quicker than if you were just taking herbal medicines and antioxidants alone.

Broccoli is a vasodilator, meaning it expands the blood vessels in the urogenital system. This re-establishes the distribution of circulation (ischaemia), especially on the prostate, enabling fresh blood to enter an already inflamed and often inaccessible part of the body. As you can see, this would provide the prostate with enough nutrition and other essential ingredients to heal, which in turn helps increase fertility and re-establish the libido.

Broccoli treatments are a good way to enhance your health

Broccoli treatments can be taken for prostate disease or for anyone who is suffering from a chronic illness and wants to improve their health. The anti-inflammatory effects can help you if you have arthritis or any condition where inflammation is a problem. The immune boosting benefits will help anyone who is worried about cancer or has an immune deficiency. Often I recommend this treatment to people who want to boost their immunity before winter, in conjunction with detox therapies or even when you are just run down and need a simple and effective boost. Make sure you get organic fresh broccoli or make your own sprouts at home.

Broccoli treatments have two effects. One is the anti-inflammatory action. The second is increasing your immunity. These properties are what make broccoli treatment a powerful tool when treating prostate disease and all other conditions where your immunity is compromised or inflammation is a big player in your illness. Broccoli has an anti-lithogenic effect on prostate, gall and kidney stones. This means that the stones can be softened and broken down with the addition of broccoli to your diet. For the anti-lithogenic effect, you need a large quantity of broccoli in the diet for at least two months.

The broccoli treatment should last for 30 days and can be added to your normal diet with no contraindications to any medications you may be taking. You should use all of the plant, including the stem, flowering tops and leaves. Or you can use sprouts.

You need to have 250 ml of fresh raw juice each morning and again in the evening on an empty stomach. Once you have had the juice, you can drink 250 ml of water over the next half hour or so but wait half an hour after the juice before you eat or drink anything else. If you have the sprouts, you will need roughly 100 grams of these twice a day. If you are taking other antioxidants and herbal medicines you can mix them with your broccoli treatment. Eating steamed or raw broccoli in meals is also beneficial. If you do not want to follow the strict treatment of juices or sprouts, then you can have 500 grams of broccoli either raw or steamed, added to your regular diet each day. This is not as intensive as the juices and sprouts; however, it will still be an awesome healing regime.

Kidney disease

Kidney failure is rare; however, diabetics and those with a genetic pre-disposition to kidney failure need to take extra care to look after these vital organs. Parsley is a number one herb for protecting your kidneys, as are corn silks and asparagus. Keep acid-forming food low in your diet, these include; alcohol, coffee, protein foods and toxins. Become familiar with your allergies as these can also exacerbate any kidney problems. Immune boosting herbs, especially wheatgrass juice, are also good to take for improved kidney health.

If you even suspect that you have problems with your kidneys then take the time to be tested properly. There are blood tests and also other scanning methods that are essential for diagnosis of kidney disease. If your kidneys do not work properly then you are creating a very acidic and toxic environment within your body because the poisons and meta-bolic wastes are unable to be eliminated properly through your blood stream. If your blood is toxic then you can rest assured that the rest of your body will also be rapidly increasing its percentage of toxins. This in turn puts you at risk of many other debilitating illnesses. Never be nonchalant when it comes to kidney disease.

Diuretics

Diuretics as herbs work to release extra fluids from your body. If you find that you have a fluid retention problem then magnesium is the number one supplement to help bring your body fluids back into balance. You could also take celery seed, especially taken as a tea daily, it will naturally eliminate any excess fluids that are in your body and act as a safe diuretic. People on diets sometimes take diuretics, this can become dangerous as you are always at risk of dehydration when these are taken in excess.

Avoid cystitis

Cystitis is another common problem. This can be caused through poor elimination from the kidneys and can eventuate in uric acid crystals that irritate the bladder lining and can eventually cause kidney stones. If you think you are suffering from this problem or are prone to cystitis, then watermelon juice is the best summer cure. Also taking large amounts of garlic, some cranberry juice and herbal diuretics can cure the problem before it turns into stones. Barley water is an old-fashioned cure for cystitis and so is lemon juice. Keep the fluids up and keep urinating, this is your best plan of action. Eat beetroot and asparagus through the day, or better still make juice from them.

The other common form of this complaint is called honeymoon cystitis. This occurs with a lot of sexual activity and an infection starts to climb its way up towards the bladder. Take the same precautions for this type of cystitis as the other. Make sure that you drink plenty of fluids whatever the cause of cystitis. This is one condition that is better cured very fast! If you even suspect you have this problem up your intake of natural antibiotic foods such as garlic and onions. Flush it out quickly and boost your immunity with some extra prebiotics and probiotics.

Libido is related to the kidneys

Keep your adrenal glands in good health and your kidneys will be healthy. Then if your kidneys are healthy the chances are that you will have a good libido too! There are some good adrenal balancing techniques you can use daily to help keep these little glands functioning well. The adrenal glands are located at the top of each kidney and they are responsible for the secretion of hormones such as DHEA, cortisone and adrenalins. Adaptogenic herbals are wonderful to help with your adrenal glands and, if they are looked after, your kidneys will be less stressed. Rehmannia is the number one herb to help strengthen your kidneys and build up your blood when you are stressed.

CHAPTER THIRTEEN

Bones and muscles

Exercise is the most important activity you can pursue for healthy bones and muscles. Imagine if you didn't have any bones? You would be a worm, incapable of humanly functioning, in fact we'd all be on the ground writhing around like slugs! So don't be an exercise slug, get up and move, for stronger bones and muscles.

One of the roles of your bones is to store calcium, as this is needed by every muscle in your body, every time you move. Bones stay strong because 98% of the calcium in your body is stored there, waiting to be used for muscle function. The other 2% of calcium is in the blood, ready and waiting for that burst of energy needed to put the calcium to use. Your bones and muscles are the foundations of your body size and shape. These are the vital parts that make you look good; if either is weak and not functioning optimally, you would physically look noticeably different.

The muscular skeletal system is in many ways the system that you need to work on the hardest to stay in shape. You need to not only watch the nutrition to these areas of your body, but you also need to work physically hard to keep them healthy. Today, people do too little daily exercise, we drive cars and take transport everywhere, we push trolleys full of groceries, or type away on computers and buy online. The leg work is taken out of life. We are physically unfit compared to past generations. In other words, unless you actively go out of your way to look after your bones and muscles, then you are at risk of poor health, which in this case means that bones become weak and brittle and muscle turns to fat stores.

The primary supplements needed for the muscular skeletal system are essential fatty acids. These work for the membrane growth of all cells in your body and we all need strong muscles and bones. You also need to take calcium and magnesium as well as other broad spectrum minerals. Exercise depletes your body of nutrients, so you really need to ensure that you are getting a well-rounded supply of good nutrients in your food and supplement regime. Talk with a Health Care Practitioner to work out your plan of health for exercise and fitness.

Too much acid in the body depletes the calcium in your bones. This includes coffee, alcohol and protein. It has been noted that women who are on high protein diets long term have a higher chance of getting osteoporosis. This is a condition where the calcium has leached from the bones after menopause and is not being replaced, leaving the bones rather brittle with actual gaps of air within. These bones are very weak. There is also a noticeable bend in the upper back of women and men who suffer from this degenerative and avoidable condition.

For your Wellness Zone please consider the health of your muscles and bones. Look at any genetic problems or personal factors that may contribute to osteoporosis, such as hysterectomy, early menopause, genetic history, acidic system, food allergies or illnesses and lifestyle afflictions, such as bulimia or anorexia, that may contribute to poor bone health in the future. Eating disorders are not limited to younger women, many women in their 40s and older are suffering from bulimia and anorexia because they want to stay thin and think they look good. These can be silent illnesses that are well hidden from the prying eyes of friends and family.

The best foods for bone health are kale, almonds, dark green leafy vegetables, comfrey, spirulina, magnesium supplements and fish with edible bones including sardines and salmon. Do some weight bearing exercise every day and increase those muscles and tone. The nutritional profile of pregnant women is very important for the future health of their children's bones. Make sure that you eat good bone and muscle building foods if you are planning to conceive or are pregnant.

Comfrey is bone building food

You can not underestimate the need for strong, healthy bones as you age. The root of the comfrey plant needs to be peeled before you dry it, then make a powder that can be used as a tea or sprinkled on your meals.

Comfrey is a wonderful food to help keep your skeletal system strong, many women have avoided osteoporosis by this simple plant being added to meals. You can also use the fresh leaf. Either make a tea using about 10 cm of a leaf per day or you can finely chop half a young leaf and add it to your daily salad.

Comfrey has been used traditionally as a herbal remedy for any condition where you have broken tissue. It is renowned for binding the skin and accelerating healing. It is very useful for any broken bones and can be used in salads, teas or you can apply it topically as a poultice or cream. Comfrey can cause hepatotoxicity if taken in medicinal quantities. However, it is safe to use topically as a cream or even to have small amounts as food and teas.

Joints are a big problem for many people

There are many types of arthritis and joint problems that can occur with your body. Auto-immune rheumatoid arthritis often has hidden agendas, with food allergies and other health problems as its precursor. However, the main form of joint problem is wear and tear from years of living in your body. With any form of arthritis or associated illness you need to clear your body of excess acidity and try to create a good eliminative pathway for excess lactic and uric acids to pass through your body.

Every time you move you are creating lactic acid, just as a by-product from muscle action. And every time you digest protein foods you are creating uric acid from the natural digestive processes. These acids tend to gather and get caught around your joints. So, the first priority for anyone wanting success with anti-inflammatories is to create good elimination pathways for these excess acids and then you will give your body a better chance to relieve the pain associated with inflammation. The liver is another organ that you may wish to cleanse, this helps to clear the inflammation as quickly as possible.

It's not surprising that many people suffer from these inflammatory conditions and if you are in this situation then address it with as little medical intervention as possible. Glucosamine is popular to help rebuild the cartilage and also to dissolve any little bone spurs that may have grown which will make life more uncomfortable. The herbs gotu kola and celery seed are both good as anti-inflammatories and pain relievers. Hops, *Boswellia* resin and devil's claw are also good herbal anti-inflammatories. Also hypericum, gotu kola, hops and capsicum extract applied topically can relieve pain and inflammation.

The lowdown on anti-inflammatory

These are agents inhibiting the effects of chemical mediators of inflammation. The two main groups of anti-inflammatories are steroidal and non-steroidal.

Actives involved are salicylates, saponins, flavonoids, alkaloids, iridoids, fixed and essential oils and tannins. Steroidal compounds prevent the release of arachidonic acid from membrane bound phospholipids, this will inhibit the production of pro-inflammatory leucotrines and phosphoglandins. The problem with many anti-inflammatories is that they block the pathways of healing in a cascading order so that other functions are affected other than the inflammation. Talk with your Health Care Practitioner about this problem if you are going to take anti-inflammatory medications.

Pharmaceutical non-steroidal anti-inflammatories are mainly silicon-based drugs like aspirin. Herbal agents involve a host of chemical compounds acting in a variety of ways, e.g. there are numerous compounds including many flavonoids that inhibit histamine release from mast cells. Other compounds include PAF inhibitors, whilst boswellic acid from *Boswellia* is a selective leukotriene inhibitor (it does not influence the cyclo-oxygenase pathway which can lead to disruption of blood-clotting mechanisms, a major problem with most pharmaceutical anti-inflammatories).

Inflammation can also cause headaches, in which case feverfew can help. Other anti-inflammatory herbs available are; willow bark, chickweed and devils claw. Hops is another anti-inflammatory you may want to add to your diet for arthritis care.

Inflammation is the precursor for many illnesses including arthritis and cardiovascular disease. You need to keep inflammation down and this can be achieved through diet and exercise. Drinking green tea or taking the extract is excellent for reducing inflammation on a daily level. If your body is acidic it is more likely to be inflamed. Keeping your system alkaline is another way to help avoid inflammation.

Inflammation is often a precursor to auto-immune diseases and these can be environmental or genetic. Make sure you have a good nutritional profile and take care to avoid inflammation, as left unchecked it can cause havoc to your Wellness Zone.

Rheumatoid and Osteo arthritis can both be relieved with the addition of omega-3 to your diet. This is because omega-3 has an anti-inflammatory effect on both auto-immune and allergic inflammatory conditions.

CHAPTER FOURTEEN

Weight management

A re you confused about the current offerings in the ever increasing market place of weight reduction? What supplements to take? What dietary choices will lead to ultimate weight reduction? And what is the best individual plan to help you get to your goal weight quickly?

Here we look at the new trends which clearly lead to choices of protein based low carbohydrate diets, low-fat diets or cleansing regimes. Once you decide which eating plan you wish to follow, you can then choose additions, such as stacks, guggulsterones, thermo-activators, carb blockers and specific hormonal controls and herbal supplements, to help you on your way to a new slimmer self.

In a world where we want dietary aids to do everything, the technology is surely getting close. In one stack (supplement combination), you can now achieve the following: promote conversion of fat into muscle, reduce appetite, increase metabolism of fats and carbohydrates, increase muscle bulk, strength and firmness, block weight gain by inhibiting storage, eliminate carbohydrate cravings, block fat absorption, increase lean muscle mass, boost energy and endurance levels and block carbohydrate absorption, all in one little pill!

Metabolic syndrome is a big problem

Stress will make you fatter faster, and it is the biggie when it comes to gaining weight. When you become stressed, as your body magically finds a way to add a few pounds of fat whilst you are looking the other way. Cortisol levels increase with stress. Activity can occur on a cellular level with stress and these all lead to inflammation, insulin resistance and fat accumulation.

There are two types of stressed individuals. The ones who get really anxious and the ones who get really apathetic. In both instances you need to ensure that you have given your nervous system support and that you are addressing the stress issues in order to avoid the subconscious reactions our body has to stress. One of these reactions is to get satisfaction from food and, you guessed it, the most satisfying foods are the ones that have a dopamine or opium like effect on the brain. This is the reward, the satiated feeling you get from eating when you are under emotional stress.

The way to keep the fat away in this situation is to support the adrenal glands and to eat protein-rich foods that offer the body satisfaction without the huge blood sugar spike that is often gained from high GI carbohydrate foods. Or if you are going to eat carbohydrate foods, stay away from the sugar type carbs and go for the wholegrain cereals and savoury foods. The herbs panax ginseng and withania are good to take in times of stress to help keep the fat away.

Remember that not everyone responds well to every type of dieting. You are an individual and losing weight is dependent upon where your body naturally stores its excess fat. If you store fat in the abdominal area then you will require different foods and a different style of weight reduction plan to anyone who stores fat in the peripheral areas such as the thighs. It can get complex as different endocrine and nervous tissues are involved with weight reduction for different people.

Talk with your Health Care Practitioner and they will help you find the simplest way to manage weight for your constitution and problem. Today science is continually finding new answers to old problems, and some of these answers are very natural, painless and simple. It is all about understanding the machine you are in and knowing what is the best exercise plan and the best fuel to help you achieve optimal wellness.

Be aware of the obesity risk

If you get depressed, then you are at risk of putting on fat. This happens hormonally as well as through the foods you consume. Often people do really well whilst they are on a diet and achieve their desired weight, only to find that once the diet is over, the fat has rebounded and gone straight back where it came from. There are key times in our lives when fat cells develop, when we are at puberty, when we are pregnant and once again at menopause.

Once a fat cell has been developed it will never leave your body. It stays with you whether it is expanded (full of fat) or whether it is contracted (empty of fat). Throughout history our body has become a refined machine that has learned to store fat when there's plenty of food about, and to take off the fat when we hit starvation mode. Part of this starvation process is the slowing down of your metabolism. This is natural.

Logically when your metabolism is fast you burn more energy. Now faced with the possibility of starving to death, your body will choose to slow its metabolism down and burn as few calories as possible to stay alive. Imagine what happens when you spend your life dieting and losing weight, only to rebound again and put the weight back on, then diet again to lose it again and then yo-yo your way through life. Yes, what happens is that your metabolism will virtually shut down and you will accumulate more fat in those fat cells as your body will fear starvation and death.

However the problem today is that we are no longer starving. We no longer have to live in these seasonal food cycles that our ancestors relied on so heavily. Yes, we have too much food and too much of that food is refined and synthesised so that it's like putting pure fuel into an already full tank. Except unlike the tank our fuel won't spill over the edge. Instead, we have those lovely little fat cells that just love accumulating, they love being full and they will happily store all the extra fat and make us bigger people.

There are so many sad consequences for those who allow this to happen to their bodies. For one, did you know that the organs become paper-thin and the digestive tract becomes especially stretched? All those extra fat cells, full of lovely fat need feeding and looking after. So, our poor heart is stressed, our organs are stressed and we are really very, very toxic indeed. But try to tell an obese person they are toxic and they will be highly offended.

So the body is full of fat: the organs are stretched to beyond capacity with all this extra fat to look after, we are toxic as fat is toxic and we are now going to become inflamed as this is such a stress on everything and we really can't cope. Then to top it all off our blood sugar levels are hitting the roof, our triglyceride levels are furiously high and we can't stop eating. Guess what? We've hit the cycle of obesity, and to make things worse we feel so rotten and unmotivated that it's near impossible to find enough energy to sit up and change the TV channel let alone go for a half hour cardiovascular session.

Oh, I wish I wasn't so hungry ... Yes, you are not getting leptin into your system, nor are you on leptin overload. This is a hormone that's secreted from the hypothalamus to tell your body you are full and to stop eating. In people of normal weight, this hormone works fine, it tells you that you are full, so you listen and stop eating. But in obese people it just keeps on sending the signal, but for some reason you are on overload and don't hear it at all, so you still feel hungry and when you feel hungry you want to eat.

Add on fat cells daily and you will feel all the worse for it. If you keep up this nasty little cycle then it won't be long before you are only eating certain foods, such as very refined carbohydrates, lots of sugary foods and sweet treats that become the mainstay of your diet. You just get bigger and then you feel worse and worse. By the time you wake up to what's going on you are suffering from metabolic resistance or syndrome X as it's known and you are really in trouble, with probably high blood pressure, diabetes type two, obesity and cardiovascular disease brewing on the side-line.

It's up to you to keep the fat away. Look at your hormones first

You may be in this cycle and wonder how you can come out the other side and keep the fat away. Or you may have been through this cycle and wonder how you can keep the fat away. Or you may be anywhere in between. Let's face it, over 60% of adults in developed countries are overweight and heading to obesity now, it seems to be the scourge of our society at the moment.

To keep fat away you must keep your androgen and oestrogen levels in balance. This is especially important at menopause. If you are concerned about these levels, please get tested. Saliva tests are the most accurate and will address this issue first before you try other strategies to keep the fat away. Insulin resistance is another key hormonal area that needs your attention. Also make sure that your thyroid hormone is working well.

The herb astragalus is known to have an effect on the master hormonal secretions. This involves all hormones. Adaptogenic herbs such as liquorice, withania and ginseng are also beneficial in balancing these hormones. Tribulus and turmeric have a reputation of balancing androgens and oestrogens.

One of the best ways to keep fat away is to increase
your resting thermogenesis

Thermogenesis is the breakdown of macronutrients from the mitochondria in your cells. The process involves the uncoupling of proteins, which cause protons to leak from the electron transport chain in the cell. This causes a percentage of energy to escape as heat, instead of being locked into ATP.

There are two types of thermogenesis. Obligatory thermogenesis is the natural heat created by metabolism to sustain life. And facultative or adaptive thermogenesis is used to increase the metabolic rate on demand. The proton leakage for thermogenesis accounts for about 20% of our thermogenesis.

There are certain activities that increase thermogenesis such as eating essential fatty acids in sesame seed oil, coconut and fish oils. Thermogenesis is induced by thyroid hormone function, sympathetic nervous system function and by the pleasurable tastes when eating food. It is decreased by insulin resistance, starvation and fasting.

If you suffer from visceral obesity then your thermogenesis will be lower until you are able to lose that bulge around the belly. Visceral obesity is when you accumulate fat around your waistline, this is the unhealthiest place to accumulate fat as it increases your chances of many chronic illnesses.

Did you know that the largest user of energy in your body is thermogenesis? This is the type of energy where your body burns fat just by sitting around and functioning as normal. You lose more calories through thermogenesis than through exercise on a daily basis. So, in order to keep fat cells away you need to up your thermogenic energy output.

Energy expenditure can be divided into three major categories

1. Resting energy expenditure which is the one we want to increase to keep the fat away. When you have a low basal resting metabolism then you are sure to gain fat in the long term.
2. Physical activity. If you have daily physical activity, especially aerobic activity for 30 minutes or longer in each 24 hour period, then you are ensuring that your basal thermogenic activity level is increasing with time.
3. Thermogenic activity of digesting food. Now to keep the fat away from your body, you need to keep the fat out of your mouth so that the thermogenesis of digestion is a non-fat storing experience!

To have good resting thermogenesis it's also important that you have good muscle mass. Research has shown that individuals with lower fat mass and higher muscle mass burn energy more efficiently than individuals with higher fat mass and lower muscle mass. So, it makes sense that you will want to increase your muscle mass with some weight bearing training and exercise several times a week to increase your muscle to fat ratio.

Exercise is as effective as diet to keep fat away

We used to think that we only needed to have aerobic exercise three times a week for 40 minutes for aerobic fitness and good health. We may need as much as 30 to 60 minutes of aerobic exercise most days to maintain weight. This is not to lose weight; this is just to keep fat away!

Did you know that if you follow this regime then you could really have your cake and eat it too! It has been shown that you don't need a restricted diet plan and that exercise is as effective as diet when it comes to keeping fat at bay. Exercise will increase your metabolism, and this will keep your weight down if you have a reasonably healthy but not a calorie restricted diet.

Exercise causes fat redistribution, decreasing abdominal and visceral fat. Exercise improves glucose tolerance, insulin sensitivity, lipid parameters, blood pressure and fibrinolytic activity. Exercise also improves your ability to maintain fat loss after a diet. Did you know that low intensity exercise increases fat oxidation? The down side is that exercise can increase your appetite. So, don't go eating up large after exercise.

A good strategy is to have a scoop of quality protein powder in a glass of water before you exercise. This will help to keep your appetite at bay afterwards. Protein is known to preserve or increase fat-free mass as well as reducing fat mass and improving metabolic profile. So, keeping the carbs down and the protein up when you get hungry, could result in less fat and leaner muscle tissue.

Alcohol will dull your sense of proportion

Naturally, when you have a large meal, your body will compensate for the size of that meal by requiring less in the next meal, thereby you will naturally eat less. Not so when you have alcohol with the meal. For some unknown reason, your body loses its ability to decide on proportion when alcohol is consumed with a meal and the following meal is not necessarily lighter. In fact the condition is called 'long-term passive over-consumption'.

Alcohol consumption correlates with BMI whereby those who actively consume more alcohol then others have a higher BMI and are more likely to be obese. This may be because you lose your sense of proportion with food when you are drinking alcohol with meals.

To keep the fat away from your body, you need to make sure you control your food portions when you drink alcohol. You also need to make sure that if you do overeat at one meal that you compensate for this at the next meal and eat less. Awareness is the key here. Eat less when you drink and learn to say *no* when you have had enough. Also remember that alcohol has virtually no nutritional value, it is truly just empty calories helping your fat cells to grow.

Omega fatty acids help keep the fat away

Omega-3 fatty acids such as wild fish oil help prevent fatty liver, increase thermogenesis and block the action of lipogenesis. Insulin increases lipogenesis, which is the storing of fat in your body. Steroid regulating elementary binding protein (SREBP) stores fat. And, when you take wild fish oil, this action is stopped in its tracks. This process all occurs in your liver cells and we need to stop SREBP.

Sesame oil, coconut and fish oil all increase liver fatty acid oxidations through the up-regulation of the gene expression of paroxysmal fatty acid oxidation enzymes. Sesamin is the active of sesame which has been shown to enhance ketogenesis, inhibit fat synthesising enzymes, decrease lipogenesis, act as an antioxidant, reduce endotoxin damage, act as anti-inflammatory, decrease triglycerides and raise HDL.

Magnesium is a key to keeping fat away

Magnesium is a cofactor in hundreds of enzymatic reactions including phosphotransferases and hydrolases such as ATPases which are centrally important in the biochemistry of the cell, particularly in energy metabolism. Many people are deficient in magnesium and this mineral is central to avoiding inflammation, repairing adrenal stress and helping the recovery of all cells after exercise. If you are overweight and lack magnesium then you could be missing a link to increase your metabolism. Research has shown that obese people get an increase in resting metabolism when they take extra magnesium. Improve your ATP production and your thermogenesis by taking sufficient magnesium.

What supplements are available to help lose weight?

Anyone who is on a weight reduction programme may be more susceptible to lowered immunity as the diet regime continues. Cat's claw works very well for weight loss programmes. Consider taking a good multi-vitamin mineral tablet, or a green food such as spirulina, barley and alfalfa daily. These green foods can also help reduce your appetite. Boost your intake of nervous system support supplements such as the B vitamins and consider taking hypericum.

Chitosan

This is a dietary fibre derived from shellfish. It attracts and binds fatty acids, carrying them out of your body. This is a localised digestive tract aid that will absorb between 8 and 12 times its weight in fat, preventing it and also cholesterol from being absorbed. You need to consume the chitosan at the same time as consuming the fats for it to be optimally effective.

The downside of chitosan is that it also takes away essential fatty acids, and you need to create a regime whereby you get adequate absorption of essential fatty acids when adding chitosan to your programme. Therefore you will need to take this supplement at a separate time of day to your essential fatty acids.

HCA's

Hydroxycitric acid serves as an appetite suppressant and inhibits the actions of the ATP (adenosine triphosphate) citrate lyase enzymic conversion of carbohydrates to fat in the liver. This product is often included in stacks. The herb brindleberry contains this constituent. HCA could reduce fat production from 40 to 70% for up to 12 hours after eating.

Chromium picolinate

Chromium helps regulate insulin, helping maintain blood sugar and cholesterol levels that result in less fat being deposited to cells. This creates an increasing lean muscle mass. It has the advantage of being an appetite suppressant, especially curing sweet carbohydrate cravings.

The chromium alone is not easily absorbed and is best taken in combination with amino acid derivatives such as picolinic acid from tryptophan in picolinate versions.

Pyruvate

Glucose is broken down in your body by pyruvic acid. The idea behind these pyruvate supplements is that the body will have increased levels of pyruvic acid and this will enhance the cell's ability to generate energy. The aim is weight loss, reducing weight regain, decreased appetite and reduced fatigue.

Carb blockers

These help control the down side of high carbohydrate intake. Many of the products contain a white kidney bean derivative, phaseolamin, which was designed to block the body's action of alpha-amylase enzymes, which results in less starch breakdown. This is supposed to create less absorption of carbs into your body. It has also been suggested that these starch blockers also reduce blood sugar and insulin levels after meals.

White kidney bean is gaining popularity as a carb blocker. However remember that when you block carbs, you are also blocking nutrition. Be aware of getting optimal nutrition absorbed into your blood stream. This means that you cannot take carb blockers with every meal and the meals that you choose to take carb blockers with, will have limited nutritional benefit.

Gugglesterones

Guggle has been used in Ayurvedic medicine for centuries. It has now entered the new generation weight loss market with properties derived from its bark. It is reputed for increasing the thyroid glands actions and is stimulant free. Guggle may also preserve or increase the metabolic rate and provide substrates for the production of neurotransmitters involved in weight loss and metabolic functioning.

Herbal supplements

Some herbal supplements that may help you support your weight loss regime are available in tea form and there are numerous supplements on the market that boast effortless weight loss support. Brindleberry is used in many preparations for its appetite-suppressing abilities and HCA. Kelp, which will work in the same way as Guggle, increases activity in your thyroid gland. Kelp can increase your basal resting metabolism rate if used in conjunction with exercise as well as offering nutrients and blood cleansing benefits.

White willow bark has the ability to increase the circulation and transportation of the other aids. It is included in many products for this ability as is capsicum which is renowned for its benefit of potentiating the effects of other herbs as a circulatory stimulant.

Gymnema is a herb that will help to block the sweet taste buds and the absorption of carbohydrates, this herb can also help with the body's utilisation and receptiveness to insulin. Guarana seed gives a dieter the boost of the stimulating effects of caffeine as well as providing tonic and diuretic actions. This herb will naturally suppress your appetite as you are bursting with energy.

Panax ginseng is a good herb to take when dieting as you will need to balance your adrenals, protecting your body against the effects of stimulants.

Often when dieting, your bowel movements are slowed down and not as regular as desired. Herbal laxatives can be beneficial when taken in moderation and for short periods of time. The herb senna is a mild and effective laxative, increasing peristalsis and bowel movements. You can purchase various combinations of laxative slimmer's tea to take daily and ensure regular elimination.

Brindleberry

Brindleberry is probably the best herb to suppress your appetite and keep it suppressed between meals. If you take 5 grams of brindleberry 20 minutes before each meal, you probably won't eat as much and will certainly feel more satisfied and full between meals.

Dandelion

This is a gentle herb, yet effective for dieters on the low carb diet. Dandelion cleanses both the liver and kidneys as well as helping to remove excess fluids. With these diets, where we are burning our own stores for fuel, it's important to keep the eliminative organs well flushed.

Black walnut

Black walnut will add extra motion to your large intestine and help eliminate build-ups in the bowel pockets as well as helping to eradicate parasites.

Capsicum

Add a little capsicum to your meals and your metabolism will increase for up to four hours after the meal.

Kelp

Kelp is another herb for dieters that increase your metabolism. Kelp contains lots of iodine and we all need that for effective thyroid functioning. Also all seaweeds help remove heavy toxins from your blood and liver. This will help eliminate problems such as cellulite and toxic build-up.

Citrus seed extract

Citrus seed and peel extracts are good to suppress the appetite and also can help eliminate built-up debris in the digestive tract. Grapefruit is a good citrus to help cut fat in your digestive tract, it is also good to help eliminate parasites.

Amino acids

Body builders have been using amino acids for many years to sculpt and tone body mass. This is always in combination with exercise regimes and there are now many products aimed at weight loss that contain isolated amino acids. The main ones sold for weight loss are L carnitine, L-methionine, Inositol and Tyrosine.

Stacks

The ever increasing combinations of new generation weight aids created in specific synergies for maximum weight loss benefits. The primary purpose of these stacks is to create thermogenesis in your body. The body has built-in regulators that control how quickly we burn calories.

As we age the thermogenesis gradually becomes blocked, creating weight gain because our resting metabolism is lowered.

These stacks may contain any the following: hydroxycitric acid (HCA), chromium, L-carnitine, L-methionine, inositol or choline, guarana or caffeine extract, willow bark, ginseng or stimulant herbs such as capsicum.

Your diet kit—where confidence is your biggest asset

You will need a determined attitude to succeed. You will need to look at your past dieting choices and really be honest about why you have the need to lose some extra kilos. Once this is achieved you can buy a notebook to write down all foods eaten, exercise completed and any other pertinent notes.

Find a set of scales and discipline yourself to weigh in once a week only, get a tape measure and measure your waist, hips, thighs, upper legs and upper arms, repeat this once a week as well. Record your weight and measurements. Get someone to take a photo of you in your bikini or underwear before you start the diet. Place this picture on your dressing table or fridge so that you will stay motivated. You will also see that you are looking better each week if you are sticking to your chosen regime.

Gain invaluable knowledge about the diet you are undertaking and the choices you can make. Research as much as you can about the different programmes and processes. Each of us is individual and we can only make a wise decision about weight loss once we have a clear understanding of our choices. You can purchase books, CD's or DVD's and even have your food delivered to your door if you join certain weight loss groups.

Confidence in yourself is your biggest asset to weight loss and maintenance. Don't buy into the multi-marketed concept that you need all the help you can get. This is not true, what you need is confidence and the belief that mind rules over matter. If you are disciplined in your choices and determined to succeed, you will be successful. Dieting is one of those times in life where a positive outlook is the only outlook. You still need to ensure that energy burnt is higher than energy consumed for effective weight loss.

Some dieting techniques can be dangerous if you only consider the short-term benefits of weight loss and don't consider your long-term health ideals. Before you undertake any form of drastic weight loss regime, make sure you are aware of the consequences. And this is where research is invaluable.

The protein diet

There are many versions of the protein diet. Basically you eat protein complete foods such as eggs, fish and various animal and dairy products as the mainstay of the diet. You are restricted to the grams in carbohydrate you consume daily. The carbohydrate intake is reduced dramatically to less than 30 grams per day to create and maintain the state of ketosis in your body which ensures that you are burning your own body fat instead of the energy derived from carbohydrates.

There are certain foods that are considered 'free' foods that you are able to consume without restriction. These are often high-fat foods such as cheese, cream and meats but these free foods also consist of lettuce, cucumber, asparagus, spinach, bok choy, kale, cabbage, beans and small amounts of mushrooms, tomatoes and onion. Every other food is measured in grams of carbohydrate only.

This diet takes 48 hours for your body to enter the state of ketosis from the onset of your diet regime. You will need to purchase keto sticks from the pharmacy and have a book on hand that describes the Glycaemic Index and the carbohydrate values of foods.

Some advocates of this diet say that you must restrict the high-fat foods, as this will create problems with fatty liver and cholesterol levels. Others state that the high protein diet is very successful when high-fat foods are consumed. You will need to read some of the books and decide which way you need to go. This diet is not for everyone. Many people become constipated and need to either have colonic irrigations or laxative herbal tea blends to create bowel movements. Generally it is successful if undertaken over a restricted time frame and alternated with a cleansing diet.

There have been reports of gradual weight gain after the diet is discontinued. Others end up actually weighing more than their original weight due to the fattiness created in the liver from the high-fat content of some of these diets. These are some of the possible side effects that you may want to consider.

It's really worth going the low-fat option if you undertake this diet, as you will then gain many of the benefits of ketosis without some of the fatty build-up in your liver that occurs when you eat fat. Ketosis is actually the body's way of eating unwanted matter including toxins, fats and degenerated cells.

There are watered-down versions of the high protein diet where you eat low-fat proteins and a limited amount of carbohydrate grams per day. This diet does not put you into ketosis; however, combined with new generation weight loss aids and exercise, they are becoming extremely popular. This is one way that you can avoid possible kidney damage which may be exacerbated by the higher protein dieting. Basically keep the carbohydrates off the menu. No wheat, no pasta, no rice, no potatoes, no pumpkin, no sweet potatoes and no foods that have any sugar in them at all.

Who would benefit from this diet?

If you enjoy meats and feel energised after eating protein foods, you don't have allergies to dairy and are able to go without fruit and vegetables for a restricted time. If you don't have a fatty liver, arthritis, gout, auto-immune conditions or cardiovascular problems and feel reasonably healthy without any medications or health restrictions.

The protein diet does put extra strain on your kidneys, liver and cardiovascular system. The extra protein running through your kidneys actually wears the nephrons out faster than is desirable. This type of dieting can also exacerbate such problems as gallstone formation, gout, auto-immune diseases and other weaknesses that can be waiting beneath the surface.

So, unless you are in top shape this type of dieting is best avoided from the perspective of acid alkaline balances and long-term health consequences. However, strictly speaking with weight loss, you can get some fast and good results if it is followed in a fat conscious format.

Keep the carbs down and the protein balanced

When you eat carbohydrate foods your body is busy metabolising them at the expense of oxidising fats. Low GI carbohydrates cause low satisfaction and overeating, which naturally creates fat storage. The herb white kidney bean extract is now used as a starch blocker. If you take this herb before meals, research has shown that it blocks the absorption of carbohydrates by up to 50% in the small intestine.

Carbohydrate causes serum tryptophan release which increases brain serotonin levels and elevates your mood. Sweet foods stimulate an opioid response, which is why depressed people like to eat carbs. They make you feel better. But carbs cause a spike in blood glucose levels followed by a dip which makes you feel hungrier faster. Often you will eat more carbs before your body has digested the last meal properly, therefore you will be overeating and Voila! ... fat deposits.

Protein on the other hand keeps your blood sugar levels stable and this has the effect of more energy without the mood swings. Protein also doesn't turn directly into fat cells in your body. When you eat the protein it enhances the body's ability to oxidise and burn its own fat.

Dietary choices to keep fat away from your body

There are many concepts of dietary choice and you need to find a plan that works for you. Not all diets are created equal, the main aim is to have a sustainable diet that fits into your lifestyle, allows you flexibility and adheres to some basic principles, such as the fact that you need to consume less calories than you expend. This is a good rule to follow each and every day.

When you want to keep the fat away there is no room for big slices of fatty bacon with eggs and toast and butter for breakfast. There is no room for chocolate mud cake as a regular addition to your diet and there certainly isn't room for alcohol to be consumed every day. You can have these items but they need to be in moderation and you need to treat sweet, processed foods as extra special treat foods, not as part of your everyday diet. Drink alcohol in moderation and keep saturated fats out of your diet as much as possible.

When it comes to perception of food it really matters when you think that a food is good for you and when you perceive that food to be delicious in the process. You will then receive the most benefits and health from eating that food. However when you think of a food as being unhealthy, as being fattening and as being bad for your general health, then hello, your body thinks it is too.

So, when it comes to eating, let your conscience do the thinking and act on what it says. Balance is the key here. If you eat more at one meal then make sure you eat less at the next. Trick your body by going on a long walk right when you thought you'd better sit down and eat! Eat at regular intervals during the day, and have smaller servings that are delicious and of course contain your favourite foods. Just be aware of the hidden sugars in foods. These can be found in fruit and vegetables as well as in processed foods. Try to have your beverages such as tea, coffee and other drinks without any added honey or sugar as this will spike your blood sugar which could lead to exhaustion later in the day.

Keep sweet foods away from your mouth as much as possible. Replace sugar with stevia. There are some good herbal supplements you can use to keep your appetite at bay, so use them. These include hydroxycitric acid, gymnema, and brindleberry. Use green tea extract and ginger as part of your plan to keep the fat away. Also the herb bilberry, the extract from the leaves is high in chromium which helps keep blood sugar levels even.

Low carb diets and why they work

Low carb diets have been all the rage for the past few years. It's simple, all you need to do is eat certain foods that are low in energy producing glucose, you will be a new slimmer self miraculously within weeks. Never to be a roly poly again. That is until you get back into the habit of eating carbohydrates and put on all the pounds shed as quickly as they were lost.

There's no need to put those kilos back on again if you follow an eating regime that will keep your weight in balance. This is the concept behind the Glycaemic Index and eating according to the principle of slow burning foods that will allow your body to make fuel from sources other than glucose.

These other fuels come in the form of proteins and fatty acids

When the body doesn't have enough fuel from carbohydrates, and therefore is unable to breakdown these into glycogen, it must seek fuel elsewhere and elsewhere is the storage of fats in muscle tissue, such as your waistline or thighs. This all makes sense since we are either in the process of burning fuel or storing it for a later day when we may be in need of extra glycogen which is the main fuel currency on a cellular level.

Keep those carbs off the menu

So we prefer to live off carbohydrates. The more refined and processed, the more efficiently our body will kick into action and process them into adenosine triphosphate, which is the cellular energy currency enabling all functions to proceed smoothly in our bodies. Every second we are making fuel and burning fuel. Our body will sacrifice all else to keep the brain alive and functioning well. Our body is the most miraculous organism completely focused on keeping its energy levels optimum and its organs well supplied with nutrients and replacement cells.

However, our body doesn't give a hoot whether it's a size 10 or a Size 20. Actually it quite likes having fuel (fat) in reserve and certainly doesn't care what we look like in the mirror.

Take control of your diet

This is where modern science has come to the rescue on the diet frontier. However, there are many interpretations of the low carb diet and often we consider it as a high protein diet when this is technically not the case at all.

The aim of this style of dieting is to place the body in a state of gluco-neogenesis, this is the term for the body making fuel from sources other than carbohydrate based fuels. These other fuel bases are fats and proteins. Naturally, our body will go into this state when we're starving; however, there are downfalls to this style of fasting diet as it decreases metabolism over time and throws our body clock out of kilter, which results in a slower metabolism and more capacity to store fat effectively.

At least with regular eating on a low carb diet we will increase our metabolism and keep stoking the body with fuel, which encourages further fat burning. The only tricky part with this style of dieting is that we need to be very strict with ourselves and completely disciplined in what we eat. This means keeping our carbohydrate levels down to under 20 to 30 grams each day and ensuring you are burning the fats and proteins instead of storing them as extra fat.

How to get thinner sooner

The way gluconeogenesis works is that the first energy pathway, gly-colysis, must be exhausted of fuel, therefore there can be no glucose in the system. Glucose is derived from monosaccharides, disaccharides and polysaccharides. This includes most vegetables and fruit, all cereals and their products, and is hidden in items such as nutritional supple-ments and alcoholic beverages. You need to get these fuel sources out of your body before your body goes into another cycling system of gluconeogenesis, where it will actively seek out proteins and fats to fuel the system and keep it operating effectively.

Healthy scientific alternatives to lose weight

Gluconeogenesis occurs in the liver and utilises most amino acids and all fatty acid storage. With this process in operation you will be able to delete the storage of fats and lose weight. However, this doesn't necessarily mean that it's good to eat a load of protein and fat to lose the weight as some dietary experts have touted over the years.

If we eat a lot of fat, it can create a fatty liver and decrease the effectiveness of our detoxification pathways and all other liver functions. If we eat too much protein, we can create havoc with the acid alkaline balances in our system, and conditions such as kidney damage and arthritis may appear. So, the trick is to put your body into gluconeogenesis (a state of ketosis) and keep it there, without unnecessary health consequences.

Your low carb diet kit

Glycaemic Index chart

If you are on a low carb diet, you need to get hold of a Glycaemic Index chart that will show you exactly how many grams of carbohydrate are in each morsel of food eaten. You will also need to ensure that you are in a sound state of health to begin with, otherwise it's best to contact your health professional and get their support and advice on this type of dieting.

Ketone sticks for good measure

Ketone sticks are available in most pharmacies. They come in packs of 100. You will need to use these sticks every day regularly to measure whether you are burning fat or fuel. Ketone sticks are best used about half an hour after each meal and then again first thing in the morning and last thing at night. You may wish to measure the level of ketones in your urine between meals and after snacks as well.

These little sticks are the only true indicator you can have to show that you are not burning carbohydrates through the day.

Stock the fridge with free foods

Free foods are foods that you can eat without fear of going out of ketosis. These are mostly light green leafy vegetables, yoghurt, meats and dairy products such as eggs and cheese. Some people eat a very well-balanced, nutritional and low-fat diet whilst remaining in a moderate state of ketosis whilst they lose weight.

Avocados, pumpkin, onions, ginger, garlic, mushrooms, tomatoes, egg plant, tofu and sprouted lentils are all good base foods which ensure sufficient fibre and nutrition in your low carb diet when combined with fresh eggs, seafood and meats.

One of the secrets to a successful low carb diet is to keep the fridge full of these low carb, nurturing foods and stay away from the carbohydrates. Don't even have chocolate or bread near the house whilst on this diet, as you can easily be tempted to have a taste which is enough to pull your body out of its energy producing pathway gluconeogenesis and swing back into glycolysis, which will take hours if not a full day to reverse again.

Herbs

The low carb diet is the perfect diet for you to take any appetite-suppressing and cleansing herbs to help your body run more effectively.

You can get fat on a low carb diet

This is true and fairly simple too. If you are very good and are eating fresh vegetables and protein foods, you may wish to add some delicacies such as bacon, cream, delicious cheeses and fatty meats into your diet. This is actually fine and you will continue to lose weight eating this way, however you must be very strict on yourself.

If for example you go out to dinner and have a delicious coconut cream curry with green vegetables and a few wines, you will be borderline ketosis. If you don't go any further than that, then you will remain burning energy, even if only very slightly, from your fat stores. But, if you decide to have sweets, an extra wine, or a slice of bread, you will no longer be burning your own energy and you will be back in the position of possibly storing fat. It's that easy.

If you make the decision to go onto this style of dieting then you need to make the commitment to stick with it for a period of time, perhaps two weeks or longer. It's actually okay to have a glass of wine, beer or whatever, so long as you are measuring your intake of carbohydrates and ensuring that your ketone sticks are staying in the levels from trace to moderate most of the time. Basically, it's up to you. Don't blow it for the sake of some garlic bread or an extra wine!

Keep your energy high with low carb dieting

If we place our body in gluconeogenesis, naturally our inclination will be to preserve energy and slow down. This is the typical pattern with fasting, you will feel a real decline in energy levels for a few days as many toxins are released from your system and excreted and fats are used as fuel currency.

However, when you undertake the low carb technique of dieting you shouldn't feel a decline in energy levels. In fact many people feel more invigorated and healthier than they normally would when following this type of diet. You never need to feel hungry either as this style of dieting allows you to fuel up often and burn fat effectively. Therefore you are increasing your metabolism which may even give you further inclination to exercise more regularly and lose extra kilos that way.

An easy low carb plan

When you go on a low carb diet please ensure that you get enough protein but not too much. Now this is a grey area, about half to 1 gram of protein for each kilo of body weight is the maximum per day. So this means if you weigh 70 kilos you would aim for a maximum of 70 grams of protein in a day. One egg equals 10 grams of protein and each hundred grams of meat equal 20 grams of protein. Tofu is the same as meat and all meats are fairly equal. This will give you a good idea of how much to eat.

Protein powder is a good source of complete protein and as you know you can buy protein snacks especially designed for these low carb diets. The following diet plan is easy to follow and can be utilised effectively even when you're working through the day:

Breakfast

Eggs of some sort or protein powder made into a smoothie drink.

Mid-Morning and Mid-Afternoon

Make yourself a dandelion tea or a cup of coffee with half milk and half water. This will stop sugar cravings and keep you satisfied until the next meal. Fresh fruit and vegetable sticks are also good options here. If you do get hungry, nibble on nuts and seeds. They are not only nutritious but also very satisfying. with balsamic vinegar or lemon juice can also be eaten between meals. Avocados are super nutritious and contain many HDL's which are beneficial for taking cholesterol out of our system.

Lunch

Some type of protein again, either; fish, chicken or red meat with green vegetables and other non-starch vegetables. Or some soup made from meat and vegetables.

Dinner

Tofu, seafood or meat with green vegetables again. Have loads of bok choy, spinach and beans. They are very good for us and also very low in carbs. Keep your intake of wine controlled, ensuring you stay under your daily threshold for ketosis.

Yes, you can have steaks with cream sauce and those oysters Kilpatrick are allowed on this diet … but you need to be careful every day. There are many books written especially about low carb diets, and you need to be well informed and consider your options before you undertake a diet of this sort. There are some medical conditions and medications that would prohibit you from this type of dieting. Check with your Health Care Practitioner first if you are concerned about your situation.

Plan your time well

When you decide to follow the low carb way of eating, make sure you plan your diet well and be prepared in advance. It's a good style of dieting for when you're at home in your usual environment. You will be more likely to succeed under normal everyday conditions than if say, you are away on holiday.

Don't worry about weighing yourself all the time. The best thing to do is to gauge your weight loss by the fit of your clothes and your own personal comfort levels. After all, we only need to lose weight for health and not technically for beauty reasons. When we do lose weight for health we will be beautiful anyway. Plan at the beginning of the diet how much weight you want to lose. It's better to be a comfortable weight and size and be able to maintain it, than to fanatically diet down a size and be disappointed six months later when you put the weight back on again.

Tell friends and family that you don't want to eat certain foods before you sit down to eat with them, this hopefully will encourage them to support you and not try to tempt you with that piece of black forest cake when you are simply enjoying a coffee. Don't plan the low carb diet for your birthday or Christmas either, it's usually too difficult, and probably won't work.

Be positive from the beginning

Tell yourself that you will be successful. The power of positive thought is very strong and we need all the positivity we can muster up when faced with chocolates unexpectedly in the middle of a diet. Remember that the low carb diet can be used for shorter periods of time and you will be able to maintain your desired weight by controlling your intake of carbs on a daily basis. Once you understand how the diet works and what foods are able to be eaten freely you will be able to utilise the diet in your everyday life. Just remember the Glycaemic Index and all will be well.

The low-fat diet

You can indulge in the delights of sushi, juices, delicious salads, tofu and any foods that are low in fat. The more fruit and vegies the better. This diet is almost the opposite of the high protein diet, where most vegetables and fruit are out of bounds. The only thing you need to measure here is fat. You will need to read the labels of all processed foods vigorously and keep your fat intake as low as possible, preferably under 30 grams total per day.

With this diet you will only be able to consume essential fatty acids in supplement form each day, i.e. evening primrose, flax and fish oils. You will be watching calories and ensuring that you burn more than you consume. Many of the most successful commercial dietary formulas have been based on this concept. The new generation of low-fat diets are becoming very sophisticated. You can be under the guidance of a support team, have your blood analysed and a diet tailor-made to suit your circumstances. This balanced diet would take into account the recommended daily allowances for each food type.

You will need a calorie counter and a comprehensive list showing the amount of fat each food contains. The advantage of measuring fat consumption is that generally people who lose weight by this technique are able to maintain the weight loss because they learn a balanced and life-long eating programme.

Who would benefit from this diet?

Vegetarians, people who are not prepared to restrict dietary intake to the extent required for the protein diet, people who are on medications or have health problems, people who enjoy a variety of foods and are conscious of cholesterol and fat levels or those who want sustainable dietary changes that will be maintainable. There are no inappropriate strains on body systems from following this type of diet and generally it is more alkaline forming to the system, allowing you to lose desired kilos without harming yourself. Generally, once people have experienced this type of dieting, they are able to apply it to after-diet lifestyles easily.

The cleansing diet

You prepare your body for a cleanse by eating clean, unprocessed foods for a few days. Then you consume nothing but fresh vegetables and fruit for a period of time depending upon your circumstances and health status. You can even consume only water and herbal teas as your cleansing programme. If you choose to fast on water and herbal teas, then your body will go into ketosis and eliminate toxins and use body fat for energy. This dietary strategy is well combined with either of the other popular methods and allows a break in routine from other diets. This way of reducing weight is wonderful as it gives your body a complete rest and provides a fast way to release stress and toxins. Many people take this option over a long weekend or during annual holidays as a way to unwind and rejuvenate.

Often this diet is a good precursor for the other types of diet mentioned. If you are suffering from hormonal weight gain from menopause or pregnancy, this is a good kick-start to any weight loss programme. The wholesome vegetarian detox diet is one good option here. The following chapter, 'The Detox Zone', goes into details of many cleansing options that are valuable when you want to lose some weight.

Who would benefit from this diet?

Anyone who wants to kick-start a weight loss or maintenance programme or if you are over working your body and have a chance to rest and rejuvenate for a weekend. In between bouts of protein dieting you can take juice cleanses to eliminate the extra acidity in your body created by this dieting style. This is a good way to detox the body and eliminate problematic conditions, enabling your body to utilise elimination pathways.

This dietary choice is often best under the supervision of your Health Care Professional should you decide to use it as the main way for weight loss. It is not suitable for people who are grossly obese or are on medication.

PART II

THE DETOX ZONE

CHAPTER FIFTEEN

Methods of cleansing and detoxing

A detox cleanses your body of built-up poisons and any chemicals or waste matters that don't belong. The process of detoxing is quite literally allowing these build-ups of unwanted matter to be released into your digestive tract or bloodstream and then allowing them to leave your body. The residues and toxins in your body that you want to remove are the materials that will eventually cause sluggishness of the metabolism, or illness and disease.

It's important to detox your body regularly, and the many people who undertake a regular cleanse certainly have a lot of energy and enjoy the best health possible in their given situation. So, for your Wellness Zone, look at the options for detoxing and see whether any of it takes your fancy.

Detoxing can be as light or a serious as you want to make it. You can do a wholesome vegetarian detox plan that enables you to still work and enjoy many foods, the 'any morning' detox that enables you to gently and regularly flush unwanted build-ups from your system, or you can choose from many other detox styles as outlined below. We are all individual in our choices for cleansing our bodies, and you will need to experiment, adapt and even create a few of your own tricks to detox comfortably and effectively.

Today we are presented with an astounding array of commercial choices for detoxification; this is a sign of the times and in the future this will only increase. Don't get confused by the masses of information out there, detoxing is a natural bodily process that occurs every night when you sleep, each time you are sick or when you have a healing crisis. You need nothing to detox properly except yourself, and some pure fresh water, a place to rest peacefully and some silence.

The reason why detoxing has become such a big business issue is that more and more people are living in the cities. They are living on commercially grown foods and are having ever increasingly busy lives where they don't have time to rest, let alone start a veggie garden!

The world is full of toxins and poisons that are saturating our bodies. Petrochemicals, medicines, environmental poisons, air pollution, chemical residues and modern lifestyle choices all add up to a huge amount of toxicity entering our bodies unconsciously.

The common foods that congest your body include coffee, alcohol, sugar, flour from wheat, meats, processed and pickled foods, frozen commercial foods, and often food prepared away from home in commercial environments. It's sad that the only water we consider good enough to drink is commercially packaged (in plastic) spring water from some foreign place! What happened to good old clean healthy tap water! Not today folks, just drinking that is reason enough to detox!

Wherever you live, don't think you are avoiding poisons in your diet. The planet is polluted, and each of us needs to detox our own environments if we plan to stay as healthy as possible.

Your detox schedule

There is technically no right or wrong way to detox. What you need to remember is that this your health, your Wellness Zone, and it's your choice how to detox. You can go fast, slow or anywhere in between. It's one of those experiences that can only be determined day to day and sometimes even hour to hour as to whether to drop a detox programme or continue it. If you start a detox and say you'll do it for three days, you have the privilege to stop at any time you want, for any reason that you like! You don't have to stick to that 'three-day schedule', and you haven't let yourself down if you stop after two.

You can't determine how long you will want to detox until you are in the process, tuned into detox mode and able to determine hourly how you feel. Your body knows when it's the right time to stop a cleansing programme, when you have done your best and when it's time to relax and live again. You can also continue a detox plan for longer than originally intended if all is going well. Do what feels right at the time and do what's best for your body and your Wellness Zone.

You don't need to go out and spend bundles of cash on detoxing. Remember that less is best with detox and that you will clear those toxins out of your body with just love, light, clear liquids and rest. However, anything above that brings the detox into a different level. Depending upon the state of your health from the beginning and how seasoned you are at detoxing, determine whether you eat brown rice and fresh vegetables or whether you are going to live on carrot juice and spirulina. It's all personal!

Once you start this process, you will note the whites of your eyes become white again. It's great to note a clear system, disappearing mucous and the end of poor dietary habits (if somewhat temporarily). But the best part is that after you have been squirming in detox mode for a while, you will become so effervescent and vibrant as your body becomes clear and you have powerful and beautiful mental clarity, cellular health is another added bonus.

Think about all the goodness cleansing programmes bring you, don't rush into a big plan for cleansing as small regular detoxes are the best way to start and build your mind and body up to longer and more disciplined practices.

If you start with a cleansing day each week, say Monday (a good way to start your week), just have fresh fruit and vegetables, soups and juices all day. Try to avoid tea, coffee and alcohol. Do this every week for a month or longer and then, if you feel inclined, go for two days. It's that easy. But just imagine the increased health with only one day of cleansing regularly each week. Your body will definitely thank you for it.

Why take a detox?

Why would you benefit from having a cleansing detox? If you suffer from any illness, detoxing can help your body heal faster, making your system uncongested and clean. Medicines work better in a cleaner system and also the body has more room to get better faster because the residues, toxins and wastes have been eliminated, allowing the body to function optimally under its condition of illness.

If you have a chronic illness or condition, infections, HIV, cancer, auto-immune diseases, obesity, metabolic resistance, tuberculosis, lupus, hormonal imbalances, depression, bowel diseases or any manner of illness that requires constant medication and looking after, then you need to detox, and you need to give your body the best conditions to heal itself. Yes, given the right environment, the body will heal itself faster when nurtured properly.

Basically, we all know that with a little bit of assistance in the right direction your body can and will heal itself naturally most of the time. However, when you have a body that is full of built-up and almost invisible slush, slurry and toxic matter, you will have to remove that before your cells can vibrate at the right frequency, with the right tools and unhindered energy to repair yourself.

If you really want to recover from an ailment, then taking a regular detox cleanse and placing your body in a good position to self-heal is one of the kindest and most self-loving acts you can undertake. Your Wellness Zone can be enhanced or deteriorated, depending upon how you choose to keep the inside of your body, cleaner or dirtier.

A clean inside makes light work for all bodily functions. However, when you are full of congestion, mucous, toxins, medical build-ups and many other foreign invaders, imagine how much they will slow you down when you really need help in healing. Likewise, if you have regular cleanses and your body is clean within, then the chances of you suffering from chronic disease are far less than if you were congested. Therefore you will be in an optimal position for healing when some illness does occur. Detoxing is natural and logical for those who want optimal health; it's just a matter of choosing when and how to do it.

When to detox?

Choosing a time to detox is entirely up to you. Only you know your Wellness Zone, and only you know when to stop having a regular diet and to start a lighter fresher diet to eliminate the toxins from your system. You can go into spontaneous detox whereby you find yourself craving lighter foods or even specific cleansing foods like carrot or lemon juice and not wanting food. This is good; it may last a day or so, and then you can go back to normal eating again. You just need to listen to your body, go with what your mind is telling you and really get serious when you need to.

The moment you feel sick you need to instantly stop your normal diet and start a cleanse

This can last from one meal to many, depending on what is wrong with your body. In fact, it's best to not wait until you are sick to detox, slot it into your existing schedule. Maybe decide to detox this weekend because you've got nothing better to do. If you feel you need a detox, slip it into your life, sooner rather than later. Plan the diet and the foods around your daily regime, but remember it's harder to detox when you are travelling to and from work all week.

You can always come up with an excuse why not to, and it's always easier to just get on with life and avoid the detox plan altogether. This way we can continue with our current dietary plan without the extra worry of restricting ourselves further. It is initially harder to make the commitment to detox, but in the long run, you will be so grateful that you did, as you will enjoy greater vibrancy and extended health.

You can eat well most of the time anyway! To eat fresh unprocessed natural foods is the key to good health. To eat processed foods as a regular part of your diet is to poison your body regularly. The best food you can eat is fresh homegrown foods prepared with the best ingredients.

You need to detox when you have been eating out a lot or eating a lot of processed food. Another good time to detox is just before and just after a holiday. Holidays always take us out of our digestive comfort zone and enter our systems into the wild and unexpected. This can be good ... but, it can also be fattening, and it can add fatty acids to your liver and internal organs.

Parasites are something that can be picked up almost anywhere. So, a regular parasite cleanse is required by everyone!

Cleansing attitude is the key to success

To succeed or not to succeed? That is the question. This is true in many levels of your Wellness Zone. However, when it comes to cleansing, there's nothing as important as an attitude for success or failure. If you enter a detox with a forced attitude, whereby maybe someone else has told you that you must do a detox, cleanse or weight loss programme because your health depends upon it, then you will certainly be starting off on the wrong foot.

If you need to lose weight, design a programme that will work with your lifestyle choices. If you need to get healthy, then get the right attitude. But don't ever do a cleanse because someone else told you to. This is a negative motivating force and will not get good results. Only do a detox because you want to improve your own health and because you want to improve and enhance your own Wellness Zone. Self-responsibility is the only really productive path to wellness. We can consult, take advice and get the opinion of others about any health issue. However, at the end of the day, it's our own decisions, or lack of, that make up the true healing and health of our body. It's no good to leave the decision of our health care to anyone else.

If you cleanse regularly, it is a clear signal to your own body that you are taking the responsibility to cleanse yourself and that you are prepared to do the best for your own Wellness Zone. If you enter your cleanse with a strong and positive attitude then chances are you will be able to keep up the strength and personal discipline needed for a successful conclusion.

Cleansing can be cyclic, and you can find yourself really motivated for a few months and then suddenly you can't be bothered detoxing anymore. You may choose to juice cleanse, water fast, have a simple daily detox or eat only fruit and vegetables for a few days. These are all good detox options that can be done regularly or sporadically depending on your needs.

There is a time and place for each style of cleansing. It may be right for you to have complete water fasts. Each and every time you detox is perfect. If your attitude is right, you will really enjoy the experience, and if it gets a bit tough then you have the determination to succeed, determined to rid yourself of those toxins and residues of poisons that could create havoc with your future health. You wash away all kinds of mental, emotional and physical rubbish. Cleansing has many layers, and these are only revealed to you as you live the experience. Each and every detox is different depending on your life and attitude at the time.

Many people feel fantastic on day three of any complete water fast. That's always the favourite time, when you feel completely elevated from the physical, yet could run a marathon at the drop of a hat because you feel so great. But to get to day three is a personal and physical challenge that can only be achieved with a certain attitude and mindset about water fasts. It is not right for everyone, and you may or may not be open to the complete water fast technique of detox. Respect your individuality and take your detoxing to the levels that you feel comfortable with, this too will change from detox to detox.

Often you will fast before any major decisions are made about any issue of importance. Well, that's another great motivation for cleansing, especially when you are involved in business and need some time to think. It's a clearer head that thinks on peppermint tea and carrot juice than the one that's loaded with coffee and wine! A heavy stomach is also the best formula for a sluggish mind. So, keeping your stomach empty and your mind clear is a good formula for the successful scholar!

How to deal with hunger when detoxing

Whenever we decrease the amount of food we eat, our stomachs react by sending a message to the brain that it's not satisfied and you will want to eat. This can be a physical sensation or it can be purely 'mind over matter'. Many people in this world have become either too thin or too fat because of their own thoughts.

So, when you feel hungry, the first question you need to ask yourself is, 'do I feel hungry because I am actually physically in need of nutrition?' or 'do I feel hungry because of some other mental reason?' (such as feelings of deprivation, emotional stress or emptiness on another level in my life). Oh, what a loaded question. So, now you need to think about the answer. And when you are on a cleanse you will probably be feeling a little of each.

You should only eat as much food as the size of your clenched fist; this is apparently the size of your stomach. When your stomach becomes distended (stretched) it sends a message to your brain that it's time to stop eating. However, technically you should stop eating before your stomach sends this message as these receptors may be a bit slower than what you can swallow. If we all ate this way, then there certainly would be no obesity in the world, so long as the food wasn't rubbish, i.e. white flour, processed fats and sugars.

When you feel hungry, the quickest solution is a glass of water. That usually abates the feeling of hunger for a few minutes, and certainly long enough for you to think about what is good for you to consume and what is not. Fibre, pure oat bran or rice bran fibre are things that you can add to your glass of water or juice, and these will help to fill you up when on any detox. This mixture is filling but not absorbed into the body and acts like a broom to sweep away any parasites, mucous and other poisons in the digestive tract. It also stops your metabolism slowing down when you are on a liquid cleanse.

When you are on a detox it's good to think about how your body actually works so that you are able to understand the process of detoxification. It's good to drink or eat regularly, every hour have at least 200 ml water, plus something else like a juice, smoothie, salad or chopped up veggies and dips. This will help to keep you feeling satisfied.

If you find that your reasons for hunger are clearly emotional and you really feel upset about something in your life, try your hardest to diffuse the issues and go for a swim or a walk and take a bath or shower.

Water, and placing your body in water, is the fastest way to change your energy to a more positive frame. Whenever you throw your body under a cold shower, or plunge into a cold river or the ocean, there is an instant shift in energy, and you will find you feel much better. During a detox you will want little ways to distract yourself from the fact you are not eating, and water is a lovely distraction.

Hunger during your detox is yet another personal issue that needs to be addressed as it occurs. Don't be so strict with eating times and eat when you need to. If you are on pure water or pure juices then do as mentioned and add a tablespoon of fibre into a glass of juice or water and drink it straight away. In fact, this is a good idea for all of us. Imagine if we had 15 grams of pure fibre each day mixed in a drink. Our bodies would be functioning very well indeed. Fibre is one of those foods that are underestimated and really help you lose weight, kerb unnecessary hunger pangs, flush and sweep your digestive tract and certainly keep your large intestine in good health as well as help manage cholesterol and triglyceride levels. There would be a lot less colon cancer and digestive tract cancers in the world if everyone increased their fibre intake.

When to end your detox

If you have been on a detox, any detox, then you need to follow certain protocol at its conclusion. This protocol is to ease your way out of the detox with healthy food choices and small serving sizes.

The fact that you have made the commitment and followed through with the detox warrants some respect. So simply be gentle on yourself with your diet for a day or so afterwards. Don't break a detox with deep-fried fish and chips followed by a carbonated drink; your body won't thank you for it.

Any detox that has gone for less than 24 hours and has involved eating some foods, however small the amount, and has not been a pure liquid detox, can be broken with just a normal meal. Try to keep it simple, not too much meat protein, and not too much alcohol and remember to chew your food slowly.

Any 'liquid only' detox needs to be broken in a special way. This involves having a very small meal of grated cabbage, carrots and other vegetables first, and the meal following this should be a vegetarian one, with no nuts or seeds. If you are on a liquid detox for four days or longer, then you need to boil some fresh tomatoes with a little sea salt, apple cider vinegar and onion. Add a cup of water and make a tomato and onion soup. Add one stock cube instead of salt if you like and you can also add garlic but no artificial flavours or toxic MSG.

Have this soup at the point you decide to break the fast, and this is okay to do between meals if you like, then wait at least one hour and have the shredded vegetable salad. You can also drink smoothies with fresh fruit, protein powder and water. Have no meats, nuts, legumes or dairy products for the next 24 hours and only eat the wholesome vegetarian detox plan, after that you can eat as you wish. This will ease your body gently out of the detox and allow you to settle back into normal eating plans. You may find that you are attracted to different, more natural and less processed foods after a cleanse. This is because your body has had a taste of these delicious options and actually prefers them to other dietary choices.

Many people fast on water alone for four to seven days and note that when they break the fast the taste of food is delicious, and they are suddenly starving. You will also notice that your mind is very clear which you can attribute to the detoxing plan. When you have juices or water fasts, remember that you are treating your body to a rest and that sometimes it's hard to keep up the energy required for work and daily activities. This is normal, and you should rest as required.

You are free to break a fast when you feel it's time; this is determined by how you are feeling. You can always break a liquid cleanse and move across to one of the lighter options if you wish, you will still be doing your body the world of goodness. Also, there are no physical restrictions on how often you can detox. Sometimes you may be really keen to detox and ready for the next one very soon after the last. Other times it might be a struggle, as for one reason or another you just can't get motivated for the experience. So, make the most of your enthusiasm when you feel it and detox as desired.

How can smokers or people on drugs detox?

It's not easy to clean your body when you are constantly adding poisons through smoking or other drugs. Basically, if you are a smoker or have other addictions, then you need to minimalise your use of these whilst on the detox plan. You are advised to seek supervision from your Health Care Practitioner because you may experience more nasty side effects from detoxing.

Stay inspired and try to focus on improving your Wellness Zone if you want to detox. Go with the healthy vegetarian detox for a few weeks and see how you are feeling before you endeavour to go on juice cleansing or fasting detox methods. Don't water fast if you are a smoker or use drugs or have any other addictions or medications that could affect the process. Detoxing can be tough with these limitations, and you could do with some supervision and help to ease the experience and get maximum benefits with minimal side effects.

Start off with a simple and easy detox plan, and you should do well in the process. Don't rush yourself as there could be many toxins that have lodged themselves in your body over the years, and it may take some time to get them out. Remember, however, that detoxing is still your best method for a good, future Wellness Zone.

If you find that the detox is too hard, then stop for a day or so and start again. Don't rush yourself. Often this is a long-term solution which needs to be taken steadily. If you are in this category of addiction and want to detox, then take a small amount of milk thistle every day with a small amount of hypericum, providing they are not contraindicated by your drugs/medicines. Also, drink lemon juice with honey as a regular beverage for a week or so before the detox to loosen up toxins and flush them steadily through your body.

Is your liver dirty?

Just existing in this world is reason enough to have regular liver detoxes, as a healthy preventative and protection for your body you would do well to consider scheduling in two or three cleanses per year just for your own wellness. We are all inadvertently exposed to various toxins. Take a moment to think about what ones can be eliminated from your world, and what ones are unavoidable? It's not hard to see that it's important to consider cleansing as a vital routine, a bit like doing the washing. If you don't wash your clothes eventually they will be putrid! If you don't cleanse your liver, eventually it will be so congested and dirty that you will want to avoid the smell yourself!

Do you suffer from waking up in the early hours of the morning for no apparent reason and have difficulty going back to sleep? If so, you may have problems with liver function and require a good detox to get you sleeping well again. Do you have a roll of fat across your abdomen that is stubborn and refuses to budge even with consistent dieting? This is another indication that you may benefit from cleansing your liver of old and unwanted toxins. Simply look in the mirror and check the whites of your eyes. Are they white? Or are they turning more creamy or yellow? If they are not a clear white then perhaps you are carrying excess toxins through your system, and your liver is not functioning optimally.

Keep your liver healthy

Anyone with liver disease will do well to have regular cleanses to help liver function. Taking herbs and following a cleansing programme has helped many people with chronic liver disease come back to good health again. If you drink alcohol, eat processed foods or are exposed to any toxic chemical residues, the first place to consider cleansing is the liver. Start slowly and then increase the intensity as time goes on. In fact, anyone who suffers from any chronic illness would do well to think of liver cleansing as a mandatory action for future wellness.

Imagine squeezing a dirty wet sponge and watching the filth come away, then imagine yourself rinsing that sponge in fresh clean water and squeezing it until it is squeaky clean. This is one comparison to your liver. Our liver is the main filter organ in the body, and it has so many diverse functions including general metabolism, filtration and organisation of many other bodily functions.

The liver is where you will first accumulate environmental toxins that have been ingested through the atmosphere and food. So, it makes sense that the liver is the first organ to keep clean, ensuring many other smooth and uninterrupted processes occur in the body. If you have a clean liver, then you will have clean healthy blood flowing through your veins. This results in clean organs and also clean cells. So, therefore keeping your liver clean is fundamental in having good energy levels and maintaining the best possible Wellness Zone for yourself. Liver cleansing is relatively simple when it is undertaken on a regular basis. However, if you ignore your body for long enough you will start to show signs of liver overload, these include lethargy, bloating, bad temperament and skin eruptions amongst others. Taking a detox is the best way to cleanse your liver.

Herbs can help

Drink dandelion tea instead of coffee at your local café. This will cleanse your liver and boost kidney function.

A special detox herbal blend contains the following herbs: milk thistle, dandelion, globe artichoke and black walnut. This tonic can be taken as a total detox plan for 7 to 30 days, just one teaspoon (5 ml) before each meal, or more gently one teaspoon (5 ml) each day before a meal.

Milk thistle is the premium liver-cleansing herb, and it helps in many detoxification pathways in the liver. This herb is helpful as it significantly contributes to the reversal of fatty liver, cirrhosis and high cholesterol levels. Milk thistle can be combined with turmeric to bring oestrogen levels back in balance and also assist in cleansing heavy metals and industrial toxins from the liver. Milk thistle makes the whites of your eyes white again.

Often grumpy people have a toxic liver, so if you are feeling a bit angry, impatient, unhappy or generally disgruntled, then a liver cleanse may settle you down and make you smile again! Milk thistle is traditionally prescribed for all manner of liver problems including hepatitis, alcoholic liver conditions, toxicity in the liver caused by heavy metal exposure and also for gall bladder protection as this herb assists in the prevention of gallstones.

Milk thistle may be taken in very small amounts over a long period of time to help prevent liver damage and gradually repair the liver. Alternatively, you can take the extract in therapeutic doses for a specific time frame, as required for a liver cleanse, combined with foods to help flush the toxins from your liver and repair the damage. Another way is to take this herb three or four times a year, as each season begins, spend two to four weeks taking a suitable dose of milk thistle along with a controlled diet to allow the liver to gently flush and cleanse. Added daily to your diet, milk thistle can be a powerful hepatoprotective.

It all depends upon your external environment and your eating habits as to how much and when you need to take a liver-cleansing herb. Anyone who drinks alcohol would do well to have 5 to 10 grams of milk thistle extract mixed with water upon retiring after an evening of alcohol consumption. Also, if you have been working in an environment where toxic dust, pollutants and chemicals may have been absorbed through your lungs, skin, water or food supply, you would do well to have a daily dose of milk thistle.

Add dandelion to your blend for gentle cleansing, and this herb suits everyone! Not many people are opposed to taking dandelion in fresh salads, and it can be taken in extract form for blood cleansing, digestive tract toning and also liver and kidney function. If you are able to grow some dandelion in your garden, it's excellent to chop up the fresh, less bitter, smaller leaves and mix them with your salad greens. Make a dressing with lemon juice, and you will have the perfect liver-cleansing salad to add to a meal.

Dandelion is good for chronic skin diseases, constipation, abdominal bloating, lack of appetite and all manner of digestive sluggishness. It also works well as a diuretic and assists kidney function, including the healing of cystitis.

Black walnut gets in on a cellular level and sneaks up on the parasites, toxins and nasty cancers and helps eliminate them from your system. This herb can be taken in therapeutic doses for about 30 days at a time before you need to give it a rest as the naphthoquinones can make your peristalsis lazy. Therapeutically you can take black walnut daily to cleanse your digestive tract of parasites and to get into your organs and start to cleanse on a deeper level. Small non-therapeutic doses of black walnut taken over a long term, such as one year or longer, will get into your cells and do some real work. If you only have a very small dose added to your daily tonic, then it can get into those cells and help eliminate any poisons, foreign bodies and toxins.

Globe artichoke is the premium herb for your gall bladder and of course cholesterol management. Your gall bladder stores bile that has been secreted from your liver, it waits there to get the message that you have eaten and then the bile is pumped from the gall bladder into the small intestine for the emulsification of fats and the aiding of digestion. Now, if you think about other wastes that can be transported to the gall bladder, such as cholesterol and oestrogen and other yucky wastes from a congested liver, you will understand why this herb is important in your detox blend. It helps your gall bladder to be thoroughly cleaned, and that will delay, arrest or even eliminate the build-up of crystals that can form gallstones. Globe artichoke is also used to help treat high cholesterol levels and reduce high triglyceride levels, making it a cardiovascular protective herb as well.

Cellular detoxification

Each and every cell in your body needs a spring clean. This is a different approach to the digestive tract and related organ detoxification such as bowel cleansing and liver cleansing. Cellular detoxification can take months or even years to accomplish if you take it slowly and ensure that you do not stress your body too much in the process. Sneak up on toxins inside the cells and clear them out so that you have less strain on your body and are able to create healthier cellular energy.

If your cells are clean, then you will naturally have more energy. The only way to get your cells clean is to have clean blood and organs, and that means you need to have a clean digestive tract too. It's an ongoing process that needs to be vigilantly adhered to in order for you to have a proper detox.

You need three months of detox for every year of your age, and in other words to be strict you will need to detox for one year for every four years of your life. If you are 40, you will need regular and consistent detoxing for ten years to ensure you have an optimally healthy body. This of course is the extremist perspective, but bear in mind that it's a really healthy and wonderful feeling at the end of a week when you have only had soups, juices, vegetable salads and fresh fruit for seven days. You will feel as though you have achieved something marvellous and healthy for your Wellness Zone. You only need to do these one week cleanses two or three times per year. Even do this once a year if you have never done it before. Make the time and create the discipline to detox, you won't regret it.

Cleansing is a very personal support for your Wellness Zone. It is a way for self-acceptance, self-love and self-respect. You can't respect yourself optimally when you are a toxic waste dump! However, when you make the effort to get rid of all those built-up toxins and wastes from the past, then you make a firm commitment on the physical level to a better tomorrow and a healthier Wellness Zone.

For optimal and efficient cellular detoxification you can undertake any of the detox plans mentioned in this book. However, to really get in and cleanse on a cellular level, add spirulina, wheatgrass or green barley shoots to your detox. These green foods also create an alkaline system which helps keep your body in optimal health and minimalises the risk of getting many illnesses.

The benefits of fruit and veggies in your detox plan

Different fruits and vegetables contain antioxidants, nutrients and cleansing properties that can be used to specifically target the system of your body that needs cleansing. All fruit and vegetables are good options to base a cleansing diet on, raw is best, taken in juice format or eaten in salads. Fruit and vegetables are also good for you cooked and steamed in the winter months.

Add some lemon juice, sea salt, fresh herbs, spices, honey, garlic, ginger, parsley, seeds, nuts, olive oil, flaxseed oil or good vinegar to your fruit and vegetables for extra flavour and texture.

Almonds can be soaked overnight and added to juices and fruits in your cleanse as they are high in calcium and also nourishingly filling.

Apples are good to help with gallstones and arthritis pain. Green apples contain malic acid, and all apples contain pectin, which helps reduce gallstones. Apples also help reduce parasites in your digestive tract and are good for diarrhoea and digestive disturbances.

Apricots are high in iron and a good juice for women to help prevent anaemia. They are also good to help coughs and winter colds, apricots reduce inflammation in the digestive tract and can help reduce migraine headaches. Taking pure apricot juice regularly through the day when you have a winter cold or flu can be very soothing. Apricot seeds can be eaten in small amounts to help prevent cancer.

Artichokes are good gall bladder and liver food and help reduce cholesterol levels. Fresh artichokes are good, steamed until soft and then marinated in garlic, olive oil, sea salt and apple cider vinegar. Place this in the fridge and add to snacks and meals as needed. Raw globe artichokes are a premium gall bladder and cholesterol-reducing food when added to juices each day.

Asparagus is premium kidney food, allowing stones to break up and reducing acidity in the body.

Avocado is high in essential fatty acids, including beta-sitosterol, which can help with prostate problems. Avocado is a complete food which is nourishing and gentle on the digestive tract when there are digestive disturbances. Avocado is best eaten raw. Cut the fruit in half then add other vegetables and salad dressing for a nourishing and delicious detox meal. You can also juice avocado with other fruits and vegetables, this is very filling and a real energy boost for those on a liquid diet.

Beetroot is the food of the bowel, anti-cancer and blood cleansing. If you have low energy, this vegetable is wonderfully strengthening for all systems of your body. Cooked beetroot is also delicious on a detox plan. Cut the beetroot into two cm cubes, coat with olive oil and bake in a moderate oven for two hours. Once cooked, sprinkle with sea salt and a little fresh garlic then squeeze lemon juice over the hot beetroot.

Berries are good to help keep your cardiovascular system strong. They increase vision and help reduce macular degeneration. Berries are also good blood cleansers and are high in antioxidants. The darker the berry, the stronger its benefits. Blackberries and mulberries are good fresh or frozen. Eating one tablespoon of berries each day on your detox plan will act as a lovely antioxidant and also help strengthen your veins and arteries.

Bitter melons are eaten in many parts of the world as an antioxidant and balancer of blood sugar levels. When you add the leaves or the fruit of bitter melon to your juices and salads on a detox then you are balancing your own blood sugar levels enabling you to have the endurance for the detox plan. The bitter melon also helps arrest the development of HIV/Aids. Small young melons and their leaves are good combined with your juices and food.

Broccoli is the food of the prostate, helping reduce inflammation and any problems associated with prostate disease. It is high in antioxidants and helps to reduce blood pressure and detoxify the liver. Steaming broccoli is a good way to enjoy the vegetable and get the maximum health benefits, and it is also very good juiced with other vegetables. Cooked broccoli is good kidney soothing food, and when you are on a low carb diet plan you can help protect your kidneys by adding a good dose of broccoli, or other green food to the diet.

Brown Rice is a premium detox food, there have been many detox plans built around brown rice as the basis. There is a mono detox plan where you eat pure raw brown rice and water. Soak each cup of biodynamic brown rice in two cups of pure cold water for 24 hours and eat exclusively for a day or longer. Do not cook or heat. You can mix this regime in with other detox plans as required. This is very nutritious, and brown rice hulls are one of the best fibres available. Brown rice is filling and can be a good addition to any detox plan incorporating this nutrition with the cleansing properties of other plants. Brown rice also tends to absorb toxins and putrid waste from the digestive tract helping to eliminate them from your body.

Cabbage is an excellent prebiotic; it is good for hyperthyroidism and is an antioxidant. Cabbage is good for sweeping toxins through your digestive tract, allowing parasites and built-up mucous to be removed gently. If your metabolism is too fast, then adding cabbage to the detox plan will help slow it down.

Try baking it in an oven in the traditional recipe of stuffed cabbage which is an excellent winter detox meal. Marinating cabbage in salt for two to four weeks is the process to make sauerkraut, a traditional prebiotic food. Simply take the cabbage and slice thinly, add one cup of salt to each full cabbage and place in a bowl with a heavy object, such as a brick (covered for hygiene purposes) over the cabbage. Make sure you are able to seal the bowl so that air doesn't get in. The cabbage will ferment over time resulting in this delicious prebiotic that is a good addition to any detox plan.

Carrot is high in beta-carotene and is the premium liver-cleansing food. It helps to regulate blood sugar levels, reduces inflammation in the whole body and is good energy food to help increase your stamina. Carrots are great juiced, although this can be rather high in sugar as there is about 4 g of sugar per average carrot. Carrot juice is an excellent liver food as it helps the detoxification pathways operate optimally. Steaming carrots with honey, fennel and ginger is good warm detox food.

Celery helps reduce uric and lactic acids in your joints and organs, and it also helps reduce fluid build-up and oedema in peripheral parts of your body, such as the ankles and feet. It makes a good kidney tonic and tends to balance stomach acidity. Add some celery into your morning juice, and you can also dip fresh celery into vegetable sauces for detox plans, or even make a delicious tea with celery seeds and hot water. Use one teaspoon of celery seeds for every 200 ml of boiling water and allow to infuse for five minutes.

Cranberries are good kidney and bladder food; they are beneficial for an acid system and to help balance the acid in your blood levels. Take dried cranberries and soak them in water overnight then add to morning breakfast fruits or eat the fresh berries whole. Dried cranberries can be added to salads for zest and a flavour burst.

Garlic is your premium antibiotic food and will help to strengthen and cleanse the blood, reduce cardiovascular disease and anaemia, cleanse the liver and kidneys and increase your energy. Roast full bulbs of garlic in the oven then peel away the skin and eat, or dip it raw into pesto or other dips. Raw garlic can traditionally be rubbed into the bottom of your feet before bed to help detox your body whilst you sleep.

Ginger is another antibiotic food, and it also balances fluid in your body, removes uric and lactic acid, helps reduce the pain of headaches and arthritis and increases circulation. Simply slice the ginger thinly and add to any salad, steam or stir-fry or add to a roasted vegetable combination on your detox plan. Ginger juice is also delicious with many other fruits and vegetables.

Grapes have been used in mono cleansers for cancer treatment as they can go deeply into the cells to reduce acidity in the body and take away toxins. Grapes can be used to help reduce inflammation and help cleanse the blood and liver. Black grapes are specifically used for immune juice cleanse diets.

Grapefruit is a dieter's best friend, as this fruit helps break down fat in your digestive tract and then helps to remove it from your system. Grapefruit helps remove parasites, especially the seeds when eaten; it also helps reduce uric and lactic acid in the joints and can help stop the formation of gallstones. It speeds up digestion and can get your digestive tract moving when it is slow.

Horseradish is good to help all types of mucous problems and upper respiratory tract problems in your body. It helps to dry up the mucous and reduce head colds. Also, good for lungs and increasing the production of bile in your liver. Fresh horseradish is delicious sliced and added to detox meals. The juice can be strong, so test for flavour first before you add to your juices. The Japanese horseradish wasabi is a powerful respiratory tract cleanser and a great addition to any detox plan when you want heat and variety. Don't forget that sushi is good detox food, and the addition of wasabi can help to clear excess toxins from your body.

Lemon is the number one fruit for cleansing your entire body. It is not acid-producing in the body but actually helps to reduce acid, dry up mucous, relieve arthritis and cleanse your joints of built-up acids. Lemon cleanses the liver, gallbladder, kidneys, digestive tract and lungs. Fresh lemon juice can be added to hot or cold water throughout the day on any detox plan. You can add lemon juice to any sliced fruits or vegetables, and it will help to stop them from going brown through oxidation.

Lentils and *beans* of all sorts can be soaked and added to your detox plan if you are able to eat wholesome foods and are not on a strictly liquid detox. Lentils add protein and other essential nutrients to your detox; however, you need to soak them for at least 12 hours and rinse well before cooking slowly and properly until they are soft.

Soft lentils aid digestion and also help eliminate toxins from your system. Under-cooked lentils can create disturbances in your digestive tract and liver when on a detox programme, and you would be better to avoid them and eat other protein sources unless you plan to cook them well. The idea of a detox is to be gentle on the body and lentils are not generally a gentle food, so keep the quantity down and the lentils soft to maximise the benefits of your detox.

Lettuce is good to soothe digestion and cleanse the blood. Fresh garden lettuce that has gone to seed is good boiled in soups or freshly juiced. Beware of commercial lettuce as the leaves are frail and can easily hold poisons and sprays for long periods of time. There are many varieties of lettuce and generally the more bitter the flavour, the better they are for your digestion.

Lychees are a cleansing fruit, and they are light. Eating lychees in the summer months is a lovely refreshing detox.

Mangoes help reduce constipation and are high in iron, and they are very cleansing for the whole body and a good addition to your detox plan as they really keep digestion moving whilst cleansing the body. When you add mangoes to your detox plan, you are increasing your energy levels because they are very filling and revitalising.

Mushrooms have different medicinal properties, and you can add them to your detox plan to increase nutrition and immunity depending upon the type of mushroom. The dried reishi mushroom is good for immunity. Mushrooms are also considered as the vegetarians' meat and often act as a good substitute for meat in meals whilst on a detox plan.

Olives are good to help keep your immunity strong. Fresh olives that are marinated in good vinegar, sea salt and olive oil are a good addition to your detox plan. Stay away from olives that have been marinated in chemicals and table salt. Fresh olive leaves are good added to juices; you can also slice these and use them as edible garnishes with your detox meals.

Onions protect your cardiovascular system, act as prebiotics, increase circulation and aid digestion. Raw and cooked onions have their place in your detox plan. Raw onions work as excellent prebiotics and help to kill parasites and other toxins. Cooked onions help reduce inflammation and are nurturing to your digestive tract. All onions added to your detox plan can help cleanse the blood to reduce arteriosclerosis and act as cardiovascular protectors. Peel the skin from an onion and steam for 15 minutes until soft, then slice it in half and sprinkle with some fresh herbs, spices and feta cheese for a delicious detox meal. Alternatively, add a whole onion to your juice for a hot and spicy experience.

Oranges are good liver-cleansing food and help reduce constipation. Slice an orange in half and add a sprinkle of fennel seed and a touch of sea salt for a summer treat. You can make orange and almond cakes for a sweet treat to break the tediousness of your detox plan. Boil two oranges (with skin on) in three cups of water and two tablespoons of honey for half an hour, you may need to add more water if it becomes too dry. When cooked, blend together, ensuring you have two cups of the liquid, then add one to two cups of pure almond meal to the mixture and stir until you have a stiff batter, in the same way you would make cake batter. Add two teaspoons of quality baking powder, place in small muffin tins and bake in a moderate oven for half an hour until cooked.

Papaya (Paw Paw) fruit and seeds are used as digestive enzymes and for digestive balance. The plant and leaf are used as an antiviral and antimicrobial. Taking the juice of paw paw leaves mixed into your daily juice is a good antioxidant and can cure many illnesses.

The seeds are delicious raw and taste peppery. They are good added to dips and sauces on your detox programme. Many people shy away from the seeds, thinking they look gross, but be adventurous and try them, you'll be surprised at how good they taste. Mix the fruit and seeds with lemon juice as a pre-dinner snack, not only will this help your digestion, but it will also kerb your appetite.

Parsley is high in all minerals, especially iron and chlorophyll. Parsley cleanses the body and also gives you premium nutrition; it is especially good for your blood and kidneys. Sprinkle parsley over everything all the time when you are on a detox plan. You can also add it to juices and soups as needed.

Peppermint deodorises your digestive tract and helps increase bowel movements. Peppermint tea is a free food on any detox plan, including the pure water fast. Peppermint leaves are delicious sliced and added to meals. There are many types of mint, and all have different medicinal properties. When you grow mint in the garden make sure that you keep it contained in pots as the different varieties tend to intermingle and eventually turn into a jumble of hybridised sameness when planted directly into the soil. Many people grow different mints at different ends of the garden to stop this from happening. Mint is always better raw than cooked, once it is cooked the flavour deteriorates.

Peppers are intestinal cleansers and stimulants. They help to reduce arteriosclerosis in the cardiovascular system and also reduce the incidence of constipation and help remove parasites from the digestive tract.

Pineapple is anti-inflammatory and also has digestive enzymes that help with stomach digestion. It contains the enzyme bromelain that is used to help reduce the inflammation associated with sinus and allergies. You can make a good digestive enzyme blend by juicing pineapple with an equal measure of apple cider vinegar and storing it in the fridge. Take a tablespoon of this blend before meals as a digestive aid. The fresh juice is good in small amounts; however, too much can create acidity and digestive disturbance.

Prunes are high in antioxidants and help reduce the build-up of putrefied matter in your digestive tract. They help with bowel movements and prunes are good to relieve sore throats and other acute infections. You can easily soak dried prunes overnight and add them to your juices. Make sure you remove the seeds before putting prunes through the juicer.

Rhubarb increases the secretions of bile in your digestive tract, helps increase bowel movements and is also a good nurturing digestive food. A freshly cooked rhubarb and honey dessert is tasty, nurturing and a good evening food that can mean the difference between your detox plan being abandoned or continued. Slice rhubarb stems into 1-inch pieces and boil in water with honey to taste. Once cooked and soft, simply drain away excess water and place in a casserole dish. Cover with raw oats that have been soaked in apple juice for half an hour and sprinkle with some coconut and a drizzle of olive oil. Bake for half an hour until crunchy on top and eat with fresh or coconut yoghurt.

Rocket is an excellent liver and kidney cleanser, aiding digestion and helping secretion of bile from the liver.

Sage can be added to juices and salads to help increase memory, reduce hot flushes and also acts as an antimicrobial.

Seaweed in its many forms can be highly nutritious and added to soups, casseroles, sushi and salads. Seaweeds can help speed up your metabolism and add minerals to your body; they are also energising and cleansing. Seaweeds take deep-seated toxins out of the liver, especially the hard-to-get ones that could cause you illness in the future.

Seeds of many varieties are good nutrition as well as good sweepers for your digestive tract when on a detox plan. Sesame seeds help increase your resting thermogenesis as well as adding valuable nutrition to your diet. Sunflower and flax seeds are high in essential fatty acids. Make sure you get fresh seeds as the rancid ones can create havoc with your liver and digestive tract.

Liquid detox plans should be seed-free. However, if you are on a juice cleanse and insist on having seeds, simply soak them overnight in water and run the whole lot through your juicer with other fruits and vegetables. You may lose some of the seed's value, but you will also be gentle on your digestive tract and not compromise the liquid status of your detox plan.

Spinach is good detox food for women who tend to be anaemic and for those who need more energy. If you are on a long juice cleanse then make sure you have some spinach daily to help your mineral levels.

Spirulina is excellent as it provides your body with nutrition at the same time as getting into the cells and neutralising and eliminating the toxins. Spirulina also helps make your body less acidic. Taking 3 grams of spirulina a day through any detox is a way of ensuring you maintain energy levels and have some complete nutrition. Taking the spirulina may slow down the detox process but will also ensure your body is maintained whilst it's busy detoxing. It is 70% complete protein and high in B group vitamins and chlorophyll.

Sprouts are living, raw and nutritious. Add sprouts to your detox plan and if you are on a juice cleanse, juice them. It's easy to make sprouts, and you can sprout just about anything that grows. Fenugreek is a very good seed to sprout for a detox plan as it helps eliminate excess mucous and cleanses the lymph nodes in your body. Alfalfa, the father of foods, is nutritious and cleansing. Many other foods will sprout like; snow peas, lentils and barley, wheatgrass, mustard, fennel and turmeric, anything else you care to experiment with is good too.

To sprout seeds all you need is a glass jar, a rubber band, some fine gauze and water. Place the seeds in the glass jar, rinse with clean water and shake off the excess liquid. Place the gauze over the lid and hold it there with the rubber band. Turn the jar upside down and let the water drain away. Rinse with fresh water every day until the sprouts are ready. The process of sprouting is easy so long as you remember to keep the sprouts watered daily. Sprouts can be added to many meals and are living proof that raw foods are healthy. In fact, sprouts are one of the few truly living foods that are easy to grow, accessible and good prana (Lifeforce foods).

Tomatoes need to be ripe for antioxidant properties, vitamins and the cleansing properties for bowel, liver, prostate and kidneys. Cooked, vine-ripened tomatoes are an excellent antioxidant.

Turmeric is an excellent additive to any detox as this helps cleanse your body, soothe digestion and eliminate excess oestrogen in the liver. It is a premium anti-inflammatory and antioxidant.

Watermelon is the best diuretic, helping balance fluid levels in your body. Watermelon is also a good kidney and liver food. Fresh watermelon juice can be used to reduce fluid retention and help eliminate deep-seated toxins.

Wheatgrass is a super power-cleanser for all organs in your body. Used for cancer prevention, all-round cleansing and as an antioxidant.

Yams are good to help balance progesterone and oestrogen levels and are good in soups, salads and even juices.

Of course, there are many more foods that are excellent and nutritious, and these are just a few ideas.

CHAPTER SIXTEEN

Special detox plans

The 'any morning' detox

This can be done on any and every morning if you want! This detox is simple, pure and easy. All you need to do is eat fruit or have juices in the morning, then have lunch as usual! This cleanse is perfect for any busy person who wants to feel good about having a detox plan, yet has a lot of stress and business in their life that may be stopping them from undertaking longer and stricter types of detoxing.

When you think about it, this detox is a natural flow-on from the fasting you have done all through the night when you are sleeping. Your body is already relaxed and cleansing itself as part of the daily process. Then instead of loading your body up with food, you place yourself in the position where you are actually sweeping those toxins out of the body gently and naturally without too much effort.

What you need for this detox

If you take 3000 mg of magnesium powder the night before, then you may also be assured of a good morning bowel movement which will be even more cleansing. Magnesium in such a large amount can cause diarrhoea, so perhaps you would like to take a smaller amount on your first detox and work your way up to this amount over time when you know your body's response to the magnesium. Don't take any extra herbs with this 'any morning' detox. If you do normally take a daily nutritional supplement, please place it aside for the morning and have it with your lunch instead.

You will eat (or drink) only fresh fruit and vegetables. Fruit is stronger at cleansing than vegetables, and citrus fruits are possibly one of the strongest cleansers you can have. Morning is a perfect time to enjoy the lushness of fresh fruit. Lemons are an excellent start to the day because of their many effects in cleansing cells. They help reduce the uric and lactic acids, they create alkalinity in your body, and the humble old lemon reduces all mucous. Plus it's a fabulous detoxifier for liver cells, helps with fluid retention and does just about everything you'll ever want a cleansing fruit to do.

When you wake up, instead of having a cup of coffee or tea, boil the kettle and add the juice of one lemon with a teaspoon of honey to a cup and fill with hot water. Drink this brew instead of your regular caffeine-based drink.

For breakfast you can fill up on as much of any type of fruit as you like. Try to keep the 'any morning' detox a pure fruit cleanse if you have lots of fruit around. This is because fruit feels luxurious to eat, and it's a real treat to have as much as you like. If you are diabetic then you'll have to monitor your fruit intake or have a vegetable-based cleanse as fruit does contain a lot of sugar. If you need to have vegetables, carrot and celery with lime or lemon juice are good, so long as you watch the sugar content of the carrots.

When you do the 'any morning' detox, it's literally that, any morning. You can decide spontaneously to do this cleanse. Perhaps you have no fruit or vegetables in the house. Then drink a cup of warm water with one tablespoon of apple cider vinegar and a teaspoon of honey as your start-up drink. Then drink herb teas until you can get out and pick up some fruit from your local store, or if you are lucky enough to have fruit trees in your garden then make the most of the seasonal varieties.

Old-fashioned parsley that just grows freely in most gardens is good to chew on, or make some tea from. This is an excellent blood cleanser as well as a diuretic for reducing fluid retention and inflammation. A lot of our diseases and illnesses are created from too much inflammation in the body. Taking this lovely 'any morning' detox regularly will help you keep inflammation at bay. It's a gentle and easy way to regularly cleanse.

Try to do the 'any morning' cleanse at least one day a week. You can do it on a weekend morning when you are free to roll around the house and laze about, or you can do it when you have been out to dinner the night before and feel overloaded with rich foods. This 'any morning' detox is perfect whenever you want to lighten up and get rid of a bit of toxic load. After any cleanse, even this little easy one, you will find you have a clearer mind and are able to think better about any projects or ideas in your mind.

You may also find you have more physical energy in the afternoon than normal after this 'any morning' cleanse because your body is literally rejuvenated, even though you may be sticking to your regular schedule. This is one of the beauties of this detox as you can just get on with your day. It's short enough to be non-intrusive, but in effect, it has extended your regular overnight cleanse by five or six hours, this is beneficial in loosening up and eliminating some extra poisons from your body.

The 'any evening' detox

This detox is another easy way to regularly give your digestive tract a rest. Pick a night, any night, or every night if you want to lose a few kilos and simply be very strict in what you eat. The 'any evening' detox is about soup, salad and juices again. All detox plans offer you the option of fruit, vegetables and fresh herbs and spices in the form of salads, stir-fries, soups and juices. All you need to do is replace dinner with these foods in any form you wish.

What you need for this detox

Start the 'any evening' detox in the late afternoon, after you come in from work or about 4 pm is the perfect time really. If you get thirsty just have water, herb teas and juices. If you get hungry, just have fruit, vegetable salads, stir-fries and soups.

'Any evening' detox soup

1/2 bunch celery
five carrots
eight cloves garlic
three onions
500 grams of mushrooms
500 grams of pumpkin
500 grams of zucchini
two low salt veggie stock cubes
two capsicums
one small chilli
one tablespoon of balsamic vinegar

one tablespoon of sesame oil
Cut all ingredients to about 2 cm pieces, Place in a crockpot and add
stock cube, oil and vinegar. Cover with boiled water and leave on
low for eight to ten hours.

If you are unable to cook in a crockpot, then boiling the soup in a steel
pot on the stove is fine too. You can even place the ingredients in a casserole dish and bake in the oven for the afternoon. It's delicious any way
you choose to cook it! If you cook it in a saucepan, braise the vegetables
for half an hour in the oil and allow the flavours to blend and then add
the boiling water for further cooking. This makes a delicious soup.

Add other vegetables that are in season too, especially fennel if you
can get it! This is a recipe that can have any or all vegetables replaced
with others depending on your taste and what is locally available. Don't
be strict in following the recipe as you can add lots of spices, herbs and
flavours that are natural and to your liking. You can even make this
soup using one or two vegetables such as carrot and celery soup, or
mushroom and onion soup. The choices are limitless.

When you go to eat this soup, you can add a heaped tablespoon of
brewer's yeast, some sesame seeds or tahini and lots of chopped up
parsley. You can also add seeds, kelp or pepper. Slice up some fresh
herbs or chilli, or squeeze the juice of a lemon, lime or orange over it.
What's more … you can eat as much as you like of this soup, on an 'any
evening' detox day from 4 pm until you go to bed.

Don't drink alcohol, tea or coffee in the 'any evening' detox. This is
a detox night, and you will feel wonderful when you wake up the next
morning knowing you have done the best for your body.

It can be beneficial to take 10 ml of herbal detox extract in the evening, also
eat lots of vegetables at this time of day as they are nourishing and comforting foods and tend to be more filling than fruit. What's more, if you
eat fruit in the evening, you tend to be up urinating a lot during the night,
which is not a good idea if you want a good night's sleep.

The 'any evening' detox is wonderful and easy after you have been
working hard and feel like you need a rest. If you are very tired this is a
good detox as you can go to bed feeling lighter than if you had a heavy
evening meal with alcohol or tea or coffee. Eat fruit or vegetables only
in the 'any evening' detox plan, drink only herb teas and water, or juices
of course. Nothing else to eat and you'll be refreshed in the morning.

You can tie this 'any evening' detox in with the 'any morning' detox
and wake up the next morning to purely fruit and vegetables until

lunchtime if you like. That will extend the detox in a simple and easily achieved manner. For seasoned detoxers you can just flow it on, with fruit until lunchtime and vegetables for lunch and all evening. Keep it up for a few days and watch those extra kilos melt away along with those unwanted toxins.

Another really delicious and light 'any evening' detox meal is to take one scoop of quality protein powder and place it in the blender with cold seasonal fruit and about 100 ml of water. Blend in mango, pineapple, strawberries, apples, cherries, grapes, oranges, lychees or even plums. This is delicious. If you like the taste and find that a few hours later you are craving food again then simply repeat the process. Make sure you only add one small scoop of vanilla flavour protein powder in each drink and make about 200 ml at a go. This way you can have one, two or even three drinks through the evening.

You may enjoy this meal better than most evening meals on a hot day. It's filling, light and rejuvenating. The blender is a wonderful tool for detoxing. If you don't have any protein powder just have the pure fruit blended with a little water, water doesn't affect the taste, and it just makes the fruit less thick and more drinkable.

The cocktail detox hour

The 'any evening' detox can also be treated like a cocktail hour detox. Get your head around the idea of sitting back and enjoying canapes and cocktails whilst detoxing. Create some really nifty cocktails out of cleansing fruit and vegetables for a fun evening.

What you need for this detox

For your 'cocktail hour detox' you can make a pitcher of juice with some fresh tomatoes, celery, carrot, onion, garlic and lemon juice. Then add chilli, extra pepper and celery sticks. Get some good glasses, ice and enjoy! Add spicy sauce to this one, and you will have a mocktail, or use a lot of tomato and lemon and make it a Bloody Mary. If you like it hot, simply add extra onion and garlic.

To really pep up your 'cocktail detox hour', cut up sticks of celery, carrot, capsicum and broccoli; you can use lots of different raw vegetables. Place them on a platter and add some coconut yoghurt laced with mint. Some light cream cheese or ricotta, fetta, cottage cheese, mashed avocado and a tad of sweet chilli sauce. Or make a dipping sauce with balsamic vinegar and a touch of olive oil and garlic. Blend some roasted capsicum with garlic and a little sea salt as a dip or blend some roasted eggplant with a little lemon juice to make another delicious dip.

You can have your cocktails and canapes as an evening cocktail hour, feel great and enjoy your detox even more. Better still, invite some friends over and make a night of it!

You can make this a fruity cocktail hour detox too. Simply blend your favourite fruit with ice and make some non-alcoholic daiquiris. Watermelon and mint blended with ice or try fresh pineapple juice with a drop of coconut essence for your cleansing pina colada. What about lemon juice served in a cocktail glass with salt around the rim, just like a Margarita, or a Martini with fresh icy cold cucumber and lime served with a tasty olive or two!

The evening detox dinner party

Invite your friends or family over and have a detox evening together.

What you need for this detox

For drinks, use juices listed in the evening cocktail hour detox and veggies dipped in a variety of sauces for canapes. Follow this with a delicious cleansing soup such as pumpkin, mushroom or a cool tomato or cucumber soup.

For the main course, make a vegetarian feast with stuffed or roasted vegetables and a salad. Desert can be fresh seasonal fruit, or you could make some really healthy, fibre-filled muffins or hot fruity pies. Then, for a nightcap, have dandelion coffee and a herbal elixir. What a delicious vegetarian feast.

Make your 'evening detox dinner party' into four courses as this always feels more decadent then three. Use good crockery and cutlery and decorate the environment with flowers, candles, music and ambience. Get everyone to dress in a theme or formally so that you can make the most of the fun evening detoxing together. Maybe everyone could even bring a dish to contribute to an evening of cleansing, therefore creating minimal work for the host!

You can celebrate detoxing with your friends, and everyone will go home feeling fabulous!

The 'lunch only' detox

This is often the hardest time of the day to detox. In the evening you can make yourself a small, super-healthy dinner and sneak away to bed early before the temptations of the outer world lure you to the fridge for some toxic treat. And, in the morning, it is easier to start the day off with the right intentions. But to follow it through and have the personal discipline to cleanse through the middle of the day can be really difficult.

Lunchtime or late afternoon is usually the time of day in any cleanse where you could easily quit for a good coffee and a tasty, off-limits snack. Many people find coffee to be the biggest daytime detox destroyer. For others though, this is the most logical time of day to detox as there are no other people to prepare food for.

What you need for this detox

The 'lunch only' detox is a healthy detox in the middle of all your daily busy activities. If you are planning to have a 'lunch only' detox, then try to keep the coffee and tea intake low through the morning. If you must have these things, then limit yourself to one or two and replace the others with water or juice.

When it comes to lunch, have salad, soup, vegetables or fruit only. Remember though, delicious fruit salad might taste good at the time, but two hours later you'll be slumped across your work like a jaded rose and as the afternoon wears on you'll just become more irritable. So, if you are going to have fruit salad for the 'lunch only' detox, divide the amount you would normally have as one serve into four or five portions and snack on it regularly every hour or two through the afternoon. This way, you should easily make it through to dinner without feeling deprived.

One of the most filling and delicious lunchtime detox treats is pumpkin with vegetables. Steamed pumpkin with roasted assorted vegetables, such as eggplant, capsicum, tomato, garlic and onion, can be enjoyed either cold or warm. Drizzle it with olive oil and some apple cider vinegar, and you are on a good lunchtime detox that's filling. It's good to add this treat to some green rocket, lettuce, parsley and snow peas, and you can also add sesame seeds, herbs, kelp or other natural toppings. You will eat well and be able to feel energised through the afternoon.

Always make a double serve of any food you have for the 'lunch only' detox because many detox foods are light and you may want to eat regularly through the afternoon. This is important if you are busy, stressed, emotionally tired or under a lot of pressure in any way. Food is nurturing, and you don't need to feel deprived when you have the 'lunch only' (or any other) detox, you should feel satisfied with the food and the knowledge that you are doing your body a healthy turn.

Soups are good; you can make up a big pot of your detox soup and heat it up by the cupful as required through lunch and the afternoon and thereby sustain your energy levels. Add some chilli, brewer's yeast, a squeeze of lemon juice or even a dollop of plain yoghurt to your soup for variety.

Old-fashioned coleslaw, without the rich mayonnaise but dressed with cider or balsamic vinegar, fresh lemon juice, sea salt and olive oil is delicious. You can add many extra vegetables to this salad, and you wouldn't even recognise it as coleslaw, except for the cabbage in the mixture. Add grated apples, raw pumpkin, beans, spring onions and rocket, really just about any raw vegetable you have to add is delicious. Add a teaspoon of raw runny honey to this salad; there is something quite delicious about balsamic vinegar, olive oil and honey mixed together as a raw vegetable salad dressing. Or add parsley and garlic, the chlorophyll in the parsley counteracts the smelliness of the garlic.

You may want to extend this 'lunch only' detox to dinnertime if you are feeling really motivated. If you choose to do this, just remember to keep up your fluids in the form of hot or cold water with cider vinegar or lemon added, or perhaps you can drink herbal teas. Some teas like ginger are delicious on a cold day, whilst peppermint is a favourite summertime tea.

Remember there are certain foods that, no matter how you look at them, are not detox foods and should be eliminated from your diet whenever you detox. These include all processed and commercial foods that contain any artificial colours and preservatives. The salt in the preservatives is likely to contain anti-caking agents, and the vinegar is likely to be the cheap and nasty white stuff and any other preservatives, you don't want to know about anyway.

Other foods to avoid are all white flour products; in fact, make it a blanket rule to avoid wheat in each and every detox. Have rye, corn or gluten-free type flour if you have the wholesome vegetarian diet detox, also eat brown rice on this detox. Generally, with the 'lunch only' detox you will want to extend it into your day either through the morning or the afternoon.

Any carbonated drinks are to be avoided during detoxing, except of course lovely naturally carbonated spring water. All sugar is banned from your diet when detoxing, including all foods that contain added sugar. Only natural fruit sugars in the fresh fruit and vegetables you eat are allowed and a little honey because it has properties that help your body remove excess mucous which is a necessary part of any detox, the honey must be raw.

The wholesome vegetarian detox

This is a delicious and sustaining diet that allows you to get healthy and become energised whilst detoxing at the same time. You can easily sustain this way of eating for several months if necessary. Many people use this as their mainstay diet in life and only diverge from it on occasion; anyone with chronic illness would do well to do the same. To stay really healthy, you would emphasise the fresh fruit and vegetables and keep the carbohydrate foods to a minimum.

A good idea with this detox is to avoid all starches and cereals every second day. This means that you can have rye, corn or potato breads and gluten-free cereals and grains every second day, on the other day you don't eat these foods at all. This is because often illnesses feed on sugars in your body and for chronic illness you would do well to avoid all sugars as much as possible. Even cereals and grains break down to base sugars in your body that are then used as fuel. Toxins are not eliminated as quickly when you have excess sugar in your system.

What you need for this detox

Only foods from vegetable and plant sources are eaten, and these are used in healthy combinations that supply the body with balanced ratios of all nutrients. There is no dairy in this diet, except for fresh cheeses such as ricotta and cottage; this is because it is a detox diet and cheese tends to encourage mucous, which is what we want to eliminate.

You can eat all the nuts and seeds you desire. Each day as part of the plan, you can have 15 grams each of the following: sunflower seeds, sesame seeds, almonds, flaxseeds and pumpkin seeds. These can be added to any meal at any time.

No eggs, no meat, no processed foods, no coffee and no tea, except herbal teas, also including dandelion tea/coffee which is actually very palatable. Don't have any really cold foods, drink water at room temperature, have no iced foods or very cold salads, have these freshly prepared and as close to room temperature as possible.

You are allowed gluten-free bread, brown rice and any lentils, chickpeas or other vegetable-derived substances so long as they are whole and unprocessed. This includes tofu and tempeh which you can eat as much as you like. Have no gluten foods, including all wheat-based barley and rye.

Every waking hour you must drink at least 200 ml of herbal tea, juice or water. This is easily achieved when you have one drink every hour that is a standard size, you can also have any of your vegetables and fruit as juices, and you are able to have juices for one to three meals a day, as desired.

Alternately, you can have your food steamed, cooked in low-fat wok style, or as a casserole or stew type meal, depending entirely upon your desires. You are allowed to eat starchy vegetables such as potatoes, yams, kumaras and turnips.

You can have any nutritional supplements as recommended, and these will depend on your health status and the desired outcome for this detox. It can be used by healthy people wanting a good sustainable and nourishing detox plan, in which case you would add many herbs that are targeting detoxification pathways in your body. It can also be used by people who are ill, with benefits for a myriad of illnesses, including HIV, arthritis, lupus, chronic fatigue, cardiovascular disease, diabetes, coeliac, food allergies, multiple sclerosis, tuberculosis, liver disease, kidney disease, menopause, infertility, viruses, chronic illness and bowel disease to name a few. Use specific herbal and nutritional supplements to help heal your specific condition. This is a great recovery detox when you are getting over an illness.

There are no portion controls on this detox, you can eat what you like, when you like, providing the foods are within the range of the wholesome vegetarian detox guidelines. It is an excellent diet to help eliminate toxins. You can't have alcohol on this detox, and you certainly won't want to smoke; however, if you are a smoker, an alcoholic or have other addictions, this is a beautiful detox diet plan that will help you eventually eliminate the addictions from your life with the help of your Health Care Practitioner and some herbal and nutritional substances.

Make sure that you stay on this detox as long as necessary when you need to cleanse your body. It is the delicious and easy detox plan that will see your energy recover and your body rejuvenate, and your body thank you for it.

Many people do this detox during the week, then on weekends follow a different diet. This way, you will be able to enjoy going out and having a few drinks on the weekend, then spend the working week cleansing your body with the wholesome vegetarian detox. Others vary it by making it non-vegetarian and incorporating various animal protein sources like protein powder, eggs, organic chicken, wild ocean fish and some red meats depending upon their personal choice and dietary needs. Often with chronic illnesses you need to incorporate protein into the diet, so this adjustment would provide the ideal diet plan.

In fact, if everybody followed the guidelines for the wholesome vegetarian detox plan and adapted it to suit their own needs, then we would certainly have a healthier world with less demand for the junk.

CHAPTER SEVENTEEN

Water

We all know that we should drink water. But do you know why? Here is the lowdown on water in your body. Where is it located? What are the percentages? What happens when you become dehydrated? What happens when you drink too much water? Why is water so important anyway? Read on, and you may find yourself swilling with enthusiasm and really seeing some healthy results.

H_2O

Water—H_2O, two parts hydrogen to one part oxygen—is the real deal. Then we can add in any particles that have attached themselves along the way, such as minerals, toxins, and synthetic chemicals that just love a little H_2O to go.

There are hydrophilic molecules which just love to attach themselves to hydrogen atoms and are water-loving, these readily dissolve in water such as sodium-based chemicals. Then there are hydrophobic molecules which are repulsed by water, such as lipid-based molecules which require some form of mixing or emulsification to blend with water.

The way molecules are attracted or repulsed to water is important in your body as this determines how nutrients are absorbed and assimilated through your system. Water is the essence of life; this, above all else, except for the air we breathe, is the most important factor for your health.

There are negative and positive ions within your body. Many trace minerals and elements are only useable in your body when they have been converted to this ion formation. This occurs when minerals dissolve readily in water: we need to drink water so that there is sufficient fluid in our body for this process to occur, along with the many other processes involved with hydration and metabolism.

Where is the water in my body?

The total amount of water in your body is dependent upon your fat content. Adipose (fat tissue) is only about 10% water as opposed to many other body tissues. An overweight person's body fluids may only be about 55% whilst a lean person may contain as much as 75% total water for their body weight.

There are fluid compartments in your body, both inside and outside the cells. About 40% of your water content is found inside your cells, and another 20% is found outside. An average 70-kilo person would have about 45 litres of water in their body with 15 litres located outside the cells (extracellular fluid) and 30 litres inside the cells (intracellular fluid).

Blood accounts for about 4 litres of the extracellular fluid (5% of the bodyweight) and water in your connective tissue accounts for about 9% of this weight. Another 4% of water is located in your bones and collagen. Other extracellular fluid is located in the digestive tract, cerebrospinal fluid, eyeball, pleural, pericardial, peritoneal and synovial fluids, plus of course the thyroid glands, sweat glands and cochlear endolymph.

So, now we know where fluid lives in our body, we know it constantly needs to be replaced and we know that this process happens most obviously through the foods we eat and the beverages we drink. The fluid in your body is always on the move; old molecules of water need to be constantly replaced by new. Water that enters your body passes into the gastrointestinal tract and is absorbed through the small intestine where it visits the liver for filtration before moving on to the rest of your body.

Blood cells take up new molecules in less than one second, and brain tissue takes up water very fast, exchanging the old for the new in less than every two minutes. These molecules are constantly being replaced, with the old molecules entering the blood and being taken around the body to be filtered by your kidneys and liver cells, ensuring that the most toxic molecules are excreted or taken out of action.

You lose about 3 to 6% of your body's water each day. Therefore, a person who has 45 litres of water in their body would lose 1.5 to 3 litres every day. This water loss needs to be replaced; however, our bodies have some awesome mechanisms in place to bring water loss right down to zero in times of non-replacement. This is how you can manage to accumulate fluid in your body at times when you are not drinking enough water, and your body automatically slows down the water turnover cycle.

Keep your water cycle going simply by having a glass of water each time you urinate and try to drink a glass of water every half an hour during hot weather as you will lose fluids from sweat in the summer as well as in the urine cycle.

Water carries toxins out of your body

There needs to be a minimal rate of urine formation to allow the removal of toxins and water-soluble metabolites. Urea is formed, as amino acids are broken down and excreted as urine; this is almost like ammonia and is very acidic in the body. Many other, potentially toxic by-products enter the kidneys for filtration and excretion through your urine, so it's essential to keep the water cycle going in your body for toxicity removal and natural detoxing.

A lot of water is evaporated from your body in sweat and exhaling breath, as vapour is derived from the respiratory tract surfaces. Water is also lost through skin evaporation other than sweat because the skin surface is not completely dry, and the cells contain moisture. Water is also lost through faeces.

The rate of water loss from sweating is variable depending on: your personal thermoregulation and metabolism, the environment, the amount of exercise you do, stress, sweating and other factors which may lead to a loss of between 1 and 5 litres a day. If you find that you are sweating more than usual in hotter weather, take this into account with your water intake and add an extra 1 to 5 litres of water to your diet. Don't panic, though, water comes in many forms, you don't always have to drink it in its pure form.

Where do I get water in my diet?

Water is in all of the foods you eat. Examples here are: a rare steak is 40% water, whereas a well-done steak is 25% water. An apple is 85% water. Most fruit and vegetables are high in water, with watermelon sitting at over 90%. Cauliflower, strawberries, marrow, beans, mangos, rock melons and broccoli all sit around the 90% water content level. Cereals, breads and drier foods obviously contain less water, even a glass of milk is 90% water. So it's not that hard to get your daily quota of this essential ingredient.

The regulation mechanisms

Obviously, you can't regulate exactly the amount of water you take into your body, so magically your body will do this for you. Yes, your intake can vary considerably from day to day, and the rate of loss can also vary. However, the water percentages in the body do not vary, they are stable, and there are some interesting mechanisms in place that control this process.

Your hypothalamus is the coordinating centre in your brain for the feedback information to regulate water in the body, and this receives input from detectors such as the osmotic pressure of your blood. The greater this osmotic pressure, the greater is your need for water intake. The left atrium of your heart also has a detector which influences the water balance in your body. When water levels are low, this is reflected in reduced blood pressure, which in turn reduces the pressure in the left atrium.

Psychological factors also impinge on your regulatory centres in the hypothalamus. Sight, smell and taste of foods can also influence these activities. A reduced level of body water is detected as an increase in the osmotic pressure in your blood and as a reduced pressure in your left atrium as already mentioned. The main response to this is to increase water retention through the collecting ducts in your kidneys, and this will reduce urine volume and return larger amounts of water to your blood. This mechanism is the release of anti-diuretic hormone (ADH) from your posterior pituitary gland. This hormone increases the permeability of the collecting ducts and allows a greater rate of water reabsorption.

The second mechanism for increasing water retention (or decreasing water loss) involves the kidneys alone, without the influence of the hypothalamus. Once reduced blood pressure is detected in the kidneys, the enzyme rennin is secreted, which promotes another hormone called aldosterone from your adrenal glands. This hormone acts on your renal tubules to promote the reabsorption of sodium ions. Where salt goes water follows, so you can imagine how this mechanism quickly reverses water loss from the kidneys reducing urine flow. The downside here is that you will be recirculating all those nasty toxins through your system until you are able to have enough hydration for the kidneys to choose to let them out again through the urine.

The third mechanism that ensures you don't have a water deficit in the body is the thirst response. The greater your water deficit, the greater your thirst will be. This mechanism can easily be ignored with mild dehydration; however, once your body has reduced urine output, and it continues to do so, then you will become more and more thirsty. Thirst is part of the homeostatic regulation of body water, but unlike the other two mechanisms it is not automatic. However, if the sensation becomes extreme and dehydration threatens our survival, the ability to control thirst becomes impossible. These three mechanisms for controlling water in the body area will be reversed when there is sufficient water in the body or when our intake becomes excessive.

It's really good to see why we need to drink water and why it's so important to keep our body fluids in balance. Many illnesses and diseases can be avoided when we are sufficiently hydrated. When I talk about hydration I want to say that clean, pure hydration is the most important factor. Imagine all those water molecules clogged up with salts and sugars from refined foods. For new cells to be healthy in all organs, you need to give them the right nutrients, for this, water is the main carrier, and the water needs to be clean.

Our body has the natural ability to make water molecules from the metabolism of protein in the liver, and our body is able to filter out many of the poisons and toxins through our liver and kidneys. But let's make the job easier by eating clean foods and reducing the workload on these organs. Enjoy your water and make time every day to put your health first.

The pure water fast

If you want to do the 'pure water fast', then start with one day and work your way up in time. This is the strongest way to detox, you eat nothing, and you will eliminate poisons and toxins from your body swiftly.

What you need for this detox

Wake up one morning and have water only. Make sure the water is good water and not tap water from a town supply with additives. Rainwater or spring water is good; however, in the world today some people can't trust the water in their environment. Get the best water you can and drink about 2 litres in the morning and 2 litres in the afternoon. That night, have water for dinner, and go to bed early. You will only be starving for the first 24 hours. After that gluconeogenesis kicks in and you start to eat your own body fat.

Your body will be feeding off its toxins and body fats until they are gone, and eventually, if you stayed on this fast for long enough, you would be eating your own muscle. We don't want this to occur. So, no more than 72 hours on a 'pure water fast' unsupervised, and this only for a very healthy person who is a well-seasoned cleanser and who isn't taking any medications, anyone else should have assistance.

As it is literally the fastest way to detox, it can also be the fastest way to headaches, diarrhoea, nasty feelings from the past coming back to haunt you and the fastest way to get gallstones if you are prone to them. This is because your gall bladder needs a supply of bile regularly, and fasting rests the body as nothing else will.

You will feel good in your mind as you require personal discipline. Flesh is dumb, so when you do a water fast you have to ignore and repel feelings of hunger. You will only stay hungry for the first day. If you continue to fast, you will probably feel sick and be resting a lot on the second day, as toxins, released from your cells, are swirling around in your bloodstream. Then, on day 3, the elation starts to kick in, and you feel blissful and full of energy. This is when you should end the fast; you are on a high, and if you wish to continue cleansing go to a pure juice cleanse or one of the other detox methods that are easier on your body.

Technically, a water fast is the only true fast. Every other method of detoxing is classified as a cleanse. Don't expect any bowel movements whilst on a fast. Your whole digestive tract will stop. This is necessary. If you wish to have a series of colonic irrigations, this is a good time to do that. Only have three in a row, one every day for three days and you will feel fabulous. Some people recommend three in one day, and this could be a wonderful treat as it will give you a fabulous cleanse. Or you may wish to have the traditional ten colonics in ten days, as recommended by some Health Care Practitioners.

Fasting is literally resting your body. So, please don't take any laxatives, herbs or other nutritional supplements whilst on a water fast. You can have peppermint or fennel tea throughout the day. This is deodorising for your body. You can also add a dash of lemon juice to your drinks as this will help to clean out the acids and toxins. Apple cider vinegar added to drinks can also help, but you may find it makes you feel nauseous and accelerates the detox whilst on a pure water fast.

If you suffer from headaches, feel sick or totally wiped out, then you may be taking things a little fast. Slow down the pure water fast with a glass of carrot or red grape juice. Then you will have three or four hours grace and just slow down the detox enough to relax again and let those toxins that were causing the feelings of overload to pass through your urine.

Please make sure you drink at least 200 ml of liquid each waking hour during the day on the 'pure water fast'. The more water you drink, the more toxins will be diluted and more quickly eliminated from your body.

Many people have their 'pure water fast' from Sunday night until Tuesday morning on water and peppermint tea only. You will feel fantastic for the rest of the week and never have to worry about obesity issues. There are some weeks when you will feel tired and not really motivated to do the 'pure water fast' at all. On these weeks, stop at dinnertime on Monday night and only detox from Sunday night until Monday night. That's still 24 hours and a fabulous gift you are giving yourself if you cleanse this way each week. Other weeks you may feel so motivated that you want to continue the fast through until Tuesday night or even Wednesday morning. You need to judge this for yourself, if it's your inspiration and your feeling that the 'pure water fast' is the way to good health for you, then this is a good decision for your Wellness Zone. Give it a go if the idea appeals to you and decide how you feel. Start off with just 24 hours, then if you like it, do it again next week. After a while you can extend the time.

A 'pure water fast' is something that doesn't have to be done on a regular basis. The hardest part about this way of fasting is actually on the mental level. Getting your head around the fact that you are not eating anything, for 24 hours or longer, can be difficult at first as it goes against many traditional beliefs and customs about food. However, there are also many cultural and traditional rituals that involve the process of fasting.

Pure water fasting is the cheapest, easiest, fastest and most effective way to cleanse. Your first 'pure water fast' is a difficult but a great achievement, once you have completed your first one, then the mental barriers will be down, and you will find the next experience easier.

If you are ever in a position of great illness, then supervised pure water fasts, that are regular and controlled, can assist your Wellness

Zone. This is a good path to wellness, and your body has a better chance to fight any illness when it is not cluttered full of toxins and rubbish.

The juice cleanse

Most people love a good juice! Fruit is the most refreshing and cleansing food you can eat. Seasonal fruits and veggies, juiced or blended into delicious concoctions are all the rage these days, and almost every corner has a juice bar. Juices can be so cheap when you use local produce, get yourself a juicer for home, and you can relish in the lushness of juice cleansing whenever you like!

What you need for this detox

Often with a juice cleanse, you need to be really in tune with how you are feeling at the time. On one cleanse you may be obsessed with the idea of liver cleansing and detoxification on that level, then you would add lots of carrot, lemon, parsley and wheat or barley grass. The list of juices and their medicinal properties are endless. Basically, you can pick and choose what you want for this detox. Stick to juices only, and you will be on your way to good health.

Digestive tract health is the first path to wellness. Juices are so easily absorbed, and even those who are suffering from a chronic illness can readily benefit from the nutrients and enhance their Wellness Zone. Juice cleansing is an excellent regular detoxifier; it is the next level of cleansing after the pure water fast. You are getting nutrition and are able to flush toxins at the same time in the simplest and less invasive manner for your body.

With a juice cleanse, it takes up to three days to get the same cleansing benefits as you would on the 'pure water fast' for one day. So it is slower. But it's also more revitalising on some levels as far as being able to maintain your daily lifestyle. You have a constant stream of energy on a juice cleanse, as you are feeding your body nutrients the whole time. You are also fuelling your metabolism regularly, so this is increasing thermogenesis and assisting in eliminating toxins very well indeed!

Try plain old-fashioned carrot and celery juice with one clove of garlic, one onion and the juice of one lemon, taken eight times a day. This is a potent potion. Add a bit of pure wheatgrass or barley grass, and you are on a zoom cleanse. You can take spirulina or maca mixed with any of your juices for an extra cleanse.

Try to get as much cellular recovery as possible whilst you are on a juice cleanse. Really visualise those cells pumping through the juices and imagine your lymphatic system flushing away all the built-up debris of the past. You can't really get these results when any food is included in the diet, only with juices or water. As soon as you eat food, your body is working again, so the energy is kind of reversed and you are absorbing more instead of eliminating. Make your policy for toxins 'better out than in', so get them out!

You can drink carrot juice until the palms of your hands are bright orange. Beta-carotene is a *precursor* to vitamin A, and it is not vitamin A, you need vegetable-derived beta-carotene to make vitamin A when you don't have enough. However, if you do have enough, then the beta-carotene will be eliminated harmlessly. All that extra cancer protection from the antioxidants makes it worth the trouble to drink large amounts of carrot juice on a juice cleanse. For variety add a lemon to each juice as this helps preserve the actives in the carrot. Different carrots taste different, little organic carrots taste so sweet.

Add juices to your normal daily dietary plan whenever you can. They are a great source of nutrients and a delicious way to avoid real food but still get the goodness and a satisfied feeling whilst having a little detox along the way.

A juice cleanse is really good when you are able to avoid the world for a whole weekend, it is the perfect weekend health kick. You can start on Friday night when you come in from the week and go all the way to Monday morning drinking up to 13 juices a day. Drink one juice for each hour you are awake. The only guideline with the juice cleanse is that you can only drink the juices of your favourite fruit and vegetables. In the morning you may prefer fruit, and then change to vegetables in the afternoon for variety.

Juice cleansing days need to be treated as special days as sometimes it's hard to get through the afternoon. A seasoned cleanser will have developed tricks to survive the afternoon hours and avoid breaking the cleanse at dinnertime, try and see what works best for you. Have fruit, juiced in any combination that takes your fancy each morning, then vegetables in the afternoon and early evening. Drink delicious herbal teas between juices and stay away from places where you are likely to be tempted away from your juice cleanse.

Drink as much water as you like, if and when you want it, but often you will find you avoid water when you are on a juice cleanse. You may want to dilute the juice with water; however, this isn't really necessary as often pure juices taste far superior to their watered-down versions.

Throughout the day, have half an MSG-free stock cube or a teaspoon of miso and mix it with 200 ml of boiling water to make a kind of 'cuppa soup'; this makes a delicious broth. Make it only once or twice a day for variety. You can also boil up a lot of different vegetables, then pour off the liquid and drink it. Place the vegetables in the fridge and make a soup or patties out of them when you come off your juice cleanse.

Use organic fruit and vegetables when available. If you are unable to get organic produce, just soak the fruit or veggies in a sink filled with water and 15 ml of apple cider vinegar for five minutes before juicing. Peel the skin off all fruit and vegetables cut off the unsightly bits and always use the freshest produce available to you at the time. Don't use rotting food for juicing. Buy or grow the best you can get and always use it as fresh as you can.

Another option for the juice cleanse is to make a seaweed broth. Take some dried seaweed, add it to water and bring to the boil for five minutes. Stay pure on this diet and don't chew anything; this gives your digestive tract a rest and enables you to power up with energy whilst detoxing.

The juice cleanse is good for three days. If you go longer, you can expect days four to five to be really low energy days as your body has adjusted to the process of cleansing and is eliminating poisons very fast and very effectively. These are the days when you will be flushing toxins and have up to 20 times the normal amount of poison in your bloodstream. Rest on these days and thank your body for its powerful eliminative ability. Days 6 to 10 are awesome, and you will be on a natural high and just want to get out in the garden, walk, swim and feel a zest for life. Stop at day 10, change to a different diet, like the wholesome vegetarian detox plan, and you will be thriving for months afterwards.

Don't take any herbal supplements when you do a ten-day juice cleanse unless these supplements are supervised by your Health Care Practitioner. It's good to take herbs before a cleanse to prepare your body and after a cleanse to restore your body. But during the juice cleanse, don't swallow anything that involves any kind of digestion other than the simple assimilation of juices.

It should be pure juice and nothing else to give your body the maximum benefits on all levels, including digestive tract resting. This is a passive detox and is very positive in health care for illness and probably one of the best ways to give your body the cleansing, rest and nutrition it requires for healing.

You must properly consult with your Health Care Practitioner who is clear about these processes. It's not easy at first, but it can become easier and even fun. Whenever you are sick, think of the juice cleanse as one of the first cures. This way, you may be able to enjoy good health and vitality without the involvement of the traditional medical systems.

There are popular juice cleansing regimes that involve coffee enemas to be used in conjunction with juice cleansing. This adds an extra dimension to your cleansing and really gets the poisons moving out of your body!

Mono juice cleansing, where you only have one type of juice, for example, red grape juice, is also a very effective cleansing plan. There are many illnesses that require medical intervention; however, there are many that can be cured with the help of Mother Nature and some time. There are many books available on various juices and their healing properties.

A juice cleanse is a little time out from the rigmarole of life, giving your body time to heal, time to look at what's going on and a clearer mind for what decisions you will make for all aspects of your future. It is caring, loving, self-respect at one of its primary and most important levels. To cleanse on juices is to allow yourself the grace of healing, the grace of time and the respect to say that your body really knows what is best. You don't need to look outside for the obvious; it all just happens naturally.

CHAPTER EIGHTEEN

There are many ways to detox and cleanse

The best thing you can do if you want to detox is to start with the easier options and work your way towards the more strict and disciplined cleansing methods through time if you choose. Remember, whichever way you choose to detox is good. It's better to make the effort with a simple programme than to try for a really strict detox and stop altogether because it's too hard.

If you can just start off with a morning of fruit or an evening of veggie soup, this is good. Then you can progress to a detox cocktail party with a few friends and have fun with the concept. Perhaps then you'll feel ready to try the wholesome vegetarian detox plan. Or perhaps a weekend of relaxing juices appeals to you. Whatever works for you is good, there's no right or wrong way to detox.

Junk food

The cleansing programmes listed here may appear very simple to someone who doesn't have a junk food habit. But there are many people who would find a day without cola or lollies a detox in itself. So, a day without these products for them certainly is a detox. For coffee lovers, a day without caffeine can be very difficult, and you may well find yourself with a headache. In this case, take it slowly and wean yourself off it. You don't have to get the detox perfect the first time around. Be kind to yourself and remember that your Wellness Zone is a lifetime plan of wellness, and you need to take it gradually and always keep up the good intentions.

Bread

Gluten-free breads are the best. But for somebody who enjoys and is used to fluffy white bread, this option doesn't sound very appealing at all. White bread is like glue in your digestive tract. It stops nutrients being absorbed, and it creates many illnesses of the bowel. Stay away from white bread as much as you can. If you do a cleanse and the only thing you eliminate from your diet is white bread, this is a good start. White bread is junk food.

Sugar

If you like white sugar, or white death, then you would do well to wean yourself off this substance before you have a detox. Raw sugar is slightly better, but really all sugars are fast GI foods and create havoc with your pancreas and the hormones glucagon and insulin. It is because of white sugar that our society has such an increase in 'Type 2' diabetes. If you could lose the taste for sugary foods and additives then you will have more success with removing poisons from your body. You will also find that you don't have so many mood and energy swings. Learn to have wholesome honey in very small amounts, at least this way you will be getting some nutrition into the bargain. Or better still try the herb stevia, which is good for natural sweetening without the negative interference to your blood glucose levels.

Table salt

Add pure sea salt to your food. This is beneficial as it cleanses the lymph nodes in your body. However, when the salt contains anti-caking agents, such as common table salt, you could be in for real trouble as these agents are thought to block the lymph nodes. Also, remember that salted foods become very hard. Think about the cardiovascular system, as all that salt passes through you are hardening your arteries and veins. That's enough to make you keep a check on quantity.

Add fresh herbs to your food as a flavour treat, and you will notice that the less salt you have in your diet, the less you will want it. Remember the saying, 'where salt goes, water follows', the fastest path to fluid retention is too much salt in your diet.

Lose weight

If you decide to have a cleanse to lose weight, know that it will take more than a good detox to keep the weight off. You may very well lose from 2 to 6 kilos a week on a detox plan, but once you go back to your old ways of eating, the weight will probably quickly return. Don't ever be conned by marketing that says you will lose a load of weight with a detox plan; this is not long-term weight loss. Each of us has between 1 and 6 kilos of putrid waste matter somewhere in our digestive tract. When you go on a proper detox plan you should eliminate that waste, or at least some of it. However, it is natural for this waste to build up again and unless you start to detox regularly this is what will happen. One of the main advantages of regular detoxing is that you keep yourself clean, and the putrid matter doesn't get to build up again. You can manage your weight with regular cleansing, but that involves changing your eating patterns and the foods eaten to be more cleansing and healthy all the time, not just detox time!

Don't worry about what others think of your detox

A cleansing programme is very personal, and it's not the kind of information that most people want to hear about. Only those who are concerned for their Wellness Zone and who want to detox will detox. You don't have to do it, but when you start you may become so enthusiastic that you will want everyone else to join you. Share the information if requested and only follow it up if the other person mentions it first and makes an effort themselves. You can never control another person's dietary habits. Parents have some control over what their offspring are eating only until a certain age or social position changes that control. But the rest of us need to make our own decisions about what we eat and don't eat.

Make the time to detox by prioritising it in your life. You may need to avoid social engagements and even plan a detox in your diary a few months ahead so that nothing interferes. Nothing is worse than you adding extra worry to your detox programme by trying to keep other people happy instead of looking after yourself and getting the most from each moment. Only talk to people whom you trust and know will be supportive of any detox plan. If you need assistance, make sure you contact your Health Care Practitioner and discuss any problems you are having with your programme.

Sometimes it's even better to stay silent about your detox and just get on with it quietly. You will find a personal strength of resolve when you find yourself in situations where others are eating and drinking normally, and you are enjoying the fresh foods allowed on your special detox plan. Because you are special, you also need to remember that every detox is special.

Vitamin C therapy

Vitamin C (ascorbate, ascorbic acid) has varying activity in the body at different levels of intake. At low levels of consumption, vitamin C is like a trace nutrient, you need very little of it to stay alive, but without any at all you die. Even 60 mg a day will prevent scurvy; however, this is the minimum, and at this dose you will not have optimal health. Most animals make their own vitamin C; however, we can't, so it's an essential nutrient and the more stressed you become, the more vitamin C you will need in your diet. It's also a very good detox tool and at moderate levels of consumption, say 500 to 1500 mg per day for an adult, the vitamin works to build health and acts as an antioxidant. Research shows fewer colds and the severity and duration of influenza is less. However, it is at high levels, say 8000 to 40,000 mg per day for an adult, that we begin to obtain therapeutic properties from the vitamin. This can be taken orally or intravenously.

At the therapeutic level, vitamin C has antihistamine, antitoxin, antibiotic and antiviral properties. The pharmacological effects of a vitamin at high concentration are what turns this simple vitamin into a powerful medicine. If your body wants 35,000 mg of vitamin C to fight an infection, 10,000 mg won't get the same results. The key is to take enough vitamin C, take it regularly through the day and take it long enough for it to work effectively as a detox tool, medicine and amazing natural answer to many simple illnesses.

If you want to have a vitamin C flush to cleanse your liver, intestines and cells of any toxins, viruses, colds, cases of flu or general illness, then do the following. Get a good quality pure vitamin C powder such as calcium ascorbate, or a good blend of vitamin C and bioflavonoids, which help its absorption. Take one teaspoon of the powder for every 50 kilos in body weight, mixed with a glass of juice. That is roughly 5000 mg per 50 kilos or 1000 mg for every 10 kilos in body weight. Follow this recipe every hour until you have diarrhoea, this is when you will be at saturation point and when many of the poisons in your body are flushed with the vitamin C therapy.

This diarrhoea is not too uncomfortable and will only last until a build-up of waste has been eliminated from your digestive tract. Now, you need to continue to take the vitamin C until you are well again. A therapeutic dose is technically a dose that is sufficient to rid the body of poisons but insufficient to cause diarrhoea again. So, for every 50 kilos in body weight, you could take 5000 mg of powder three times a day, with approximate five hour periods between doses. This would help your body recover faster and more effectively.

If you are under stress then a good daily dose of vitamin C would be one teaspoon (5000 mg) in a glass of juice, one or two times a day. It makes sense that because we don't produce our own vitamin C, we will really thrive if we take some in stressful times. This will help repair your adrenal glands, help your liver detox and also give you energy.

Conditions helped by vitamin C therapy include diphtheria, staph and strep infections, herpes, mumps, spinal meningitis, mononucleosis, shock, stress, viral infections, arthritis, polio, drug addiction withdrawal treatments, toxicity and poisoning, prostate illness and many other inflammatory conditions. It's best to work with your Health Care Practitioner when using this therapy and remember to generally incorporate vitamin C into your diet in a good daily dose that will allow it to act effectively to help prevent illness and act as a super antioxidant.

Herbal colon cleansing

The focus for good health is your colon

Many illnesses today can be avoided if we have a clean digestive tract. This involves regular colon cleansing to rid the body of unwanted toxins and waste material. Chronic conditions including; psoriasis, eczema, chronic fatigue, cancer, insomnia, obesity, depression, irritability, memory loss, arthritis, Crohn's disease, diverticulitis, irritable bowel syndrome, parasites and weakened immunity can be improved and relieved with herbal colon cleansing.

What is the colon?

The colon starts where your small intestine ends. Basically, the role of the colon is to reabsorb liquid back into your system, pass nutrients through to your liver for reprocessing and assimilation, and of course to eliminate the unneeded waste matter from the body in the form of faeces.

There are three main parts to the colon (large intestine). The first is the ascending colon that runs up the lower right-hand side of your abdomen and ends at a sharp turn left called the hepatic flexure. When chyme (liquid matter) passes up through this part of the colon it is very slushy and full of liquid as well as waste products. The second part of the colon is called the transverse colon. Here is where the liquid is reabsorbed through to your hepatic portal vein and carried across to the liver for recycling of nutrients. The chyme at this point becomes the hard faecal matter that we eliminate as waste product from the anus. The transverse colon ends at the splenic flexure, which is located on the left-hand side of your abdomen, just under your last rib bone. The descending colon is where the eliminated matter rests until peristalsis (smooth muscle movement) pushes it out of your body, passing the rectum and anus.

Auto-intoxication can create health problems

The colon is very important as it is the base where your body either passes clean fluid back into the system for recycling, or it passes toxic fluid back into your system for recycling at the transverse section. There are many small pockets in the colon, which is about two and a half cm round. These small pockets are where old, putrefied waste accumulates and creates trouble for your health.

When we pass clean fluid back into the liver, this eases the stress on our body and allows for a healthy system. However, when we pass toxic fluid back into the bloodstream from the colon, we can create auto-intoxication, which is dangerous to your health as it allows your body to recycle dirty and unhealthy liquids. This adds stress to the whole system, including your liver and kidneys, which have to filter the toxic matter.

If we just go about our normal eating habits and don't bother to cleanse the colon, then eventually you will have a build-up of waste matter that compacts itself against the colon wall and all fluids that are reabsorbed into your body will have to pass through this toxic compacted filter. Auto-intoxication is when you pass waste matter back into your body that technically should have been eliminated a long time ago. This compacted matter along the colon wall can become a breeding ground for unfriendly flora, parasites and mucus as well as uneliminated waste matter. These parasites excrete their own toxins and wastes which you then recycle through your body. Imagine the damage this can do on a cellular level. The healthiest solution is to eliminate your own waste quickly, keeping your body healthy without this added burden which can lead to all manner of chronic health problems.

Herbal colon cleansing techniques

For the best results, combine your herbal colon cleanse with a reduced diet containing no processed food, alcohol, caffeine, heavy proteins, wheat or cereals. Intestinal cleansing involves sweeping the digestive tract clear of putrefied and accumulated waste using fibre such as oat bran and rice bran combined with water and some cleansing herbs.

The idea behind intestinal cleansing is that you spend a week or two taking a simple and unprocessed diet containing mostly fresh fruit and vegetables. Often you will only consume juices or raw foods. The diet will depend upon your physical health and lifestyle at the time and can vary from water fasting to a delicious vegetarian diet. This intestinal cleansing has become very popular as a boost for energy and also for those wishing to have the added benefit of losing a few extra kilos.

It is estimated that the average adult has from 2 to 9 kilos of uneliminated waste matter in their digestive tract at any point in time. The intestinal cleansing method is a boost to your system as it tunes up the smooth muscles in the digestive tract increasing peristalsis, which is the method your body uses to move food through the system. If you have slow peristalsis, then you will have slow digestion, poor elimination and an increased chance of having accumulated waste, which can result in auto-intoxication as well as many other chronic diseases which result from a putrid system.

The intestinal cleanse can be targeted to any part of your digestive tract, specifically to help with; parasites, accumulated waste removal, liver detoxification, improving absorption, leaky gut repair and bowel cleansing.

Herbs can help

The best herbs for colon cleansing, in conjunction with a cleansing diet are the ones that gently sweep away toxins and release parasites and unwanted material from your body effectively and gently. Once you start to use herbs for cleansing the colon, then you will notice that you are also taking measures to cleanse your liver, kidneys, bloodstream and cells simply because you are taking the strain off the eliminative organs by recycling good clean blood.

You can pick and choose the herbs you need to help with your cleanse depending upon the time you want to cleanse and the desired outcome. Talk with your Health Care Practitioner about a personalised programme.

Black walnut is an important colon cleansing herb as it increases peristalsis by toning the colon wall with its tannin action. It removes the nasty parasites and is very high in iodine which helps increase metabolism, encouraging improved bowel function. Black walnut is acidic in action helping remove unwanted floras and alkaline-loving yeast.

The acid-producing lactobacillus acidophilus appears unaffected by the presence of black walnut, whereas the unwanted floras just disappear. Haemorrhoids are also relieved with black walnut.

Aloe vera is healing and cleansing and tonifying to your colon. Aloe is good to use for relieving inflammation and is often combined with other colon cleansing herbs to help remove the heavy, built-up mucus lining from the edges of the bowel wall.

Peppermint taken daily in the form of tea is excellent to deodorise the colon and helps relax the smooth muscle, which can relieve spastic colon.

Berberis vulgaris (Barberry) controls the overgrowth of *Candida albicans* and operates as a bactericide making this herb excellent to combine in your herbal colon cleansing programme. Berberine, the primary alkaloid in berberis, is a potent antibiotic, astringent and antifungal.

Cascara sagrada is a herbal laxative that contains bitter compounds that increase peristalsis, act as a purgative, increase the flow of bile and improve the growth of friendly bacteria in the colon. Cascara is regularly used for constipation, liver congestion, dyspepsia, gallstones, haemorrhoids, jaundice and intestinal parasites.

Slippery elm is known to have a demulcent, emollient and wound healing effect on the digestive tract. The demulcent expectorant effects of this herb assist in releasing old mucous straps from the colon lining. The bark powder of slippery elm works as a viscous fibre, lowers the bowel transit time, absorbs toxins from the colon and regulates intestinal flora.

Senna leaf contains sennosides that have a cathartic effect by stimulating peristalsis of the large intestine to bring about bowel action in six to ten hours. The sennosides are absorbed from the small intestine to act on the nerves of the large intestine which stimulates the action of the colon. The anthraquinones are absorbed, and the laxative effect can be carried to breastfed babies through the milk. Senna also causes some gripping pains and is best taken with carminative herbs such as ginger, peppermint and fennel.

Paw paw leaves, stems and fruits have been used to aid digestion and elimination. Papain as enzymes, cut long-chain proteins into smaller chains and individual amino acids whilst in the digestive tract. Papain helps digest fats and carbohydrates into useable compounds. Paw paw also acts to eliminate parasites and microbes from the colon as the protein-rich cell membranes can be susceptible to paw paw's proteolytic enzymes.

PART III

THE ENERGY ZONE

CHAPTER NINETEEN

What is energy for wellness?

The low down on energy

Energy is created in each cell of your body, and it can be abundant, balanced or deficient. If you have an abundance of energy, then you are more likely to be active and capable of achieving your tasks effectively and creatively. If you have balanced energy, you will have the ability to think clearly and act accordingly. However, if you have a deficiency in energy, then you will suffer many consequences associated with this deficiency, including ill health and lack of motivation and inspiration. We all want to have a balanced energy zone, and we all want optimal wellness.

There are many ways that we can choose to use our energy. Each moment is a new opportunity to observe yourself and see whether you are creating optimal energy or using it up in ways that will eventually lead to a depreciation or deficit. How you use your energy is a personal choice; the decisions you make today will affect how you feel tomorrow. Energy is not just limited to how you are physically. There are systems in your body that can be utilised in ways that will either enhance or deplete your energy. Think about how you use your energy and make conscious choices to help your Wellness Zone.

Energy is currency

Energy is the currency we operate on at all levels in our lives. It's an awesome and amazing life we live when we think about this currency. You can decide what energy you will use to think any thought, feel any emotion and experience any experience. All we have is our response, and that response is energy. There are so many ways to look at energy, and it deserves our utmost respect because without energy we are literally nothing. With energy, we have control of our lives and are able to decide at any point what we will do about any situation, whether good or bad.

Your Wellness Zone is dependent on how you use your energy. It's important for you to understand that energy is a free-rolling currency. There is no limit to how much of it you can attain. Every day we need to look at how we intend to expend all types of energy and what ultimately we do with this energy. It is the result of who we are, and what we do or don't achieve for ourselves.

Energy is what you need to feed your body. Break food down into nutrients, absorb those nutrients, assimilate them and eliminate the wastage. That basic currency converts to lifestyle and wellness. Your Wellness Zone is dependent upon you filtering through the different types of energy that you require each day and deciding how you will adapt that energy into your own lifestyle. This is your Wellness Zone.

How you choose to use your energy is entirely your business. However, if you use certain types of energy too often, then you run the risk of deteriorating health and wellness. This is not a good position to be in. There's an energy bank in your body, and this needs to be constantly topped up with new energy. If you use more energy than you replace, eventually you will experience some kind of consequence to your health. This can take many forms; however, the most common today are chronic fatigue syndrome, depression, burnout, hypertension, cardiovascular problems and even auto-immune diseases. Also, genetic weaknesses can come to the forefront in our lives when we have used too much energy and are not able to replace it satisfactorily.

Avoid illness with appropriate use of energy

Many illnesses and diseases today could be avoided if there were more consciousness of energy patterns, and efforts were made to avoid the types of energy that wear you down and deplete your resources. Make sure you enhance the types of energy that bring you happiness, good health and a balanced lifestyle. When we consider the primary aspects of good health for your Wellness Zone, the first thing to consider is your use or misuse of energy. If you are deprived of good nutrition and put yourself under undue stress for long periods of time, you will be a prime candidate for illness in some form.

Illness and disease are not only caused by physical, genetic or environmental factors. As you well know, illness and disease can follow quickly after emotional upsets, mental strains and traumatic situations.

Often our immunity is compromised, and we have a nervous system that is stretched and stressed through trying to take on too much. Now this concept of 'too much' is different for each of us. We all have different tolerance levels to any aspect of our health. This is where diet, genetics and attitude certainly have a big part to play in your day-to-day health and wellness.

The energy levels that you choose to focus on have a large part to play in your Wellness Zone. This is true for both the way you perceive any situation and the way you cope and respond. This is where energy is such a biggie on your wellness agenda. Often we forget that we have energy and that we soak up or project certain energies. We often forget to be aware of how we are responding to any situation. Certain people can cope with large doses of stress, emotional upset, mental fatigue, or even physical endurance, whilst someone else may not cope or respond well to the same experience.

We can learn to control our energy by understanding patterns in our own lives and learning what we can do to help ourselves become more balanced. Also, by accepting the lifestyle choices, we have made and knowing how to enhance those on an energetic level. Yes, you can change the responses to any situation if you try. It takes a bit of discipline, a few herbs, a dose of good nutrition and a mentally open and perceptive attitude to change, for this to work. If you want an optimal Wellness Zone and you want to selectively choose when and where to use your energy, then this section of the book can be most helpful.

Herbs can help your energy

Energetic herbs have the beautiful combination of being physically beneficial to the person who takes them, as well as being able to carry the energy of the medicine deep into your cells and allow the vibration to focus on the intuitive side of illness and disease. There's an old saying that we carry our memories in our bones. This suggests that every experience you ever have is stored in some unknown and highly developed system within our bones and cells.

In energetic healing, the idea is that you get to the core of these memories and release the negative and blocked patterns that are creating illness or threatening your development in some way. These memories need to be given a short sharp shift. They need to be deleted from the programme and replaced with a good healthy energy that will help you become a healthier person. If you think that you have unresolved issues, bad memories or diseases and illnesses re-creating themselves in your life, then a tad of awareness about how you can change your energy habits and some lovely herbs that are going to bring you back into balance again will help.

The way to good cellular health is through good cellular energy patterns being created and vibrating through your whole body. You can only be a happier person when you have healthy cells. There's a growing sense and feeling of wholeness and wellness when you are thinking health care on this level. You will become very selective in what medicines you choose to use, and you may also find that you will need fewer medicines as time goes on.

The way to good cellular health is through good physical nutrition that is targeted at whole-body health. We need to approach health care and energetic wellness from the top. The top is the brain and the master hormonal secretions. Then we work our way to the body and its specifics.

Herbal medicine can be used for energetic healing with flower remedies, crystals and other natural substances. Also, we use the sense of smell in aromatherapy. Nutrition has a big part to play in all aspects of health, and it does matter what you eat. If you have good food then this will be reflected in your Wellness Zone. You will vibrate to the food you eat today. Today's health truly is based on yesterday's diet!

Genetic energetic medicines

Genetics are very important when we deal with energy, wellness and future health. You see, if you combine genetic history (which shows potential weaknesses and strengths), with environment (which indicates the potential health hazards present today) and attitude (which indicates cellular health and energetic vibrations), you get a pretty good idea of what ballpark you are playing in and what needs to be done today to enhance your health for tomorrow. So, when you think about your health and the health of your future generations, please take these genetic influences into account. This way you'll be able to assess what nutrients, herbals or other medicines are required to hopefully avoid the onset of illness. This is appropriate preventative medicine.

None of us can afford to ignore this aspect of our Wellness Zone. So, if you have a family history of any illness or disease, or if you know that the environment or attitude you have is not in your best interests, please consider seeking help today to change the situation. Because a gram of prevention is better than a kilo of cure!

Each and every illness that you will ever encounter is a reflection of your energy, a reflection of how you have been abusing your body, or how genetics have come to the fore through certain aspects of your health. Medicines can be given to you based on your genetic weaknesses so that you are in a position to minimalise the impact that genetics may cause your body in time. Herbal medicine is very good in this arena of preventative care.

Use your energy well every day

If you don't consider your own health and your Wellness Zone as a top priority in life, then you are asking for trouble in the future. If you repeat the bad business of typical day-to-day grind where you aren't getting enough exercise, your diet isn't good, and your energy levels are declining then you may not have good health to enjoy the future. Stress and overdoing life are certain ways to create disease and illness in your body. You need to consider attitude and the way you perceive energy for optimal health and wellness.

Did you know that you generate more energy when you exercise regularly? Did you know that being a lounge lizard could actually be more exhausting for you in the long run than being a fit person? It's not hard to be a lounge lizard; you may be one unconsciously. Many people are very busy mentally and don't focus on physical activity. If you are not making the effort for cardiovascular activity for one hour at least four days a week, then you are a lounge lizard and are setting yourself up for illness just by the fact that you do not exercise for your body to operate optimally.

Bad business is putting your energy levels last and not considering the consequences of having a limited supply. Good business is putting yourself first when it comes to energy and making sure you create enough for yourself every day. You need to make the extra effort to move your body and generate energy; today's world has become lazy with appliances and transport systems literally stopping the need for you to work physically hard. We all know the consequences of a physically lazy but mentally stressed lifestyle as we see more and more people suffer from chronic fatigue, chronic illness and cardiovascular diseases.

Be aware of your energy each moment in time

Being aware of the way you use your energy is a powerful tool in finding your Wellness Zone and staying in it as long as possible. Your Wellness Zone is individual and celebrates the things that keep you unique. The idea is that you find your own path to health and wellness. This is not the same for everyone.

Your Wellness Zone is about being the best person, in the best health, that you can possibly be on any and every day. You need to take tiny steps. For example, you may find that you are having a hard time in a relationship or work environment. You are living predominantly in stressed and nervous energy zones, burning out your adrenals with worry each day and not replenishing your energy. This is living outside of your Wellness Zone. You would be happier if the energy was calmer and you were not so stressed and rushed. If this is the case, then you need to understand that the situation is temporary. It's okay to live outside your Wellness Zone occasionally. You can make the effort to mitigate negative effects that may occur by taking herbs and nutritional supplements and making some relaxing lifestyle choices as required when you find some time!

If you are in a position where you know your health will suffer if you keep up the bad habits for too long, then you can make the best effort to help yourself because you are aware of your Wellness Zone and aware of the need to do something about it. It doesn't remove the stress. You are treating it in a different way which ensures a different outcome and ultimately a healthier outcome if you make small efforts every day for wellness.

How you use your energy is habitual. Often we slip into a comfort zone that is self-sabotaging. Often we do the same things with our energy for so long that we don't even know we're doing it. That's why the Wellness Zone is such an enlightening gift that you can give yourself and teach your children and loved ones about. It's your opportunity and way to express your individuality, to live each day as you decide and to transcend any old patterns of energy usage that you are sick of following. It's like shedding an old skin and allowing yourself to live in beautiful energy whenever you can, anywhere, anytime!

Remember that there is no right or wrong way to use energy. You can't just stop the world and take a break from everything. However, you can slow it down, enjoy the journey and note what turns you on, what helps you and what makes for a higher quality life. These are the types of energy that help you. You can still be busy and still achieve what you need to achieve, and you just don't have to treat your energy or your body in the ways you have in the past. Let go of that energetic cellular stress and those tight shoulders and neck muscles. Let go of that nervous twitch and that worrying thought you had in your mind. Let go of the overactive energy status that can lead to many illnesses and limitations as we become older.

As they say, an angry 20-year-old may look cute, but an angry old man certainly doesn't! So, on that level, if you've been holding onto anger, pain or anything that doesn't help you live a quality and optimal existence, then let it go. You will have to let these things go one day. Whether it's today or in the future, let them go, move on and live happily, as often as you can. It's no good clogging up your mind with energy that may block the good thoughts and feelings from your body. It's important that you look at your Wellness Zone and be open minded about where you are and where you are headed.

It's all very well to think about your health in terms of energy levels. However, we need to make our life as 'well' as we can every day. In order for you to do this, you need to think about the physical, mental, emotional and soulful areas in your life that are second nature to you. So when you are thinking about how you feel and how you are addressing your energy, then you need to look and relate this to the everyday circumstances that you experience. This means that your physical self needs to be looked after in certain ways that allow you to use the energy you want in the best manner possible.

The same goes with the mental, emotional and soulful aspects of your life. You need to acknowledge the other aspects of yourself on an energetic and vibrational level. Negative energy may contribute to depression, emptiness or obesity as people feel depleted or deprived in ways they cannot explain or understand. Take a little time on the energy aspects of your life and enhance the energies that you strive towards. Have empathy with yourself and others as you become aware of how energy is used and reflected around you.

Stay in touch with your energy

You are always using one type of energy or another. You are either feeling level and in some control over your energy or you may be feeling uneven and not in control. There are many ways to think about energy. Once you have the lowdown, you will be aware of what emphasis you place on your energy zone every day. Think about it for a minute. What kind of energy do you feel now? Can you understand it for yourself? How you feel energetically is intrinsically transferred to others who are in your immediate environment.

You need to understand what types of energy you want or need to enhance your life and what types of energy you need to minimalise or eliminate for your own Wellness Zone.

CHAPTER TWENTY

Energies to enhance your Wellness Zone

Physical energy

Physical energy is cellular energy, and cellular energy is mitochondrial energy. The mitochondria is the battery of your cells; they are your mini powerhouses that live in each cell, each organ and each system in your body. So, for true health, we need to keep our cells full of good clean nutrients and make sure we are producing more mitochondrial (true physical) energy than we are using. When you are toxic with poisons from the environment or emotional or mental sickness, then that is directly reflected in your cells, which directly relates to your total health. The physical energy you generate is in your control.

Many people wonder why they become sick; they go for years following the same unhealthy habits and suffering accordingly. Often illness creeps up on us, especially when we don't expect it. The physical manifestation of illness can sometimes be attributed to the physical misuse and storage of negative, sick and inappropriate energy on a physical level. This physical energy is the final layer of energy expressed in your body. Energy needs to work its way from the other levels of mental and emotional fields before it becomes real, living and breathing in the physical.

We can look after ourselves on a physical level and make sure we have appropriate physical health in order to create and maintain an appropriate Wellness Zone in our lives. This often means sorting yourself out on other levels first. Often you need to get rid of emotional and mental hurts and old, outmoded belief structures before you can have good physical health and good physical energy. You need to be aware of your physical energies at each moment, also of contributing factors to your energy levels. You can take measures each day to ensure you are being fair to yourself and your physical energies. It's an important part of your Wellness Zone and something that needs to be considered daily.

Have you ever noticed that the more energy you use physically, the more you tend to accumulate? This is especially noticeable when you are well-nourished and feeling buoyant. However, when you step over the threshold to exhaustion, then physical energy will deplete very quickly. This needs to be monitored and kept in balance.

Good cellular energy equals healthy energy for today. It also equals optimal physical health with minimal opportunity for illness and disease. What a wonderful world it would be if we could all have good healthy physical energy. Imagine what could be achieved in one day! It's awesome. You need to have good physical energy to reach your own personal potential. Give your cells the nutrients and support they need to create your best physical energy today! This doesn't have to be the best energy you could ever aspire to, but it should be equal to or better than the energy you had yesterday.

Always think in the best way possible for you at any point in time. Whenever you get a negative thought, replace it with a beautiful physical thought of wellness. Physical energy is important; without it, you will surely be frailer and less successful in all your endeavours, and this energy only comes when you are in balance. You can burn out your adrenals, your nervous system and your general health as much as you like but ultimately one day you may want to rebalance all of that to create what is actually your born right, abundant physical energy. This will happen with a good diet, a lifestyle that suits you and good thinking regarding your own health. Only you can do that.

When people exercise regularly and take time at regular intervals to go for long walks, swims or runs, they tend to handle stress better, use less adrenal energy and also have abundant physical energy. However, when people don't exercise or make the effort for a regular routine in their lives for this type of activity, then they tend to have less physical energy as a result. The idea that you can save energy for later by not using it now doesn't work. Once you slip into physical laziness, you can stay there because we can all naturally be lazy without any effort at all! That doesn't mean that if you rest between periods of activity that you will lose energy. In fact, it's quite the opposite. People who exercise regularly tend to have a greater ability to relax and physically quieten their pace, thereby recuperating and allowing more energy for later.

And so it goes, when you use physical energy, you tend to make more, but when you use nervous or adrenal energy or too much mental energy, then that tends to deplete all energies. This downward spiral in energy stores can lead to chronic fatigue syndrome or other degenerative conditions and illnesses.

Regular daily exercise for an hour or so is perfect. The idea is to move as much as you can and to be active in your life instead of taking the less physical option. Make time to create physical energy. Walk where you can instead of driving or using public transport. Take that mountain trek holiday. Go kayaking along some awesome river this summer instead of lying around at the beach.

Energy is such a special and important commodity in your Wellness Zone; it is something that is so fundamental to your health and wellness that you should be grateful for each new mitochondrial cell that is developed to help you feel enlivened and bubbly and as physically active as you can.

The interesting thing is that if you don't have energy, then you want more. However, if you have a lot of energy, it can be easily be taken for granted. So, you need to take it in baby steps, take each day as it comes and make the most of the energy that you can muster. Look after yourself on every level. Try to be optimally healthy because nothing depletes energy like sickness, and nothing can increase energy like good cellular nutrition. So detox, de-stress, balance and readdress everything you do when you want to increase energy. It is something we all want lots of, and the only person who can give it to you is yourself. It's not a case of just deciding today that you will have more energy, you must create it, it is like the prize for all the goodness you have been doing for yourself. Physical energy is a true manifestation of being in your Wellness Zone and the knowledge that you are thriving.

Herbs and supplements to support physical energy

Keep your cells clean by taking milk thistle and dandelion regularly. Take Coenzyme Q10 and maca as well as essential fatty acids such as spirulina and fish oils. Take a special combination of olive leaf, echinacea purpurea root, black walnut and cat's claw to keep you healthy on a cellular level. In combination, these herbs are very balancing and antimicrobial and will help to strengthen your immunity. Nettle is good to increase cellular integrity.

The B group vitamins in a complex, including folic acid and Vitamin B12, are good to help support optimal development and growth of all new cells. Taking an iron supplement or eating iron-rich foods can help increase physical energy. Cooking in an iron pan is beneficial as the iron is absorbed into your food. Eating unprocessed foods is one key to good physical energy. Also if this food is unadulterated with toxins from insecticides and pesticides, that will help to keep the strain off your liver and other organs.

Many herbs will help increase your physical energy as they will put various parts of your body back into balance again, add fresh garden herbs into your meals. Your potentially weaker areas may need rebalancing before you are able to claim the prize of physically abundant energy. For example, if your hormones need to be balanced, your eliminative organs need to work well, and your digestive tract needs to be assimilating nutrients. You may also need to eat good nourishing foods and ensure that stress is managed. Take whatever herbs and supplements you need to support all areas of your being before you can expect to have abundant physical energy.

Mental energy

This is something that we all need to consider as a priority in our Wellness Zone. How many times have you had an idea and then thought 'Oh, I can't be bothered doing that'? This may be because you are finding it too exhausting to use your mental energy to capacity. Often we choose the easy option in life. This is the option when we have to think the least and relax the most mentally. This is all very nice for the present moment but, if you are honestly true to yourself, and if you really want your Wellness Zone to work in your life, then you need to readdress how you use your mental energy and make a point of using it effectively from now on.

You may make negative mental comments to yourself, or you may think long and hard about something, only to become more confused than ever. Nobody can tell you what to think or how to think it. This is where you decide what you really want to help yourself achieve your goals for the future.

It's your mental energy that makes the decisions in your life. This wonderful energy that allows you to make the decisions for success or failure in any venture you undertake. This is a very powerful energy indeed. It's the kind that needs feeding, supporting and encouraging.

Your brain loves good nutrition. Many nutrients are able to cross the blood-brain barrier and assist you in having clearer mental function. Make sure you eat protein because this breaks down in your digestive tract to amino acids that then reform and are added to co-factors and co-enzymes to create new cells in your body. Your brain is a priority zone for nutrition.

Some co-enzymes are really good brain food, and Coenzyme Q10 is one of the best. Take 100–400 mg daily for really focused mental energy in combination with protein foods and lots of fluids to keep all the electrical responses related to the master of your nervous system, the brain, operating optimally.

Yes, mental energy is hard or easy depending upon what you feed it and how you treat it. Remember that your master hormones are controlled from the brain, and every function is influenced primarily by your brain and your capacity for mental energy. Many people experience a dip in energy after having sugar and other carbohydrates. It's also interesting that many people experience a mental dip after the initial stimulating high of coffee. Mental cloudiness and exhaustion often occur after alcohol.

Sometimes the things we use to relax us, pick us up or soothe us are the very things that sabotage one of the most important types of energy we can ever wish for, clear mental energy. Mental energy is the deciding force in many aspects of your life. You can choose to change your mind at any second in time. Just because you have thought a certain way for so long doesn't mean it's the only way, and for the sake of your optimal Wellness Zone it may be outdated! The thoughts you keep today may be holding you back from that which is best for you! So, look at your mental energy. Look at what you think about. Is it a waste of time thinking what you think each day or are your thoughts wonderful and a sign of your continued growth and development as a person? Your Wellness Zone is totally dependent upon what you think about every second of every day.

Perhaps a bit of personal discipline is required on a mental level. When you are in a situation where you are unedited in the thoughts you are thinking, ask yourself why you are thinking about this now. There must be a reason. There must be something you need to learn from the thoughts you keep! We keep coming up against the same brick walls or the same lessons in life until we have mentally grasped the situation and are mentally able to resolve it. Once this has happened, we tend to be able to use our mental energy more freely without the limitation of that brick wall in the way. This must be such a common human feeling that we intrinsically all know that we need to get past one stage before we can reach the next. Therefore, sorting out your mental energy should be a priority.

You are able to visualise something and then help it become a reality simply by putting the idea in your mind and feeding it the right ingredients. A simple example is planning a holiday: you will look on the internet or talk to a travel agent; then you make decisions depending upon your budget, or you decide to go and earn the money you need to upgrade your budget break to the ideal holiday you had visualised; you make plans mentally and then physically, by booking tickets or arranging time off work; finally, often months or even years after you have made the mental decision to take a holiday, you will be there enjoying your holiday.

Or it can go all so terribly wrong, and you say to yourself 'I knew this would happen' … well did you? Yes, because you probably invested valuable mental energy into worrying about all the things that could go wrong, and you didn't prioritise your thinking by focusing on what would go right.

Use your mental energy positively and say 'It will all be fine' and with some good planning and research mentally, it can be! Well done to you if you use your mental energy well. Eat, according to the effects it will have on your mental energy, knowing what you are undertaking that day, and plan your life around this. When you get lazy, sleep and rejuvenate your mental energy, or maybe plan some slack and watch a movie.

Do you suffer from insomnia? This is a condition whereby you get to sleep either with great difficulty or too easily. Then, when you are asleep, you don't stay that way for long, an insomniac is often awake for half the night worrying about everything. If they're not worried about life, then they worry about not sleeping. This is a classic case of over-stressed mental energy.

Do you have much time for silence in your day? Do you listen to the radio or watch television at all in the day? Going to and from work with music playing in the car is a number one way to get insomnia. This is because when you are listening to any outside noise or music, you are not processing what is already in your mind that needs sorting out for the day. Instead, you are adding more energy to your mind that will need to be cleared and sorted out later.

Simply turn off the radio and avoid all noise going to and from work if you are in a stressed and busy situation. Think whilst you travel. Let your mind wander. Now when you get to work, leave the music off and when you get home again leave the television off for the evening. Do this for a few days and see whether or not you sleep better. If you do, then you are using your mental energy well. You need to take the time to process mental energy daily.

Don't you think you have enough to think about during your life without all the added external distractions of noise, clouding your thinking ability and judgement? You need time to think. Small children do it beautifully. They play in the sandpit or the garden for hours on end, processing and thinking about anything. Whatever crosses their clear little minds. Try it yourself. Go and sit on the beach for an hour or so, or climb that local mountain and sit there in silence for an hour. Turn off all the noises at home and sit, think, allow your mind to wander, then quieten it and try to achieve silence in your head.

Mental energy is cleared and enhanced by you simply creating time to process the thoughts you have in your mind and allowing your head to be decluttered of all the excess thinking matter. Aim for silence and peace of mind. Let yourself breath, think about whatever you need to think about and drift in and out of consciousness daily. Do it when you go to work or when you have a break at work. Do it when you're travelling or when you're walking.

Every moment in life is meditation; it is that exactly. Because thinking peacefully and allowing thoughts to drift in and out of your mind uncluttered is the same as meditation. You will find that the more often you allow your mental energy the privilege of peaceful thinking and silence, the less cluttered your thoughts become and the clearer you are able to see yourself and what you need to think about in your day.

Mental health comes with a clear mind and uncluttered thoughts. The ideal of living in the moment mentally, whilst consciously planning the future and being able to make the right decisions at the right time is achievable. That's a fairly big call for some of you who are cluttered with thoughts and mental chatter that won't cease. So, take it one step at the time. Think less, talk less and be aware that you don't need to think all the time. Take frequent rest breaks through the day to help stay relaxed. Nothing creates a tense body faster than an over-used mind that has been working incessantly for hours on end. You must learn to stop the mental chatter and try to create a sense of peace and tranquillity in your mind.

When you wake in the middle of the night and thoughts of the day's activities swirl in your mind, you are actually setting yourself up for more stress the following day as you are not getting the rest you require. You are spending time trying to process information mentally instead of resting and processing the bigger issues and real things in your dreamtime that need sorting.

If you spend hours during the day with issues worrying you and unresolved problems running around in your mind endlessly, then you certainly don't have the time to appreciate the present moment or to focus on the bigger issues and think clearly about your life and what really needs to be dealt with. Every day deserves some silent moments that are stress-free and reflective in a light manner. Make it one of your goals each day to experience silence and lightness. Lightness of thought, comedy in thought and peacefulness. Smile unconsciously and laugh mentally whenever you can.

When you look at your mental energy today, what do you see? Are you thinking in ways that are really helping you get the best out of your life today? If not, you need to eliminate the thoughts that are counter-productive and increase the productive ones. Remember, a journey of a thousand miles begins with one step, and that step can be made today.

Make that phone call to find out about the study you are interested in or make that visit to your Health Care Practitioner to get the nutritional support you need. Make a list of reasons why you can have a better tomorrow when you use your mental energy to the best of your capacity today. Don't be lazy with mental energy; it's the quickest way to miss opportunities in life. When used properly, it's the fastest and best energy to use to help you increase, improve and enhance what you have today.

The Wellness Zone is about you, and it's about how you choose to live. No one else thinks the way you do. So go for the individual mental twist in your life. Make your Wellness Zone a beautiful mental energy zone that helps you, that stops the mental sabotage and brings goodness into your life. You can't control anything about other people; however, you can always control your response, and your mental Wellness Zone is the first place to start doing that.

Herbs and supplements to support mental energy

You can feed this energy with vitamin B complexes. All amino acids are excellent brain foods, as protein is one of your brain's favourite nutrients. L-glutamine is very good as are ginkgo biloba and other circulatory stimulating herbs. Bacopa and gotu kola are both known as brahmi herbs which increase all mental capacity. Lesser periwinkle is another favourite brain herbal. Nervine herbs help you relax into the clarity and can benefit your mental energy when you are stressed. Try some hypericum, melissa or chamomile teas mixed in with some fresh rosemary for mental clarity. You may want to boost your mental energy with green tea and ginger.

Nobody wants their mental energy depleted with toxins, such as mercury from fillings, aluminium foil or cooking pots, which make their way through the blood-brain barrier. When your liver is clean, your brain is clear too. In fact, good clean body cells equal a good clear brain. When you've had a few days of cleansing, you are thinking very clearly compared to when you have rich foods. So for a clear brain, keep your diet simple, your body clean and your nutrients optimal. Trust in the fact that your body and mind are always reflecting your nutritional status. It's easy to be overfed and undernourished; however, it takes mental vigilance to be optimally fed and optimally nourished.

Level energy

To be balanced is beautiful!

Now here's an interesting kind of energy that we don't often think about. Level is when you are in your Wellness Zone, and there is nothing extraordinary going on in your life in any way. You are emotionally at peace, mentally quiet and relaxed, physically as pain-free as you can be and feeling energised. This is level, and this is the ultimate type of energy to operate on.

Level energy is a simple type of energy and creates a very pleasurable place to be. You are not sick, tired, rushed, emotionally or mentally stressed, and you are feeling totally and completely comfortable in your mind, body and soul. Level is definitely an indicator that you are in your Wellness Zone. It is living in the present, not cluttering your mind with the past or future or anything that is distracting.

Each of us can choose a comfortable place where we like our energy to be; this is your level zone. You may thrive on a bit of mental noise, emotional stimulus or adrenal energy and need this as well to stay in your Wellness Zone. When you are able to accept varying degrees of levelness in your life, then you will find that you come to crave certain things that create level energy for you. Some people need to exercise each day to remain level, and others need to achieve certain goals before they are truly in their level comfort zone.

Level energy is about not being volatile, overly responsive or inappropriate in any given situation. It's about facing the world head-on, in a level manner that allows you the grace of time before a response to any given situation is needed. It's that breath between the present and the next moment, the feeling that you have as much control over your energy levels and your responses as possible. This is your levelness: your level-headedness, your level emotional-ness, your level physical-ness, your balanced energies and your balanced self.

You have your hang-ups, your limits and your boundaries. However, if you want to live in your level Wellness Zone, it's only you who can change your responses to any situation. It's only you who can make your world a better place by your responses. By your level energy.

Level energy goes quite deep when you think about it. It's almost a feeling, a state of being as you delve into any given moment and literally choose your response. Sift through the old worn out ones, look at the new ones and allow yourself the grace of levelness to make the choice that will be the best one for all concerned. Yes, being level is about compassion, kindness, and understanding; it is about taking the qualities in life that actually mean something good and incorporating them into your life.

We all have our various levels of confusions and toxicity to sift through to achieve this type of philosophy. No one else can do this for you. To be in your Wellness Zone, you really need to be in your level energy zone as much as you can. So, only you know how to achieve this and what you need to do in order to be as level as you can at all times. You may be sick or recovering, and you may not have the ultimate energy levels that you desire. However, when you start thinking level energy zones, then you are on the mend. It's that simple!

Once you start feeling seconds, moments or hours of level energy, then you will know it's about pure, old-fashioned good health; it's the best energy you can ever have. It represents the fact that your cells are vibrating in the present to a contented body, and you are in the optimal position to heal. Level energy represents good cellular health, and this means that you are creating good mitochondrial energy.

To be level, you need to be focused on what you are doing now, and you need to be feeling emotionally okay in order to do this. Very often, people who are undergoing emotional trauma are unable to become level, simply because there is one aspect of their lives so out of balance. When this happens, the imbalance needs to be addressed, and that aspect brought back into perspective. Likewise, if your hormones are out of balance or your diet is not optimal, you will find it harder to achieve level energy.

But you can do it ... one step at the time. One minute of level energy is like a light going on in your soul, and you will crave this kind of energy always. People who thrive on emotional dramas have not had enough level energy experiences to appreciate it's beauty. You must want level energy enough, so much that you want to create it in your life. It's not an easy path though; it's hard work. It's about breaking conventional boundaries on thoughts; it's about prioritising your own health and every aspect of your life that leads you to level energy. If you thrive on and crave level energy, you also eventually thrive on and crave silence. Appreciation is another aspect of being level. When you operate on level energy as your prioritised energy level, then often you will appreciate what is going on in your life and take time to be grateful for what you have, where you are going and how you are living your life.

You don't have to live the perfect life to be level with your energy. You are where you are. It is about doing the best with what you have at any point in time. You could be experiencing a traumatic situation which we all do from time to time. There are times when you are in mourning, grief strikes and you are down, or other times when you may feel that you have failed or been let down. There are times when you receive information that alters your plans and other times when sickness is overwhelming. It's not all in your personal control, and you can never be so ignorant as to suggest that you can be level and in control over everything. You need to go with the great river of life. Cry when you need to cry, laugh when you need to laugh, feel what you feel, be who you are. However, also realise that level energy is the energy that is most appropriate for any given situation at any given time.

Have some grace, try to be appropriate and stay in the moment. Get yourself together and then respond to what the world is offering. Be level and stay in your Wellness Zone. Be appreciative for the goodness and do your best when you are placed in a difficult situation. Act to reduce the stresses, emotional dramas and the other aspects of your life that stop you from being in your level energy zone. When you are level, enjoy and appreciate the experience and try to stay there as long as possible. Find your level energy Wellness Zone and live there, interestingly, when you find this zone you will also attract others who are feeling level energy too!

Herbs and supplements to support level energy

The best herbs to improve an already level energy state are the ones that will support it. Melissa is good as it is a mild nervine and can just keep the edge off any stresses that come your way. Also, take nutritional supplements such as zinc and a good multi to keep you level. Herbs such as nettle when you are already level, let you go that little bit further with using your energy and add a little support to help keep you level for longer. Bacopa is good as is ginkgo biloba. You don't want herbs that will increase your energy, just ones that will potentiate what's already good and level in your day. These are the adaptogenic herbs and the herbs that maintain wellness.

When you experiment with herbal medicine, you will find that there are some herbs that resonate with your energy fields. The herbs that make you feel good and energised without feeling stimulated are good level energy herbals to take to enhance this type of energy. Some suggestions are astragalus, withania and gotu kola. You may do well to have some ginseng if you are feeling level and are using this to potential. Panax is good for men, and Siberian ginseng is good for women and children.

Positive energy

Now here's something positive! You need to think positively for the highest good of yourself and your loved ones and for the greatest good of the planet. It's all about ethical positive thinking here. You need to be in your own Wellness Zone and contribute to the Wellness Zone of others, and this will happen when you think positively. When you get an idea and think you can do it, then do it. But, when that little voice comes into your head and tells you about the failure and the negative aspects, listen, tell it to disappear from your thoughts and stay positive. Because if it wasn't for positive energy, then nothing good would ever be achieved in the world, and it is to be nurtured and treated with the respect it deserves. Start thinking positively about yourself and your life. You can never have too much hope in life no matter what anyone has told you. The only boundaries you should have in your life's potential are the ones you see and are waiting to break. You can be positive.

Positive energy is especially needed when you or a loved one is sick. You need to muster up every grain of positive energy and drink it like you were in dire need of water on some desert island. Without positive energy, all the other good things about energy are useless. The limb of positive energy needs to be nurtured on the tree of life. It needs to be watered, fed, and most of all it needs to be believed. Positive energy hates cynicism; the sceptical cynics are your worst enemy. Most of you have a sceptical cynic living somewhere in your heart that needs flushing out with a glass of pure clean positive energy, this negativity is the enemy of positive energy and it needs to go.

A little bit of healthy cynicism isn't a bad thing in life, but if it's stopping you from having positive energy, then it needs to be given its marching orders. There is plenty of room for abundant, random, kind, positive thought, and there should be no room for these to be sabotaged, so keep your energy positive as much as you can. It can be difficult to muster when you are feeling unwell, so the best way to increase your positive energy is to stop negative thoughts whenever they happen and try to turn them into positive ones. The same with your speech and your actions, try to make these as positive as you can. Speak positively to others, compliment and forgive small offences easily. If you have been living in a world where you do not think positively, then today is the day to change that. And remember, when you think in negative ways, you're really hurting yourself because you live with your own memories and responses ... Try to make every response and every thought positive. If you truly can't do this, then there are some areas in your life that need help for you to be in your Wellness Zone.

Herbs and supplements to support positive energy

You can take many herbs here. If you want positive energy, take hypericum, as it will help you to be positive. Even though it is used as an anti-depressant and a nervous system balancing herb, hypericum also helps relieve pain, and it can trigger positive energy. Ginseng, astragalus and nettle also help you create positive energy. A good combination is hypericum, maca and panax ginseng extracts; take 10 ml twice a day. If you are overweight, it is easier to be depressed than when you are within a healthy weight range for your height and age. When you are within this range, you have a greater ability to keep your body in optimal health, and you can avoid or delay ill health.

When you have a wonderful attitude that brings about positive energy, you are often open and willing to try new herbs and supplements to enhance your Wellness Zone. This is good. This is where preventative medicine works at its best. When you are within your Wellness Zone and feeling positive and thinking positive thoughts, that will enhance everything around you. Talk with your Health Care Practitioner about ways that you can have optimal health, because you deserve it!

Positive energy is the best cellular breeding ground for good DNA replication and good health for the future. All herbs can help if you are specific and you target where you want improvement in your health. It could also be said that no herbs are needed because you are so positive and vibrating positive healing energy throughout your body all the time, and that's wonderful. However, herbs can help enhance the process and potentiate your health and healing in every way. When you want to enhance positive energy, juices are very good, especially carrot juice and other juices that work on cleansing the liver.

If you feel that you want to improve your positive energy, then a good detox always helps. When your liver is congested, you can often be bad-tempered, a detox helps eliminate the built-up poisons in your mind and body! Eating light meals is another way to increase positive energy. Keeping your blood sugar balanced creates a lightness of spirit. Magnesium is good to help reduce many side effects of oxidative stress; taking a magnesium supplement can help you be positive too!

Loving energy

Loving energy is one of the most powerful energies you can give yourself and others. Loving energy is strong, gentle and kind, and it's the energy we all thrive on. As little babies we live off our parents' loving energy. As we become older we strive to maintain loving energy. We seek it in the outside world and in our relationships with others more than we seek any other kind of energy. Loving energy feeds us; it fills us with love, happiness, security and a feeling and sense of placement in the world.

Loving energy is an essential type of energy for your Wellness Zone. When you consider what you want to achieve to gain optimal wellness and health in your life, then you must include loving energy as one of the basic needs and requirements. You love yourself, you are loved by your loved ones and you love them in return. You love your vocation and your lifestyle. Or do you? If you don't love what you do with your life, then change it. Why waste your time doing things you don't love doing? If you don't have a sense of direction, contentment and joy in your daily life, then you are not applying enough loving energy to what you are doing each day. Love breeds more love; this energy just wants to consume the world.

We all want loving energy, and we all deserve to love and be loved, this is quite different from positive energy. You don't necessarily have to be positive about something to love it; in other words, love is more unconditional. Often it's something that wells up inside us, and we feel out of control with excitement, desire and passion for life, that's loving energy in play. This energy can be basal and sexual, caring and compassionate, or nurturing and energy-giving, but it is always the highest energy source you can bring into any situation. The quickest way to end any conflict is through love. Loving energy is not heated mental energy that takes a lot to muster, it's rather lazy and placid in its nature, although also very active and fruitful.

It's not hard to employ loving energy into your life. Start off by feeling comfortable in your own bones. Then you need to look at the love you have already. Who is in your life, and how do you feel about them? How do you feel about your daily, weekly, monthly and annual activities? Do you really accept yourself and are you in your own Wellness Zone enough, to love yourself and love all that surrounds you no matter what the winds of change may bring?

Loving energy is about following your interests and your passions in life. Can you believe that there are people out there who don't even know what interests them? It's all about energy and about loving yourself enough to give yourself a fair chance each and every day. If you sit around bored or not knowing what to do next, then you need to start to apply some loving energy into your day and make the most of whatever needs doing. Also, try to make the most of your relationships with family and friends.

Applying random acts of kindness and senseless acts of beauty is a good motivating start point for those of you who are at a loss about the application of loving energy. Go and help a sick or elderly neighbour, volunteer somewhere where you can be useful, get a job helping others, train yourself further in areas of your greatest interest. Learn to sing if you have always wanted to sing, learn to fly a plane or snow ski and bungy jump your way out of this rut and into your ultimate Wellness Zone.

Travel, write, read a good book, do something, do anything that will create a passion for you and tune you into loving energy. Go to a yoga class, meditate by the ocean where you feel absolute peace and joy, go to your favourite restaurant for dinner and have a glass of your favourite wine. Write a long letter to an old friend and send a photo along with the letter. Reconnect with yourself, reconnect with your capacity to give, to be compassionate, caring or selfless, be a contributing wheel in the steam train of life, or a chip in the motherboard of the world. Whatever it takes to create, nurture and give yourself and your loved ones loving energy, is what will bring you the greatest joy in life. If you are able to give, then what's interesting is, that all we desire will come to us in the fullness of time.

Loving energy is about putting your life in perspective. It's about letting yourself do what you need and want to do, each and every day, with a feeling of rightfulness and the knowledge that you are following your own path in life. It's not predestined stuff we're talking about here. There are many things in life that are mutable, changeable and adaptable. Don't for one second let life trap you into some outdated mode where you are restricted and not enjoying the life you are living. Don't let loveless energy carve a path into your day. Make loving energy your preferred and encouraged energy source at every possible moment in your Wellness Zone.

Here's a little exercise for you to try. Think about a favourite activity, if you have many favourite activities, choose one that is realistic and achievable for your Wellness Zone and budget right now. Then plan, on the physical level to do this activity. It may be something quite simple like lying in bed and reading the paper all morning with no interruptions. Or it may be more elaborate, such as a holiday, a shopping spree or a night out at the local pub with some friends. Perhaps you love going to a good movie or a live show, or maybe taking the children to the beach where you can make sandcastles and lounge around eating ice-cream. Whatever you choose, this exercise will be something that you can get excited about, plan and then achieve fairly simply.

Get a notebook and start taking notes about how you feel from the beginning right through to the completion of this project. Note the excitement and the loving energy that comes through, note how you are feeling. This kind of energy can only be healthy for your mind, body and soul, and it provides the motivation that encourages and energises you to plan your next loving energy experience. When you have experienced it once you will want it more and more often. This is the power of loving energy.

Each of us needs to feel loving energy. When you are deprived of it, you are like a flower that doesn't bloom, like a wave in the ocean that doesn't form into a beautiful tubular wholeness, the sight of which makes the ocean so beautiful from the shore. If you deprive yourself of loving energy, then you will be on the shore of life, on the side-line of the circus, backstage of your own life. This is something to seriously consider when you look at your Wellness Zone and how you want to live your life; loving energy is something we all deserve to have plenty of. Don't look for others to supply you with your dose of this energy. Do it yourself in your work, your recreation and your lifestyle. When you do this, you will attract wonderful people into your life who reciprocate the loving energy you put out yourself.

Remember, loving energy is not about taking, it's about giving, and you can't be fearful when you are dealing with it either. You must be trusting; you must take risks in life to follow your interests and your passions, maybe even break some boundaries on past restrictions that you have placed upon yourself for some long-forgotten reason. Let love be a major contributor to your life, be it, feel it, send it, but on the other hand don't let others take your good nature for granted. Use that mental, positive and level energy to decide what is right and wrong with the loving energy factor in your life.

If the love isn't reciprocated in a romantic relationship, then maybe this isn't the relationship for you? Or if you're too busy giving and feel that you are not getting anything in return and you are becoming exhausted and negative maybe you are using the energy in the wrong places. Take a really good look at the love in your life, take the time to do what you need to do to get into a level Wellness Zone with your loving energy. Remember that your Wellness Zone is very personal and it is different for everybody.

Love ... the opposite of fear, the part of you that vibrates with clarity, kindness, compassion and caring for everything and everyone you encounter, every day. Animal, mineral, physical, spiritual, loving energy is what we all need.

Herbs and supplements to support loving energy

Gentle herbs that are subtle in their action are the ones to improve your loving energy. These herbs will be chosen by you and your Health Care Practitioner for their ability to get in and heal any specific parts of your body that require healing. They can also be circulatory herbs that improve your flow of energy and your blood and lymph throughout the body. These herbs that improve your loving energy are the herbs you choose to tune into to help you get through whatever blocks are holding you up on any level that may be limiting your ability for acceptance and love. In fact, bilberry is a loving energy herb, and it increases your capacity to see clearly literally, with its vision-enhancing abilities whilst acting as a cardiovascular protective.

Other cardiovascular herbs are good loving energy herbs too, such as ginkgo biloba, myrrh and hawthorn. These herbs strengthen the vascular system and help increase circulation, which can only have beneficial effects on your cardiovascular system at all levels. Love is heart, and your heart needs good clean blood flow, and sarsaparilla is wonderful for cleansing the blood. Clean blood means that you have enough self-love and respect to keep yourself in a loving condition. Use dandelion to enhance loving energy and keep your kidneys flowing; this is a nourishing and gentle cleansing herb. It has been said that when you get kidney disease, then on some level you are literally 'pissed off' with the world, dandelion softens and releases that angry feeling, improving your capacity for loving energy.

Another good loving energy herb is avocado. It is green, it is nourishing, and it contains essential fatty acids to buffer and protect the cell linings. Any antioxidants or green foods are good to enhance loving energy. When you want to improve your capacity for loving energy, prepare your food with love, have an ever-present feeling of gratefulness and appreciation when you eat or drink. If you swallow food with love, then surely that vibration will reflect itself in good assimilation and that all contributes to cellular health with *love*!

Sexual energy

Loving and sexual energy are separate energies that may be intertwined accordingly, but when you are working with your Wellness Zone you need to define each energy individually. It's really good when you can mix one with the other; however, the truth is you can have one without the other.

Once you hit puberty and those hormones have kicked in, then sex becomes important. In fact, without it none of us would be here today! There are so many boundaries and restrictions directly related to sexual energy, and it is one of the primary energies you need in your Wellness Zone for motivation, initiative and good health and energy flow throughout the body. Sexual energy can be used appropriately or inappropriately; it is the motivator for many activities and achievements in your Wellness Zone.

All energy needs to flow, and sexual energy needs to flow to help you have the energy to do anything at all in life. Without sexual energy the world would be a very unmotivated place. Look at your personal sexual energy and sort it out for yourself. Sexual energy is your right as a human on this planet, it is a very important energy to express and even though many people don't acknowledge it, most of your life force, chi and motivation comes from this basic source, your sexuality. Have some humbleness and humanity about your methods of expressing it. Yes, have grace with your sexual energy but remember that you can be held at bay by it, because without sufficient amounts of sexual energy, you'll never achieve anything you want to achieve. It is the driving force behind all that you do, every day.

With your Wellness Zone, you need to look at your sexual energy and work out what you need to do to bring it into play. When you have misguided sexual energy, you can become angry and depressed, and you can become frustrated with yourself and everything in life. However, when your sexual energy is operating well, when the flame of sexuality is burning in your engine room, then you are on fire; your life is on fire. You are motivated and you are burning the flame of energy which will transcend and relate back to every other type of energy you require for your life to operate optimally in your Wellness Zone. Think wellness, Think sex!

Sexual energy is not all about sex either. There's loads of sexual energy everywhere that's got nothing to do with the physical experiences associated with sex. Sexual energy is in every piece of artwork you see, in every movie, or theatre production and even in every meal you eat. Sexuality is the core of creativity. Creativity is art, art is innovation, innovation is experimental, experimental is science, science is development, development is civilised and civilised society is based on sexual energy used in a constructive and productive manner. Everything that you experience, which is sophisticated, creative, technical or scientific is created through appropriately used sexual energy. So, when you see it that way, the whole world just revolves around appropriate sex, and you will also see the destructive and negative ways that sex can be used as well.

Sexual energy is a very basal physical energy that is the right of every-one. If you look at your creativity and your experimental side of life and see that something is lacking, then you will also need to address your own sexuality and see where you are contributing to this lack. Your Wellness Zone is a place where you are totally and completely yourself, and you are able to be as creative, as experimental and as sexual as you like. This is a good development.

New ideas come from this base in life, and it's a good thing to have new ideas and bring new ways to old methods. It's important that you grasp your own sexual preferences and turn-ons in all levels of life. Look at what attracts you in life. Not just people but ideas, lifestyles, vocations, careers, places, experiences. See what turns you on, and you will see the direction you need to look towards to reach your ultimate Wellness Zone. Don't be sexually isolated from the world, don't be sexually stuffy and don't get old before your time.

Sex is the energy you need to retain youthfulness, to balance the seriousness in your life with the playfulness. Look at sex as your saving grace for youthfulness and happiness, as a balancer where you can meet the world in a totally open and equal way. Sexually, we are all the same; we just express it differently. We can all have a varying intensity of the same experiences; however, we all have the ability to express this in ourselves and to the world, given the opportunity and the personal motivation to do so. Basically, if your hormones are operating well, you are interested in sex, but if you are not experiencing sexual energy in one way or another, then you are not as happy as you could be. You are also letting a part of you slip away before your time.

The experience of sex is the experience of vulnerability and openness which is important when you want to have a decent and improving Wellness Zone. Your ability to be open and vulnerable is also a wonder-ful quality to take into other areas of your life. It's a risk. And risk means that you are stepping out of a more secure zone to try something new and enjoyable and that may make your life more comfortable.

Sexual energy is expressed as a risk in many incidences. Many people will take a plunge and quit their job for a self-employment opportunity, or they will buy air tickets to an exotic and far off land just for the joy of it. These acts are sexual energy acts. Sometimes they may be impulsive, they may even be a wrong decision, but they constitute a want or a need to experience something that allows them to develop and get further ahead in their life. When you are in your Wellness Zone, and you see opportunities to be taken, you will be able to use your Wellness Zone skills to better analyse and make the right decisions. These will be based on your ability to see more clearly where the experience may lead you and whether it is to your advantage or not. This is where your Wellness Zone is an important quality to nurture, especially with sexual energy.

Sometimes people who are single make the same disastrous relationship choices they have made in the past. This is very common. People meet and in their very rampant search for a soul mate they connect with people who they would be better to have just had a platonic friendship with. The sexual energy gets flowing, a long sleeping sexual energy that has wanted to be used for so long. Now, here it is waking up and relishing in the pleasure of finally having met the one. Eventually, the relationship hits a wall as you discover the person you have been having wonderful sexual energy with is incompetent and doesn't match your energies on many other levels.

If you have been in this cycle or situation, creating your Wellness Zone can be very beneficial as you will be able to better analyse anyone who comes along and you won't be so ready to compromise your own energy values in order to fit in with someone else. If you are smart, then you will be using your own sexual energy all the time in creative outlets so that you will meet someone with similar interests and energy. Also, you won't be so quick to go to bed with the wrong people. It's all about how you use your sexual energy. If you ignore it for too long you'll end up a frustrated and desperate mess.

You may know people who don't use their sexual energy or don't use it well; they are frustrated, usually angry and often opinionated. They have the ability to create conflict in their lives unconsciously just because they have nothing better to do. Release some of that sexual energy, and you've got a whole new person; balanced, happier and less ready to whip the nearest relative or friend who comes along.

Sexual energy is the kind of catalyst energy that flows along your whole physical being. It's the energy that lets you relax, feel contented and be whatever you want to be and be okay about it. Sexual energy is something you want lots of in your Wellness Zone, it allows you to move forward in so many ways in your life and stops you from getting stuck in a corner, somewhere that you don't want to be!

Infertility is a huge issue to do with sexual energy in this day and age. If you are having trouble conceiving then visit your Health Care Practitioner and talk with them about your options. Herbal medicines and alternative practices can be used very effectively when you really want the best results!

Herbs and supplements to support sexual energy

If you are having real problems with your libido, then you need to address it from the top. The top is your brain and the master hormonal secretions that occur there. You also need a proper diagnosis to see whether you have hormonal imbalances anywhere else in your body. If this is not the case then you may have to address the drugs you are taking, your body weight and size, the dysfunction or lack of spontaneity and love in your relationship with yourself and others and also your possible level of heavy metal poisoning. In fact, impotency is so high these days due to stressful lifestyles and toxicity.

There can be fertility problems that are undiagnosed because of simple factors such as mild obesity or polycystic ovarian syndrome. Perhaps infertility due to low sperm count, or non-ovulation. Whatever the cause of your sexual energy levels not operating well, herbs can help. If you visit your Health Care Practitioner, they will possibly put you on a detox, get your blood and saliva tests back in balance again and ensure that you are really on the move upwards with sexual energy. If you lack sexual energy, the herbs to improve it are the adaptogenic herbs such as liquorice root, ginseng, astragalus, withania and balancing herbs that will really get you balanced again.

Your diet is important, you need clean water, the best unprocessed foods and you also need good supplements. If you are planning to have a baby, then detox, and ensure you are both well-nourished with hormones in balance, give yourselves a time frame of six months or longer from the start of this process before you conceive. If you don't want to conceive but just want to improve your sexual energy, then please take the adaptogenic herbs and give it a few months before you get results.

Some medications will be bad for your libido, and you will need to speak with your Health Care Practitioner about these if you need to switch medications or go off them all together to ensure good sexual energy. Remember that this is not the most important energy but if you are lacking in sexual energy, then rest assured there will be problems in other areas of your life as well. This can indicate a good health check and overhaul to bring your sexual energy into a good Wellness Zone.

You can try the herbal horny goat weed formulas if you like but if you want some serious sexual energy herbs then mix the horny goat weed with tribulus, damiana and withania and a bit of ginseng. Take daily and see whether your libido increases. Or if you are using your sexual energy for drive, creativity and motivation, try a daily tonic of adaptogenic herbs as a good tonic to keep you motivated and your drive up. Getting your adrenal glands in good repair is critical for good sexual energy levels. Make sure you are well-balanced in other areas of your life and keep your hormones in good order.

Persistent energy

How persistent are you? When you start something, how well do you apply yourself and do you get the job at hand finished? Persistent energy is an accumulation of many types of enhancing energy. It's interesting though, as without persistence you will not be able to have a Wellness Zone. You'll be just rolling around in the sea of life drifting in whichever direction the wind and tide may take you.

Persistence is an interesting energy and quality to bring into the Wellness Zone. You can be persistent in so many ways, some good, some not so good. The idea of bringing persistence into your Wellness Zone is to work out what's worth persisting with and what's not! In other words, there are some aspects of life that deserve your unreserved and determined application. There are other aspects of life that deserve to be dropped in the nearest public waste station and left there to decompose with the rest of the rubbish. Outdated, superseded concepts that deserve nothing less than your modern and wise intervention to decide what works in favour of your wellness, and what works in favour of decomposition. Organic waste that is better taken out of your brain to make room for the things that deserve your time and effort.

Now to work out what is worth persisting with in life. However, you will first need to work out some other issues, such as what are your interests and passions in life? How to use your mental energy to create positive energy? To balance the other energies and eliminate the negative, nervous and adrenal energy, so that at the end of the day you are living in wellness and only persisting with what you see as useful and helpful in your life. This is persistent energy at its best. Write a list of what works for you and what you want to persist in and write a list for the local dump. You can be ruthless. This is your life, and you only need to persist in things that make your life better, more comfortable, more loving, more real and more pleasurable.

Minimalise or eliminate unnecessary tasks that are unpleasant, painful or non-productive in your life. Minimalise the must-do, those tasks that you don't enjoy but that have to be done. Be persistent in perusing the bold, the adventurous, the groundbreaking and the enjoyable tasks.

Also, be persistent in the tasks you don't want to do, but know you need to do in order to have a better life in the future. In other words, you can't dump your studies, or your work unless you have a better plan that is realistic and able to be used effectively with this gorgeous persistent energy that you are about to bring into your life.

Persistent energy is important. Incorporate it into your Wellness Zone today. It's good to be aware when you are using persistent energy in your day. This energy can be the difference between success and failure of any venture.

Herbs and supplements to support persistent energy

Persistent energy can be tiring, and it can be stressful. This energy is often necessary to complete tasks that need to be done. The best herbs you can take are supportive and nurturing herbs that will support your mental, adrenal and physical energies whilst you are busy being persistent. So, any of the herbs for these other areas are good. Make sure you eat protein foods when you are using persistent energy as you need to increase your potential for endurance at the same time. Persistence and endurance can be one and the same, and you should support yourself with warm nurturing foods as well as plenty of drinks to keep you hydrated.

Wheatgrass juice and fresh vegetable juices can be taken when endurance is necessary. Keep away from stimulants as these tend to deprive you of persistence when taken too often. To be persistent, you really need to have every energy in a level zone and be capable of following through with your ideas and dreams. Address the supplements needed daily, as some days you will find it harder to be persistent. On these days you may need extra minerals and vitamins as well as some energising herbals such as nettle and maca.

Hormonal energy

Hormones are to be balanced from the top down. Master hormonal secretions will impact on all bodily functions, and keeping your hormones happy is one solid way to enhance your Wellness Zone.

Everyone over the age of 30 finds some imbalance with one hormone or another. You either have a slower metabolism and put on visceral fat, or lowered thyroid function. You may have lowered or raised progesterone, testosterone or oestrogen levels which cause serious imbalances in the whole body ranging from mood swings, hot flushes, depression, weight gain, to any manner of odd crawling sensations. Or perhaps you are having glucose uptake problems, insulin deficiency, syndrome X or you could be lacking sleep from melatonin depletion which comes naturally with age. You may have been so stressed that all hormones are disrupted which can lead to chronic illness.

Hormones rule; they are what we all need to stay young. Hormone production decreases with age. When you've burnt out your adrenals from too much overplay, and you have got a compromised nervous system caused by this, then your hormones are the first to go on strike and give you extra trouble. Hormones are troublesome for everyone from the 3-year-old boy driving his parent's temper to boiling point with the over-production of testosterone, to a teenager rampantly experiencing those beautiful mood swings and ugly acne experiences that we all know too well as hormonal energy. You need to keep your hormones balanced on all levels to enhance your Wellness Zone.

What are your hormones doing today? Oh, what an interesting question that one is. Well, you need to know. Get saliva testing done; it's the most accurate hormone test available today. Then when you know the balance, herbs and nutritional medicines can give you support to help you feel level again.

Young mothers often fall prey to hormonal imbalances. Whilst they are pregnant, all their hormones are geared towards the production of a baby. After the birth, when they start to get themselves back again, the hormones kick in and can leave them feeling a depressed mess, some women can have this feeling for years after childbirth. This is where herbs and natural medicines can help very much.

Men often suffer depression and cover it up with stress. This can be a deadly combination; you can become not only hormonally imbalanced, but very stressed. One result is inappropriate emotional outbursts, more common in men who would rather yell than be seen crying and expressing their feelings. Then again, hormones can make anyone cry! Have you ever been in a state where you start to cry and feel totally miserable for no good reason. Or you feel rage, pure rage, that deep anger that won't go away and didn't take much to trigger, or the feeling of unease? These can all be related to hormones. Hormones can only get worse as you age, so deal with them now and keep dealing with them always!

Herbs and supplements to support hormonal energy

There is so much written on hormones; it's everywhere. You will get conflicting advice from different Health Care Practitioners as to what to take and when. Natural hormone replacements are one avenue to follow, and some people feel completely hopeless without replacements. If you are one of these people, research every option, leave no stone unturned and make your choice wisely!

Herbs can help immensely. Women's balance blend consists of black cohosh, hypericum, Siberian ginseng and astragalus. Hot flush formula containing sage, liquorice and black cohosh can help. A good PMT blend of vitex, hypericum and cat's claw can relieve symptoms from two weeks before your period. Men may benefit from tribulus, saw palmetto and damiana blend.

There are some beautiful herbs and creams that will go well with or without prescription medications. It's all in the personalisation of the mixture, the balance between the trouble your hormones are causing and troubles coming from other aspects of your health. You need personal attention when you try to balance hormonal energy in your Wellness Zone; personal attention to detail is the key to success. From saliva, blood and other diagnostic tests, through to researching your options and then balancing diet and lifestyle so that you don't tip the scales. Let's face it, you can't put a 40-year-old brain on a 16-year-old body, so when it comes to hormones, stay young in mind and hormones and be as vigilant as you can about staying that way.

There are many herbs to choose from that can be applied topically or take internally. Dietary habit's need to be addressed and you can certainly benefit from eating plant-based foods such as soy as part of your regular diet. The arena of hormonal balancing is receiving and will continue to receive enormous attention as the population ages. Herbs are the number one solution, and you would do well to give them a good therapeutic go before opting to synthetic versions of hormonal replacements.

Nutritional medicine has a lot to offer in hormonal balancing. If you are able to prevent the problem in the first place, or at least delay the downward cascade of hormone secretions as you age, then that is your best option. For example, there are lifestyle and dietary choices you can take today to help you be more hormonally balanced in the future. Enhancing your hormonal energy is one way to help prevent many degenerative illnesses.

CHAPTER TWENTY ONE

Energies that need to be kept in control to enhance your Wellness Zone

Nervous energy

Nervous energy, as you can guess, involves your nervous system. You can see when people are living on nervous energy. They fidget; often they have shaky hands, jittery knees, sometimes they can be a little too quick in speech, have twitchy eye movements, become evasive or you just know they are plain old nervous. This energy can also be expressed as anger, bad temper or nastiness, because the nervous system is out of balance.

It's okay to be nervous at times: we will all have nervous experiences; nervous energy is part of our lives. But it becomes a health issue when it's the main type of energy used, or it is used too frequently. This type of energy is dangerous to your nervous systems and adds a lot of strain on every aspect of your body. Nervous energy is a roller coaster ride where everything is a little out of your control, and you aren't quite in control enough to put it right.

There are different types of nervous energy. If you have been abused or emotionally stressed, when someone close passes away, divorce, traumatic situations and accidents are all understandable nervous energy situations. For a period of time during and after these events, you will feel nervous energy as your nervous system is stretched, and your body is coping naturally the best way it can under the circumstances. However, after the event, if this type of energy is still used predominately, it can create all manner of havoc in your life.

People who live on nervous energy are often the ones who jump at the sound of a loud noise, or who feel upset at slight events and tend to unconsciously make mountains out of molehills. After a trauma or life-changing event, we all tend to use nervous energy as our dominant energy currency for a short time as we come to grips with the situation, sorting ourselves out and trying to get back on track. However, when we unconsciously train ourselves to live on this kind of energy all the time, then we are heading for health problems in the longer term. Nervous energy is exactly that. It's when you are using your nervous system over time, and you are very sensitive to all that surrounds you.

The somatic nervous system is the part that's in our conscious control. This is every movement like eating, walking, feeling, sensing life in the physical and controlling our responses. The autonomic nervous system is the part that's out of our conscious control like; our heartbeat, breathing, digestion, bowel movements and all the parts of our body that really operate automatically.

It's the autonomic part that is really affected when people live on nervous energy for too long. Constipation, heart palpitations, bad circulation, pains in the digestive tract after meals, lack of appetite, repeated headaches, discontent with life and waiting for negativity are all signs of nervous energy. Often these people get the shakes; they have wobbly fingers and twitching eyes. They are so busy living on nervous energy that they find it hard to concentrate on anything other than their own emotional dramas which tend to be exacerbated by time. Nervous energy is the energy of people who are addicted to drugs and also often the energy of very busy and stressed or emotionally lonely people. It's the primary energy source when you feel out of control in a situation. Stress is so close to nervous energy that it's hard to tell the two apart.

Nervous energy itself can become addictive. Women can suffer from this energy when they are bored, lonely and feeling like they are living their lives through their children. It's very common amongst business people who are under severe long-term stress and can also be the energy of the depressed housewife. When you look at your Wellness Zone and decide that you need to eliminate some nervous energy from your life, the best way to do this is to move more; exercise and get more physical.

Often nervy people tend to be thin as well or suffer so severely from oxidative stress that they are fat around the abdominal area and tend to put on weight easily. They don't eat enough, or they don't eat well enough and are always worried about things. When you exercise, you start the endorphins going in the brain, the happy hormones. Hopefully, then you will be using more physical and positive energy which will save your nervous system some strain.

The thing about living on nervous energy is that you are also using adrenal energy, and you will probably need some adrenal herbs and nutrients. Good nutritional support is important when you live on nervous energy. Even if you are only in this zone temporarily, when you experience a trauma in your life, it's still important to look after yourself. If you have been physically abused and are living in the zone of nervous energy long term and feel that you are unable to transcend this on your own, then please get some professional help. We are not all islands unto ourselves. It's important to live in love and not allow fear, paranoia, addiction or worry to overtake your life.

Nervous energy is responsive; it's the kind of energy that will respond to how much room you are willing to give it in your life. If you allow it to dominate you, then it can be like a bottle of champagne, when the bottle is not cold enough, and you pop the cork, the contents will just spill over the top and keep flowing uncontained until the whole bottle is gone and you have nothing left. Nervous energy will drain and exhaust you until you have nothing left; for yourself or your loved ones, until you are able to get out of that nervous energy rut. When nervous energy is properly contained and utilised, it is like the bottle of champagne that was placed in the fridge and chilled to the right temperature, when you pop the cork, you can pour it into your glass to celebrate living on a level plane. Your nerves and emotions are now contained in their rightful place, under your control.

Nervous energy has its benefits too. Often before an important event in your life, you can be very nervous. This is an appropriate time to use nervous energy and look at what you need to focus on for that particular event so that you can do your best. If you suffer from this kind of nervous energy, then you certainly don't have a problem, unless it leads to other health problems or becomes the dominant energy in your life. When you do suffer from intermittent nervous energy, have a supply of appropriate nutritional and herbal supports at hand and use them accordingly.

Find the place for nervous energy in your Wellness Zone today. Look at yourself honestly and see where you are, then you can really decide how you want to live your life. Are your nerves ruling you or are you the one in charge?

Herbs and supplements to support nervous energy

Ginkgo biloba, passionflower, valerian, hypericum, hops, chamomile, melissa, motherwort, plantain, goldenseal, withania and kava kava. Take herbs regularly and in small amounts when you are nervy. Take therapeutic doses of the Vitamin B group and rest whenever you can. Avoid drugs and alcohol as much as possible. Caffeine is the number one plant food to avoid, caffeine is a stimulant, and when you are under nervous stress you can potentiate the feeling with stimulants. Avoid sugary foods as these will add to nervous stress.

Anyone who is living on nervous energy needs hypericum extract each day, providing you are not on any pharmaceutical medications for depression or anxiety. Hypericum will help level you out faster than any other herb. You will also need large amounts of vitamins and minerals, as you are probably depleted nutritionally in all areas.

When you have a chronic problem and nervous energy is regularly in your life, you can become either very thin or very fat. The reason for this is that different people respond to nervous energy in different ways. The gustatory nerve runs directly through your nervous system, and some people respond to nervous energy by being incapable of eating food at all. In this case drink plenty of nutritional fluids such as soups and juices. Take supplements of spirulina, alfalfa or barley grass to help ensure you are getting essential vitamins and minerals and make sure you drink water and other fluids throughout the day. Where nervous energy is involved, some people simply forget about their need for food and the digestive tract almost becomes numb.

Then there are the ones who drown the nervousness in masses of food, and they eat anything and everything they can lay their hands on. These people are responding to nervous energy with a great need to forget all about it and drown their sorrows by over-indulging. Usually, the more sugary, fatty or carbohydrate-laden the food, the better! This can lead to all manner of illness and poor health issues, and you will need to address the underlying problems of emotional and nervous system stresses in order to lose the extra weight and get on a healthy path again.

Nervous energy affects different people in different ways. Often addictions are exasperated, eating disorders are highlighted, and emotional and mental stresses are brought to the forefront. Getting nervous energy under control is a primary factor for your Wellness Zone if you want long-term health.

Adrenal energy

Out of all your hormones, these are the ones to get you in the most trouble with your Wellness Zone, by the overload placed on your adrenal glands from too much work and too much stress. You need to make the effort to keep these glands in good health to enhance your Wellness Zone.

Adrenal energy is great stuff when you are chased out of a cave by a dragon, and it provides the perfect energy when your life is at risk of being swished by a dragon's tail or your limbs are at risk of being scorched by fire breath. For the rest of the time, you want to support and balance your adrenal glands, not stress them out!

The adrenal glands are two little pouches located above your kidneys. They are hormonal creatures who love nothing more than to secrete lots and lots of adrenaline until they are shrivelled up and exhausted. When you are secreting adrenaline you will have abundant energy and drive, and you will be operating at top speed. When the adrenal glands become exhausted, you will fall in a heap, unable to feel motivated or enthusiastic about anything. Once these adrenals are exhausted you need to repair them; otherwise, they will add a new load of stress onto your thyroid glands and other hormones. That's right, when your adrenals are dangling limp on the side-lines, you will probably have about 5% running power for the rest of your body too. You will barely recognise yourself in the mirror with extra dark circles under your eyes.

Obesity is another consequence of chronic adrenal stress that is continued for long periods of time. Many women spend their 20s and 30s as very busy people, thriving on adrenal energy, then they end up with dangling, almost non-functioning adrenals. Then possibly the thyroid gland will take over, and they use up too much thyroid hormone, which in turn burns out the thyroid gland, and they end up with various symptoms of hypothyroidism. The women then pump in heaps of extra oestrogen to make up for all the thyroid and adrenal hormones that they no longer have, to create extra energy. When menopause is reached, women tend to literally spread, and everything starts to head south. From here, you can become insulin and metabolic resistant, which tends to be a natural consequence of this pattern.

Men are in a similar position. Much of the waistline fat can be avoided if you look after your adrenal glands and avoid adrenal stress as much as possible. Visceral obesity, which is concentrated fat around the abdominal area, is often exacerbated by too much adrenal stress. You know when you are using too much adrenal energy when you are working long after you should have stopped for a rest. You will be pushing yourself beyond your physical limits and feeling low on energy, but you keep going because your internal driving force is pushing you onwards.

The best way to avoid adrenal stress is to be as relaxed as you can about life whenever you can. Try to keep deadlines to a minimum, avoid personal dramas and unnecessary stress in your life and learn to laugh. There are times when adrenal energy is what is required to push you to the finish line in an important project. If this is the case, then keep it to a minimum and make sure you take measures to recover once the event is over.

Herbs and supplements to support adrenal energy

Nothing beats panax and Siberian ginseng in combination with withania and some reishi for adrenal support and repair. When you let your adrenal glands get tired, you pay for it. You may feel exhausted and place yourself at risk for all types of stresses, including lowered immunity and vulnerability to genetic weaknesses. Boosting immunity is paramount to adrenal support and health.

Astragalus and liquorice root are good to take as a preventative when you know you're overdoing your adrenal energy. Combine herbs with L-glutamine the amino acid, also magnesium powder taken last thing at night before bed assists in adrenal support whilst you are sleeping. Remember to add rehmannia to any tonic when you want to repair adrenal glands and strengthen your adrenal energy.

Exhausted energy

Do you feel exhausted? Well, you're not alone, many people feel as though their energy levels are depleted. This is common, and unfortunately it can snowball and become worse with time unless something is done about it. Don't burn yourself out. If you think that you are about to burn out or you feel like you can't go on, if you think you need to rest, then rest. This is not something to be taken lightly in the scheme of life. When you feel tired, there is always a reason for this, and it is important that you get the rejuvenation needed so that you can go on, feeling energised again. There are different kinds of exhausted energy, but they all tell you that you are, to one degree or another, outside your Wellness Zone. You need to take measures to step up your energy now, and this doesn't mean soldiering on, putting up with the tiredness, drinking more coffee or taking stimulants to keep you awake. When you are exhausted, get the message … *rest*.

We all have days when we are tired and, somehow or another, we stumble through that day and have an early night. This is occasionally okay for your Wellness Zone. However, when you layer tiredness upon tiredness and just keep stacking it upon itself, then you can cut through your immunity. If you rely too heavily on nervous and adrenal energy, you can also make mistakes in your work, muck up your body clock and generally become a mess, which will eventually need sorting out.

You can't ignore exhausted energy forever. Sure, you can go to sleep and have enough energy the next day to get up, get coffee and get working but in the end you will have to pay the price for ignoring yourself on this level. The result is often a breakdown of one system or another in the body. Even small children at school are expected to work hard all the time; they can use up all their energy, become exhausted and then continue this cycle through their weekends and then throughout their lives. It's almost as though we are expected to be respectable by being on the go all the time. You can't avoid exhausted energy sometimes, just don't make it a way of life; this is a direct path to illness and disease.

For your Wellness Zone, you need to decide how much sleep you need each day to continue the lifestyle you choose. You need to decide when you are heading into an exhausted state and how to counteract that. You need to look at why you have become exhausted and take nutritional supplements, exercise and rest to counteract the situation and bring yourself back into balance. As with all self-inflicted conditions, there is only one person who loses when you become exhausted, and that's you!

Make sure you are riding on the wave of healthy energy and when you think that you are sinking into the murky waters of exhaustion, pick yourself up as quickly as you can and get back into the healthy energy zone. Look at your nervous system, immunity, hormones, diet, digestive tract and your sleep patterns. These are the things you need to address. You need to be fair to yourself. Make sure that when you are tired, you get the rest you need.

When you are sick, stop yourself until you are able to be better again. This means to rest your body in all ways. No rich foods; only juices, unprocessed food, clean water, herbal teas and lovely homemade soups. No exercise, no books, no TV, no computer. Just sleep, rest, sunlight, a little music, a little conversation and lots of sleep. Then when you're better and stronger again, your body will be thankful that you have rested when you needed to. Otherwise, the exhaustion can become chronic and can lead to lowered immunity, chronic fatigue and many other health problems.

One option is to take a weekend out every month to rest and detox your body; you will avoid exhaustion rather than ignoring the symptoms and paying for it later. Everyone is capable of overdoing it and becoming chronically exhausted, and this is something you must avoid and be constantly vigilant about. Know when to slow down, then when you are re-energised again you can pick up the pace. When you are tired, rest, often rest during the day as well as sleeping at night. It's your body, and it's okay for you to do whatever you need to do to avoid, delay, stop and repair exhaustion.

Exhaustion can sneak up on you; however, part of the process of finding and maintaining your Wellness Zone is to watch out for it. Keep a tab on when it wants to take you over and be prepared to dump it; with rest, nutritional medicines and herbals. It's easier to avoid now than to recover from once it's taken hold of your lifestyle. Once it has sneaked up on you, it clings like a leech and never lets you forget it's there. It will take over your day, decrease your functioning abilities and lead you to all manner of negative behaviours as you try to shake it off with caffeine, sugar and fatty foods.

There's nothing more demotivating than a room full of exhausted people, their energy, or lack of, can pull your own healthy energy down. Have you ever noticed that when you are with a group of exhausted people there is also an element of negativity in the air? They don't bounce ideas, they don't aspire to improve what they are doing, and they don't congratulate each other or celebrate their successes. Exhaustion means that you are past the stress limit for your Wellness Zone and in need of some rest and relaxation. So do yourself a favour right now, if you're reading this and feel exhausted, go and have a sleep. Rest is the best cure, every time.

Herbs and supplements to support exhausted energy

We all want to eliminate exhausted energy. Take passionflower with valerian, melissa and hypericum every night upon retiring. This will ensure you have a good night's sleep and hopefully avoid those middle-of-the-night 'wake up and worry' sessions that tend to cause insomnia and stop already exhausted people from sleeping.

During the day, a good supporting and re-energising tonic with ginkgo biloba for mental clarity, Siberian ginseng for adrenal support, nettle and kelp to speed up your metabolism and assist you in getting rid of the sluggishness that tends to develop when you are exhausted, and some echinacea root for immunity. Take this every day and night until, either your lifestyle changes or the exhaustion has been replaced with efficient, bubbling and healthy energy. If you are exhausted, you should eat small regular meals.

Magnesium, zinc and vitamins are all needed to help counteract the added strain on all systems in your body. Bilberry is good for vision improvement, and you may want to take omega 3 fatty acids. You will need to up the tempo and increase supplements when you are exhausted, especially if you are travelling and on the go all day and night. Your immunity is likely to suffer and you will be prone to all manner of illness with exhausted energy.

Take some olive leaf, astragalus, cat's claw and lemon juice regularly through the day. Close your eyes and rest for a few minutes whenever you get the chance. Also, if you are suffering from exhausted energy, remember to move your body and exercise regularly. It's a fast path to obesity when people live in exhaustion and don't take time for regular physical exercise.

Exhaustion can be triggered by many different factors. You will need to ensure correct diagnosis if there are any viruses or bacteria present in your body that are contributing to the problem. Find nutritional medicines and herbals that are specific to the symptoms that you are feeling. Try to mitigate exhausted energy when it arises to avoid chronic illness in the future.

Negative energy

This is another type of energy that is to be avoided as much as possible. Wasted negative energy is anything from thinking negative thoughts, to being around others who are negative in their thoughts and actions. Negativity breeds negativity. It is something that can start off as a little black spot in your mind and grow until it is all-consuming. Negative energy is easily recognisable; it's the kind of energy that brings you down. It has a way of cutting through your immunity, increasing your stress levels and decreasing your motivation. This is the worst type of energy if you want to be successful in life.

Let's think about today. Have you felt anger or resentment, are you emotionally upset, frustrated, rushed or even upset today? Well, these feelings all attribute to negative energy. It's up to you to transcend them as quickly as possible because they will cause physical stress on your body. This translates to negative cellular energy, which equals more stress on your body and therefore more susceptibility to illness than if you were more positive in your energy. Does this make sense to you? We are all like a sponge to the environment around us, and this environment can include your own emotions and thoughts. So, the best person to help you stay healthy and positive is yourself. And the best way to do this is to eliminate negative energy thoughts before they become dominant in your subconscious body energy patterns.

If you are around people who are negative, the best things you can do is get away from them and leave them to their own devices. Don't support negativity in others. Don't lower your own energy levels and buy into their little games and emotions. Because negative energy leads to illness and disease. Good health results from the avoidance of negativity in all manner.

Herbs and supplements to support negative energy

When you focus on negative energy, you are really wasting your efforts and could clearly be living a more fulfilling life. You see, when you are negative, you are wasting all that vital life force on nothing more than your lowest thoughts, and you are vibrating at your lowest level. So, even suggesting herbs is a waste of time, don't you think? But when you are negative, you probably need herbs and supplements more than ever, even though in your negative frame of mind you probably think it's a waste of time. You need a good herbal detox for a week or two because the best herbs to counteract negativity are the cleansing herbs that get into your liver and take away the toxins, then maybe you can start to think with a clear and positive mind again.

People who have been using drugs or alcohol in excess are often very negative in their outlook. The first and best medicine is a daily dose of carrot, celery and lemon juice, followed by cleansing herbs to work on the liver, kidneys, large intestine and parasites in the digestive tract. This cleanse is often hard on these people, and they complain daily about the headaches, diarrhoea and stressful thoughts they are experiencing during the detox. However, when it's over they aren't nearly as negative, and often there is a remarkable change in attitude after a good detox. This regime needs to be controlled and tailor-made for each individual to avoid negative side effects as much as possible.

Other herbs to counteract wasted negative energy are nervines and anti-depressant herbs which are gentle and non-addictive. Anyone who is negative would do well to eat a lot of fresh garlic, ginger and vegetables in their diet. Take them off all processed and junk food so that the body has the best chance to heal and feed them some quality dark chocolate every day. Just a small amount will do wonders to help sweeten life up a bit! Not too much sugar though as it will send the blood glucose soaring which is another contributor to negative thoughts and stresses on the body.

Sick energy

This is when you are down and out on a healing crisis or if you have been chronically sick for a long time either mentally or physically and are sick of being sick! A healing crisis is a time when you have depleted your energy supply, your immunity has been compromised in some way and it's clearly time to stop and rest. This sick energy can also be called healing energy. The aspects of sick energy are that you just feel so tired, rotten and fluey that you want to eliminate the sickness as quickly as possible. Sick energy is when all of the toxins, mucous and gunk in your system decide it's high time to get going and release themselves to the world. These little pathogens don't want to be in your body, and your body doesn't want them there either.

Sick energy can also be the energy you experience when you have been ill for a long time, when you are so sick of sickness that you just live from day to day in a state of sick energy. This can lead to many side effects including depression, also the many stresses associated with chronic sickness such as financial stress, emotional inadequacy and personal relationships being strained and compromised following long-term sickness. When you are in this situation, you need to transcend the mental limitations of the sick energy as much as possible. This is a difficult energy to live with and is often the end result of great illness.

Sick energy can take over your body if you are unconscious about what you eat and drink and think. It's far better to learn to change your tastes and desires for foods, than it is to eat unedited for years on end and have sick energy occurring all the time. Many people who have lived on wheat products, processed foods and carbohydrate overload for many years will lose a lot of weight, regain their energy and lose all the built-up sick energy simply by changing the way they eat. A more natural and unprocessed regime will help their body become vibrant and healthy.

You need to recognise that what you eat, what you think and how you act today is a reflection of what your body will be tomorrow. So, in many ways, illnesses like the flu, colds and other acute attacks are signposts that our body has had enough build-up and congestion, and it has a reason to stop. Obviously, you aren't stopping on your own, so even though it may be inconvenient to you, your body is stopping for you. This is a healthy way to view a sick energy healing crisis. Because your resources are low, when your body was exposed to some outside influence, your immunity was not able to comfortably fight it off on its own.

As you see, sick energy is the next stage in the weakened energy chain after exhausted and depleted energy. It is when there is no more escape channels for your body and the time has come to really slow down and clear out some of that unwanted gunk. For those of you who are unfortunate and suffer from chronic sick energy, such as a persistent virus or chronic fatigue or any myriad of other long-term illnesses, then you need to take every measure to find out what alternative approaches may help you and improve your Wellness Zone.

When you live physically in the sick energy zone as your primary zone, you need to do everything you can to clean out your body, detox, get strong and become as healthy as you can within your sick zone. People who are chronically ill, even those of you who are coping with cancer or other illnesses where your body's dominant energy is sick energy, you need to constantly be on the lookout for any opportunity to increase your potential healthy energy for the future. You need to think as positively as you can, nourish your body as well as you can and you need to rest and try to make the most of the moment you are experiencing.

When we are chronically ill and feeling locked into sick energy like there is no escape, this is when we need to remain our most vigilant. These are the times we need to become empowered with information, research and loving energy. This is when we need to take detox to a new level, nutrition to its maximum zone and eat the best way we can. This is when we need to pull all our resources together for the betterment of our health. Even though our Wellness Zone is at its lowest, it's very important to have a Wellness Zone plan in place, even when you are feeling sick. You will need your wits about you, to be as positive and strong and stubborn as you can possibly be, determined to succeed and determined to be well again.

This is the best hope you can have for your future health. You are the one who can make the most difference, and you are the only one who can take that sick energy and let it vibrate gently with acceptance and healing energy to enhance your health each and every day. Sick energy is hard to deal with some days, but you must remember that it will pass.

You need to be very specific when you are not well and ensure that you take herbs that deal with either the chronic or acute illness you are experiencing. Sickness, is such a present and 'in the moment' experience. Drinking lemon juice with flat mineral water or plain water with very light and nourishing foods is good when you are sick. As for herbs, there are so many you can take; it depends on your situation. Don't underestimate the power of correct medical diagnosis when you are sick. Sick is sick, and it needs fixing. You are either having a healing crisis, where you will need some serious rest and detox, or you are having a health crisis, where you will need a correct diagnosis and healing. Either way, you need to be specific.

If you know of someone else's illness and you think that you may be a candidate for the same, don't let it dwell in your mind. You may create the symptoms of an illness simply through the power of the mind. Accept that different people have different lives and that often lifestyle, as well as environmental and genetic factors contribute to diseases and illness. If you are really concerned about a condition then get it diagnosed correctly, and hopefully that will eliminate the fear from your mind.

Sickness is something that should never be ignored. You may need medical attention, and you may need medicine to help you get well again. Don't just pass sickness off as insignificant. If you think something is wrong, find out what it is and then take measures to heal yourself.

Herbs and supplements to support sick energy

Fennel, infused and blended with peppermint tea is a good 'sick energy' herbal beverage. It doesn't really matter what's going on with your body or what medicines you need when you take this blend, it settles the stomach and in some way balances out the nervous system, whilst keeping the energy moving around in your body.

Remember to stay hydrated when you are in the throes of sick energy, take whatever medical precautions are necessary and get professional help as required. Stay in bed and rest until you have passed the healing crisis. Sick energy is very physically dominating, and you must relax into it, go with the flow and trust that you will come out the other side in bouncing good health.

Chronic sick energy needs a nervous system and immunity support above all else; it also needs diagnosis, rest, love and possibly appropriate fasting. Juices, soups and easily digested nutritional medicines will help support your system depending upon the problem. Specific herbs and also lots of positive energy and patience will help you for the duration.

The combination of cat's claw and astragalus with black walnut and Chinese wormwood will boost your immunity, keep you strong and get in on a cellular level to kill any nasty viruses, parasites or mutated cells. Coenzyme Q10 at 200 mg per day with some selenium and a complete amino acid, mineral and vitamin supplement will help give you an optimal chance to heal easily.

When you are chronically sick, your body needs every bit of herbal and nutritional support you can give it until you are well again, however long it takes. Wheatgrass juice taken daily is very beneficial for sick energy as it creates alkalinity in your body, which is always needed for optimal health.

Often when patients are in hospital there are many nutritional and herbal supplements that can be given safely in combination with orthodox drugs and the diet provided by the hospital. You can talk with your Health Care Practitioner about designing an individual programme for someone who is in this situation to help maximise the healing.

Spinning energy

Have you ever looked at someone and known that they are out of kilter? There is something about them that doesn't seem quite right? They are up one minute, down the next, focused and then confused. Perhaps they are unable to stick to any task for long, have great difficulty concentrating and also may have problems with basic skills such as reading or articulation problems. Well, this is spinning energy.

You see it often in young boys and even teenagers, you can see it in every walk of life and in every clinical environment. This type of energy is such that the person who is feeling it doesn't even notice. They are often so frustrated with their lives because everything just seems to spin the wrong way! When things start to go right, they will often spin back into a daze of confusion. Spinning energy is not attention deficit disorder. It is caused by a lack of essential fatty acids, B group vitamins and minerals, including magnesium and zinc. This problem can be caused by the dilemma of malnutrition, whereby although you are eating you are not absorbing or getting enough of the nutrients you need, on a regular basis.

Perhaps these people could be suffering from coeliac disease, autism or other malabsorption syndromes. There has been a link in research between autism and gluten intolerance. Perhaps there are mysterious allergies to any number of the toxic preservatives, insecticides, chemicals and hormones that are pumped into the over-processed foods we consume. But this spinning energy is something that can be reversed with the simple commitment of specific nutrition and herbals to bring the body's energy back into alignment.

Spinning energy is a sign that everything is out of whack; it is an indicator that there could also be heavy metal toxicity in the body. There could be drug or alcohol abuse involved, or even coffee abuse! There are some people who find that once they are able to settle down and lose that constant spinning energy, they are able to change their lives dramatically.

Spinning energy can also be genetic, there are varying degrees of this type of energy, and you will need to be realistic in your approach to helping and healing when this is the dominant energy in a person's life. All kinds of havoc can be created when this spinning energy gets out of hand, so first and foremost get a nutritional plan in action and ensure that you work in, with both alternate and orthodox Health Care Practitioners as required.

Don't ever go cold turkey on any medications or drugs, find support and follow it's directions. It can take a while to shift spinning energy into other more balanced types of energies, but in most cases it can be done. There are some types of spinning energy that are best left to the professionals, but most can be helped by a holistic plan and a good attitude to your Wellness Zone.

Herbs and supplements to support spinning energy

The best herbal supplements are the adaptogenic ones. Bacopa is a terrific herb when you are trying to balance out spinning energy. Another good one is withania. Any herb that will assist in levelling a person's mind and body and aids concentration and focus will help in these situations. Essential fatty acids are of primary importance here, and these can be attained from avocado, flaxseed, deep-sea fish and evening primrose oils. Spirulina and the green superfoods are also of great assistance because they enable nutrients to be absorbed easily and assimilated in the system.

Look for allergies and chemical imbalances and have them diagnosed to see if they are the problem. Eliminate preservatives and artificial foods from your diet all the time. You cannot afford to have even a random dose of these poisons as they can take days to get out of the system again and can set off a downward cycle of spinning energy. Make sure nutrients in the diet are adequate and have large doses of antioxidants such as grape seed extract and vitamin C.

Take selenium at 50 mg per day. Remember though that the difference between a toxic and a therapeutic dose of selenium is very slim. See your Health Care Practitioner for advice.

Take Vitamin E, magnesium, zinc, essential fatty acids and silica. Make sure you have the correct balance of biochemical cell salts in the body. Drink 200 ml of water every two hours during the day, more often if possible. Address toxins, if there is chemical, insecticide or heavy metal poisoning, then you will need to clean out the liver and have a supervised detox. Nervines are also good.

Basically, there are many approaches to take and they are all dependent on the person concerned. But let's face it, the sooner you can be in balance again, the sooner your life will be successful and the sooner you will have a healthy Wellness Zone.

PART IV
THE INTUITION ZONE

The Intuition Zone contains exercises and visualisations that you may wish to record and play back to yourself for enhanced healing and relaxation.

Take the time to process at the end of each day! To have time for silence in your day is special and is something that, once used to, you will crave and seek out daily. Learn to love silence and appreciate each moment in your life that offers it, and it's a special feeling to have your mind clear with no physical noises interrupting the peace and tranquillity.

Most of us live with lots of noise, all the time. Traffic, radio, people and animal noise, or the constant hum of the towns and cities we dwell in. Even when you go right out into the bush and experience the silence of nature, it's noisy. There are birds, trees, wind and water. In fact, it's virtually impossible to have complete silence anywhere these days. Earplugs are fairly ineffective, and even putting your ears underwater in the bath doesn't offer total relief from noise as you can hear your own heartbeat! So how can you have total silence?

Well, be realistic and make the most of what silence you are offered. Accept the wind in the trees, the birds and wildlife, the pounding of the ocean, the hum of the city and the buzz of people as aspects of your personal silence. Basically, just block it out as much as possible, develop the skill of avoidance for noises that are not directly involving you and that do not require your immediate attention. This is a skill that you will have probably already developed effectively over time anyway, even if you're unaware of this skill. Anyone who works in a group situation or has regularly travelled on public transport, even a child in a classroom environment, will learn this skill fairly swiftly in order to accomplish the task at hand in a distracting environment.

Create your own silence now

Create silence deliberately in order to process your day, thinking it through thoroughly from beginning to end. Once you have mastered this art of quiet contemplation, your sleep will be deeper, your dreams sweeter and there will be less waking in the middle of the night with thoughts of the day whirling around in your mind. This is an important aspect of your Wellness Zone.

The reason why you can't stay asleep some nights is simply because your life is too busy. You have difficulty keeping up with yourself, let alone being able to process all the associated information. When your body is finally relaxed in sleep, your subconscious wakes you up with the need to process the previous day, knowing that if it doesn't happen now, it won't happen at all! So you wake up, you think and worry, you lose sleep and then you start the next day exhausted; the following day you repeat the process and become stressed and even more exhausted. Continuing this routine can lead to you making some unwise choices, like taking sleeping tablets. These may knock you out, but they will also decrease your dreaming, eliminate your processing, slow down your body on all levels and then leave you feeling hungover the next morning. Meanwhile, there has been no processing done, you operate ineffectively at your chosen work, and then you wonder why. Isn't it obvious?

Make time to process your day

It may be as simple as turning the radio off in your car on the way to and from work, and this can allow you enough time to process the important things that need your attention. Often we are so busy worrying about 'so-called' priorities that we can forget about other important aspects of our lives that require some thought and planning. Take time, either in the car as you drive home, on a train with your mobile switched off, on a plane between venues, sitting on a lounge in a quiet corner or just lying in the bath contemplating the day. This is when you can start to find solutions to problems, when ideas start to form, and you think of new ways of doing old tricks. These are the moments when you are able to come to some sort of resolution with yourself about your life.

How to process your day

First, you need to make time to process each and every day as it comes. Don't delay doing this, it will only add to your personal stress levels, and you will miss out on the great opportunity of dealing with situations in an enlightened and clear way. For example, if you have a problem in the morning, deal with it immediately, don't delay it until the next day when you are sure to have other priorities. If you take the opportunity to process the incident straight away, then you may find a unique and creative solution. More importantly, you can move on and no longer be plagued by re-surfacing issues that you haven't initially taken the time to process and if necessary, solve.

You must simply take the time to process your day. If possible, go for a long walk, sit in the garden and just think, or do it while you're cooking dinner. When and how you do it is up to you and determined by your own unique circumstances. All you need is silence, no interruptions from other people and the desire to think, reflect and sort out the demons and worries in your head.

If you are operating on level energy in your Wellness Zone, then chances are that you are already unconsciously processing your day anyway! However, if your energy levels are anything less than ideal and you are living under stress and pressure, this can lead you to believe you have no time for this thinking process. If this sounds like you, then maybe try it out for yourself to see whether daily processing makes a difference to your rest and stress levels.

Sleep well

Some insomniacs, who have learned to process their day, are now able to sleep again. Try the following 'sleep well' herbal formula for a good night sleep: valerian, chamomile, passionflower and melissa. These herbals work on your autonomic and somatic nervous systems. Take the extract with some warm water before bed, and you will just have enough time to process the important parts of your day before sleeping. This is a special formula for stressed people who need to unwind and get a good night sleep.

Another good tool for sleeping well and processing your day is to go to bed early. Have a lovely bath or shower and then climb between the sheets and turn the lights down low. Just lie there thinking about your day. You can do this regularly after a busy day, and you will find you're able to sleep better, have a clear mind the next day and will probably be less rushed.

Children have a beautiful way of processing their lives: they daydream and make up stories; they use play. Perhaps you can use play too! Just keep the silence in the background and take on characters, you act yourself and everyone else in the situation too. It can be funny as you may find yourself responding to yourself in some unorthodox ways. This can be another way to process events from your day.

Keep a journal of your day: your emotions, events, responses and how you do and don't handle different situations at different times. Decide whether you want anyone else to read these, if you don't then simply burn them when the book becomes full. This is a good way to ensure that you are transforming old patterns, when you start a new journal, afresh with new ideas, you may find that you don't repeat old habits. Writing in your journal last thing at night is a really good way to process your day.

Breathe deeply when you are processing your day, imagine that each breath in is fresh air and each breath out is old stress, removed from your system. Processing is very personal.

Recipe for sleeping well

1. Get up early in the morning each day
2. Make sure you have 40 minutes of cardiovascular exercise at least four days a week
3. Eat natural unprocessed foods as the mainstay of your diet
4. Learn to say 'no' to unwanted stresses
5. Take the time to relax and process your day every day before you go to bed
6. Eat a light nutritious meal in the evening with limited alcohol
7. Don't use stimulants, drugs or excessive alcohol
8. Drink relaxing herbal teas. To sleep well, take an herbal extract of valerian, chamomile, hypericum, melissa, passionflower in the evening before bed
9. Have a warm soak in the bath or shower just prior to climbing between clean sheets
10. Limit computers, music, television, movies, theatre and other obstructive noises and entertainment in the evening
11. Read a good book in bed before going to sleep
12. Make sure there is silence in the house when you want to go to sleep

Turn on your intuition

For your Wellness Zone to be successful and optimally beneficial for your long-term health, you may need to break boundaries on how you think about the various aspects of your life. We live in a diverse and eclectic world where there is so much to do and see.

You may wish to delve into the deep waters of intuitive healing and personal intuitive medicines. All medicine has energy, and that energy is transformed into wellness for the patient when the medicine resonates with the particular individuality of each person.

Intuitive medicine is the non-scientific part of medicine. It's what many Health Care Practitioners call the placebo effect or, in everyday terms, 'fake' medicine. The part that is so unrealistically successful that there is no scientific reason to justify the results achieved from maybe a piece of bark swallowed with ritual, or a small amount of some floral infusion taken to cure a technically complicated illness.

There is such a strong public groundswell in favour of natural medicines, and people are drawn to them because they want a personal touch. They want intuitive medicine, a solution specific to them, individually. People are no longer running away from alternative practices. They are often so disillusioned by the mainstream system that they seek out the alternative, to balance the disparity in their health care regime.

The healing arts … isn't that a wonderful term? Intuitive medicine is one of the foundations of today's medicines. Historically, medicine has been developed through the combination of experimentation and results; this is true for all types of medicine today, including what we classify as 'alternative'. Cultural medicines are very effective and to be respected for their combination of time-proven remedies, ritual and intuitive understanding of the patient.

Healing sometimes involves tricking the body into wellness. This is because illness and disease have a way of sneaking up on you. If this is the case, then the best course of action is to sneak right back up on the illness and get rid of it thoroughly. This is where herbal and nutritional medicines are very effective. Saturate the illness with the overpowering goodness from the wonderful herbs and nutrients you take, thus helping to eliminate it.

Intuitive healing is unlimited; it is accepting the situation and finding out how to correct the balance to bring the body back into the kind of wellness that enables you to live your life to potential. Intuitive medicine is literally 'you' taking responsibility for your own health care. This involves finding out what is wrong, looking at the solutions and then open-mindedly making decisions about your healing regime based on the facts presented and your own intuition or 'gut feeling'.

Intuition is that feeling when you know something is wrong and needs addressing; it's that niggling feeling that you need to act in a certain way to achieve a certain result. We all have this ability; however, it can be closed off when you don't allow yourself the freedom of open-mindedness, or when you are too strict in your beliefs on the process of how things should be done.

For example, if you will only look at a medicine that has been 'scientifically' proven to work, then you may easily miss the best medicine for your ailment. Science has not yet found all the answers; in fact, science has a long way to go to understand natural medicine and the intuitive effects of medicine on a patient. You will be giving yourself the best help when you look at all your options and consider intuition as a part of the healing process, where you learn to trust yourself and your own instincts.

Once you have looked at your options, let your intuition help guide you to make the final decision. This is an holistic 'living medical' approach to wellness. Depending upon your openness, this may be a radical or a completely natural approach. Turn on your intuition today and see how balanced your life becomes as you trust yourself and the decisions you make.

There are times when wellness defies the boundaries of science and modern medicine in its various guises. Make sure you don't miss the path to good health because you have closed your mind to one of the most important and underrated aspects of health care; the magical art of healing and the use of personal intuition to create a truly wonderful Wellness Zone.

Balance your inner self

Living in today's world can be extremely exhilarating; it can also be very stressful. It's easy to look at things from a physical perspective as we view the world around us because this is the most obvious and also the easiest way to view our lives. However, you need to recognise that there are many non-physical aspects of your life, and these are also important in creating and maintaining your Wellness Zone. You need to learn to balance the inner self with the physical situations you are exposed to.

Your beliefs and philosophies will largely influence how you see your Wellness Zone and whether or not you wish to experiment with alternative healing therapies. Personal development is about experimenting with your intuition and trusting your inner voice. This is important if you want your Wellness Zone to expand beyond the current boundaries. You need to trust yourself enough to trust your intuition because we all have the ability to be intuitive.

Many people are limited in what they perceive because of society and the way they have been led to think in the past. Environmental and societal beliefs can inhibit your Wellness Zone. Some will choose to make the planet a better place for future generations, and some are extremely ethical in both business and personal practices. These choices are usually made because people recognise that there are future generations who need us to act responsibly now for their wellness and for the wellness of the planet.

You have the birth right and personal obligation to be true to yourself, if you can't trust yourself and your own instincts, then whom can you trust? Use your intuitive ability to improve your Wellness Zone and have a healthier life filled with trusting and loving experiences. Use your intuition and trust your own inner guidance; these are your most powerful tools for good health and will enable you to get through many difficult situations.

Visualise your wellness today

This is not as hard as it sounds, find some silence then close your eyes and think, allow yourself a few minutes of silent contemplation each day to see what comes up in your mind. Even waking up in the middle of the night, feeling the stillness and just listening to yourself. You can achieve this sense of stillness and space for your intuition to open up, after you have processed the head chatter that stops you from tuning into your intuitive self.

You need to take yourself through the process of mental visualisation, place yourself in a position of trust with yourself so that you are able to let go mentally and experience the intuitive realms that are available to each of us. This process takes time, and you may wish to join a meditation class or read specific literature about this area of wellness if you want to pursue the avenue of intuitive healing. Other tools for visualisation include floatation tanks, hypnotherapy and different types of meditation.

What is a personal visualisation?

Visions are ideas that you can see in your mind. Once we have an idea, we can either follow it through and turn it into a real-life experience, or we can let the idea drop away and become nothing but a fleeting thought. If you are sick, you can visualise that you are well again; this is a positive tool in your intuitive healing regime. If you empower yourself with these helpful healing visualisations then, with the right attitude, you will have given yourself the best opportunity for good health within your Wellness Zone.

You may need to take time each day to have silence and meditation in your life, or you may need to use energetic healing techniques that are not traditionally related to your own personal experiences. By opening yourself up to new ways and experiences, you are better able to look at what is beneficial to your wellness and what is destructive. You are what you make yourself to be, and every day provides a new opportunity to invest in the future 'you'.

We all accept dreams as a natural nocturnal event, so why not daydream? Why not have visions during the day that can help you to create wellness in your life and enhance that which you are already experiencing? This is easy when the wellness you visualise is the plaster coming off your leg in six weeks, or the bouncing and beautiful baby you will hold in your arms at the end of your pregnancy. However, it's much more difficult to try and mentally melt away cancer cells, or destroy a tumour in your brain, or even to rid yourself of a virus or other illness that is lingering, painful and chronic. It's even harder for those with addictions such as drugs, alcohol or tobacco?

Visualising a time that you are healthy and not craving or bending to your addiction is a hard vision indeed, just like seeing that tumour completely gone or imagining the day you have a kidney transplant and no longer require dialysis. But it's only as hard or as easy as you want to make it. After all, a visualisation is just a thought, one that allows you to forget a bad experience or see yourself with the plaster off, that sees the kidney transplant as a success, the healthy new baby, the cancer-free body or the end of obesity. The only thing that stands between you and that visualisation is fear, let go of the fear and take a risk for your wellness. Visualise and make it happen.

This can be done on any level you want, but it's best to first realistically plan and imagine the qualities you want to bring into your life. It's like going to a personal trainer and lifting a heavy weight straight away: it may be possible, but the pain and after-effects may be enough to put you off the whole idea after just one try. You can be truly well when you have the ability to visualise it and the desire to have a healthy future for yourself in a world where your dreams can come true.

Visualisation is your number one fantasy tool to lead you into wellness; it provides relief from the humdrum of problems that life presents.

Meditation is visualisation, and imagination is visualisation, drama, theatre, movies, books and everything that is around you is really the end result or manifestation from a visualisation.

The following example is synonymous with a visualisation for wellness; it is about a garden that was created from an empty field. First, you need the field (a fertile mind), then you need the seeds (ideas), you then plant them (the visualisation/dream) and water them (keep remembering the dream and feed it what it requires, i.e. positive thoughts). You can now watch the trees grow in the field, and you can add flower and vegetable gardens, you can add seats, boathouses and a dam with fish in it. Expand the garden (your thoughts and dreams) to exactly what your ultimate visualisation can be; the only limit is your imagination! Finally, you can sit back with joy and watch the manifestation of this beautiful garden. That is how it works with visualisation; you put in the hard work and then sit back and enjoy the results.

This is possible for you and for anyone. This level of wellness, of dreaming, and of beauty in your life is well deserved if you can put in the hard yards to visualise and create the reality that you want. If you want to visualise ultimate wellness for yourself, understand that this doesn't mean that your body will be perfect, or that your life will be a fairy-tale of excellent health, as when you were younger. It doesn't mean that you will have everything your heart desires. What ultimate wellness means for you, is different from what it means for someone else. Ultimate wellness is for each of us, the best level of wellness that you can have in your given situation.

Wellness is all about quality; it's about feeling the pain today but knowing that you are working towards a better tomorrow. It's about recovery and visualisation and knowing, that you have the self-respect, self-discipline and self-love to be the best and wellest person that you can be today. And by taking baby steps, your tomorrows can only be better.

Every day you should visualise and aim towards your own ultimate wellness; it's personal, just like your dreams. Continually strive to be your ultimate best today and then tomorrow, repeat the exercise all over again. Visualise the best wellness you know how to, take a tiny step down your hallway and know that one day, with all going well, if you do your best you'll be able to walk down that hallway, out the door, down the street and into that beautiful garden that was once just an empty field.

The visualisation challenge

Every morning for a week (or longer if necessary), with paper and pen, write down what is worrying you and what is creating the pain, illness or disease in your life. Then write a list of what you would replace this with and how you want the pain, illness and disease gone.

Now, here's the challenge. Once you have these thoughts on paper, close your eyes for a few minutes and visualise your plan to replace the bad bits. Make time every day to visualise your wellness plan. Whenever you get bored, or your mind is triggered to the idea, do this positive outcome visualisation. Do it until you are not so sceptical and you really, truly feel and believe that the results are both positive and possible. Do it until you have told yourself that it's really true, reprogramme your mind to accept that visualisation can be a very helpful tool in your Wellness Zone.

There are no limitations if you don't set them in your own mind. Just trust your instincts, if it feels good for a minute, that's enough encouragement for you to keep going for another minute, then another. Eventually, you will find that you are using visualisation as an active and positive tool in your day, initially just on the occasional day, then, when you start to really notice the benefits, you will use it most days and then hopefully, every day.

The energy that is mustered through visualisation can be strong and perfectly tuned into the body so that illnesses and genetic deficiencies may be minimalised and possibly even reversed. Nobody has the right to tell you that something is impossible in your healing, or that you will never recover from a situation. Many people have put in the hard work and achieved very good health and fabulous Wellness Zones simply by adding dreaming, vision and a future garden of wellness into their daily lives.

It only takes a moment of your time to create your own future. Don't sabotage the opportunity by not allowing yourself the very best chance to be really well. Intuition and visualisation are very powerful tools when used in the best way.

Healthy body visualisation

This is a good vision for you to begin with: daydream and imagine your Wellness Zone. You must believe that it's possible; it's no use doing any visualisations if you don't believe they will help; however, one power-ful thought that is '100% believed-in' can work miracles in your life. Just let your cells experience that optimal 100% wellness for a split second, let them get a taste of the beauty of wellness, and the vibration of true health and they will begin to crave the experience.

What you are going to do in this first visualisation is to imagine each part of your body from the top of your head to the tips of your toes, release any tension and energy blocks and replace them with beautiful, relaxed healing energy. You will need to picture a beautiful clear orange light for this exercise. With each breath inwards, you will be breathing in this clear, fluorescent orange healing breath of air. With each breath out, you will be breathing out any pain, worry or energy blocks that are in your body.

1. Lie on your back in a comfortable place where you are warm. Keep your body uncrossed and straight, and this is because you will be thinking about energy in this visualisation and it needs to have a free and unblocked passage in your body.
2. Relax your body. Take five deep breaths into your lungs through your nose and with each breath out, imagine yourself sinking a little deeper into where you are lying, with each breath try to relax a little more. Close your eyes and try to breathe deeply and gently into your diaphragm. Let each breath in be slow and deep, and each breath out be just as slow and releasing. In your mind, you will imagine that you are breathing in healing energy and breathing out your worries, illness, toxins, negativity or old habits that you want to leave behind.
3. Breathe in and out for a minute or two, thinking as you breathe in, of a beautiful clear orange light filling your mind. Then with each breath out imagine all your pains, worries and negative thoughts just drifting out of your body with the air. Clear your mind and thoughts of anything else. Work your way through your mind, head cavity, ears, eyes, nose, mouth and face. Think about each part separately and breathe in the beautiful orange light and breath out all tensions until you feel as though your whole head and mind are relaxed, clear and healthy.
4. Now that you have done this to your head, move to your neck. Just five to ten breaths in and out, emptying your neck of all tensions, worries and pains, and visualise again the lovely orange light.

5. Work your way down to your shoulders, then your chest and right down your torso. Think about your body and picture it with each breath in and out, to the extent of your understanding of anatomy and physiology. It's good when you can picture the major organs such as your lungs, stomach and digestive tract, your liver, spleen, gallbladder, pancreas, uterus, bladder and genitals. Also, try to picture your glands, hormones, skeletal and venous system, your blood, your lymph and your cells. Just take as long as you need, from at least two minutes and up to 20 minutes of focusing on each and every aspect of your body. Remember that you are breathing in the lovely orange healing light and that you are breathing out all energy blocks, tensions, illnesses and worries.

6. Once you have worked your way through your body, work down through your arms and legs. Just breathe in and out; everything you feel is only held together by the power of your breathing, breathe deeply and focus on each part of your body.

7. Once you have completely worked your way from your head down to your toes, take five breaths in and out and just experience how you feel. Nothing more, nothing less. Just observe how you feel. Visualise your whole body filled with this awesome orange light.

8. That's it, get up and get on with your day when you're ready. You can breathe for as long as you like in the final stages. However, the idea is to clear your mind and body of everything except the focused concentration of the gentle breathing.

Try to repeat this exercise regularly, maybe a couple of times each week. This will help you to understand and feel the difference in your Wellness Zone, on days when you make the effort to do the exercise and days when you don't. You may find it easier to write a list of all the body parts you want to visualise in this exercise and in what order you want to think about them. Have the list by your side as you do the exercise and look at it if needed. This will help you to stay on track until you know the visualisation well enough to do it alone.

After you have completed this vision for the first time, ask yourself how you truly feel. Do you feel a bit lighter, more relaxed, maybe less stressed? Does it make you feel a little better, or does it just leave you cold? Were you unable to complete the exercise because of lack of time or concentration? If this is the case, then keep trying, at least until you are able to develop the personal discipline needed to see the first exercise through. It's not hard; in fact, any difficulty you may experience is actually all in your mind. It's only as hard or as easy as you want to make it, and the results are truly worth the effort.

Herbs can help visualisations

Words can fail us when we try to describe translucent experiences that we hold personal. Each of us will have a different response to any visualisation, and it's important that you see through your own responses. Try to be open to healing your body on a cellular level that involves more 'thought' than medicine. This is why it's important that you really give these exercises a go and see for yourself how they can alter some cellular vibration and help you achieve optimal wellness for you today in your Wellness Zone.

Herbs that help with visualisation and dreaming

With the herb valerian, you can have success in enhancing nocturnal dreams. If you take a therapeutic dose combined with melissa, then you can be in for a real treat with visualisations and dreaming clarity. These herbs can help to relax the nervous system; melissa is also an emotionally calming herb which helps you to relax into the visualisation and somehow allows your mind to feel and think clearer. L-glutamine, the amino acid, is an enhancing and clarifying nutrient if you wish to visualise and create positive healing thoughts for the future. Passionflower, hops and other nervine herbs are also beneficial for visualisation exercises as they tend to help relax and allow you to slip into a state of positivity.

When you want to be visualising and dreaming well, ensure that you have eaten light foods that don't clog up your digestive tract. Keeping a dream diary by your bed can help you to remember your dreams. If you wake in the night with memories from a dream, immediately jot down everything you can remember, then try to get back to sleep again. Talk about your dream first thing in the morning, trying to recollect it verbally, then you may remember most of it. However, the most accurate way to see your dreams and then try to interpret all the symbolism involved, is to write it down with as many details as possible as soon as you wake from that dream.

You can turn a scary dream around too, simply change the ending. It's possible to do this when you are in that semi-sleep dream state that's almost like a trance, and you are dreaming so clearly. You need to engage your conscious mind in the act, as often you may half-awake in the course of a dream. Keep the dream going, you can then change scenes as they happen, simply by changing them in your mind. You can be in a dream, wake up and then make yourself go straight back into that dream again where you can completely change the bits you didn't like. You can train yourself to wake up in dreams and do this. It's rather easy once you have done it a few times. You just need to turn the belief that dreams are out of your control around to the belief that dreams are reflecting your life and you are capable of visualising the best results possible for your own Wellness Zone.

Remember that bad dreams are a personal way of sabotaging the goodness in your Wellness Zone. You need to be aware of the messages they are sending you, while at the same time being aware of how you can turn dreams around in your favour. This is the same with visualisations. You can turn them around and make them into something that's good for you. If you find yourself thinking negative or damaging thoughts, simply turn the thought around in your mind to a more positive and healing thought.

If you don't want to go there, don't even look

When you catch yourself in a daydream, the least you can do is to make it a wonderfully good daydream. If it's negative, turn it around and make it good, practice these positive visualisations. If you catch yourself thinking negatively about anything, remind yourself of this little ditty. "If you don't want to go there, don't even look!" In other words, just don't even think about, talk about or waste your energy on something or somewhere that isn't in your plan for your Wellness Zone. This is the best way to stay on track. This includes visualisations, dreams, movies you watch, books you read, people you communicate with and places you go to. Everything.

Take yourself where you want to be and stay away from everywhere else; it's simply not worth the hassle. Follow the same principle for any therapies, healings and medicines in your life. Unless you personally resonate with the practices, the style and the belief structure of the Health Care Practitioner, either orthodox and alternative, then go elsewhere.

Don't waste precious energy with Health Care Practitioners who do not have an intrinsic common ground in the matter of their patient's

Wellness Zone. This is an unwritten law of good health practices. Do yourself a favour and learn what you can and cannot resonate with. Don't compromise, if you really don't want a medicine, or a type of medicine or therapy, say *no*, walk on and trust your intuition. Put your own physical health above someone else's belief structure, if it goes against what you want for your Wellness Zone. However, don't be close-minded and don't be so open that you hurt instead of healing yourself. Make the most of the body you were blessed with, and we only get one in this lifetime, so make your Wellness Zone your priority.

Intuitive healing, chakra breathing, visualisations and dreams can all be part of your healing regime if you choose them to be, these can enhance your Wellness Zone if and when you need them. It's not the same for everyone; your Wellness Zone is exclusively yours, nobody else's is quite the same. There will also be different requirements for each phase in your life, and it's up to you to choose what works and when. Understand your own needs and develop your own rituals and thoughts about what is best for you. Be strong in spirit, and this will allow you to follow up on any ideas you may have that are unconventional in another person's eyes!

The Wellness Zone bath for breathing and listening to your heartbeat

Run a nice hot bath, put in whatever extras you desire; some essential oil, a flower remedy, perhaps a crystal. The aim of this treatment is cellular cleansing and mental clarity. This is the bath to have when you want to feel fabulous and re-energise yourself.

Lie in the bath with your ears and most of your head under the water, keeping your nose and face out of the water. Relax, and you will soon hear a thud, thud sound, that is your own heartbeat. Listen to your heartbeat and practise circular breathing. This involves breathing deeply and slowly through your nose, feeling the breath go deeply into your lungs and then breathing slowly out through your mouth. Don't have a break between breaths and make sure the breaths are slow and long. Allow thoughts to come and go as they please.

Stay like that in the bath for about five minutes, longer if you are happy and comfortable. When you need a break, get out of the bath and lie comfortably on the floor for a few minutes, continuing with the breathing. Take note of what thoughts pass through your mind and then just let them drift away. Make sure you have a comfortable towel under you and a pillow while you lie on the floor, maybe cover yourself with another towel or soft blanket.

After five or so minutes, return to the bath and continue the circular breathing. If you have an issue within yourself that you are thinking about, then breathe in the positive aspects of what you want to create concerning the issue and breathe out the negative aspects. So with each breath in, you are creating a visualisation of what you want, and with each breath out, you are releasing the old and unnecessary thoughts and processes. Continue like this in the bath, with your ears under the water, listening to your heart beating and processing your thoughts.

View yourself as an observer in your life, if you get really upset and start to cry then just keep your mind on your breathing and continue the process. You will find that eventually the crying will subside and you will feel some release. The aim of this treatment is not to get you upset; however, if you do, then just relax with the feeling and focus on your breathing and heartbeat.

It may be wise to have this hot bath at a time when there is nothing really wrong in your mind. That way, if you do have a bad time and have the need to use this ritual for some deep cleansing, you will feel more at ease with the idea and more inclined to try it. It's a lot easier to handle this 'water circular breathing' in a trauma after you have practised it dozens of times in peaceful situations, then you can handle a few tears and a pained heart. If you try this process for the first time, straight after a traumatic event, you may find it quite difficult. Circular breathing and listening to your heartbeat, while at the same time trying to manifest positive ideals and release outdated thoughts, is something that requires practise.

You can alternate between the floor and the bath for as long as it takes. Stay in the bathroom for two or three hours if necessary. It's wonderful how time can fly during this exercise, so a leave a glass of water at the side of the bath to sip when want. You can alter this process by having cold spritz showers between the bath and the floor, go from the bath straight into a cold shower, lie on the floor for a few minutes (if you're not too chilled) then jump back into the bath again. When you think it's time to stop, dry yourself off, have a cup of herbal tea and have a good sleep or go for a long walk.

This bath is special, and you may find it helps you through a difficult day or you simply have a lazy afternoon to while away.

A simply delicious meditation
This is another way to spend a delicious hour in the bath!

Meditation is a way to open doors within our mind and allows new thoughts to enter and old patterns to transform gently. Here is a meditation you may like to try. The aim is stress release and appreciation of the good in our lives.

Lie down in a quiet place. Close your eyes and breathe deeply. Feel the air entering your nose and filtering down through your throat, into your lungs and deeply down to your diaphragm. Hold the breath there for a few seconds and gently release it out again. Keep breathing until you are only focused on the breath. Allow any thoughts that are in your mind to drift away.

Once you feel completely focused on your breath and you are comfortable that the daily thoughts have receded to the back of your mind, think about a place that you love. Your favourite place where you are always safe and comfortable. Go there in your mind. Keep breathing deeply. In your mind's eye look about the place, breathe the air, feel the energy, relax. Keeping your eyes closed, imagine that you are there alone. Now in the middle of this place, there is a big ruby crystal ball, it is about the size of a normal armchair. It is sitting right in front of you, walk over to the crystal and wrap your arms around it. Just flop your body across the imagined crystal.

Now, feel all the stress, pressure and frustrations of life slip gently from your body into the ruby crystal. Let it melt away. Take deep breaths and feel all the tension just slip away. With each breath in, you can focus on a particular stress that you are releasing and on each breath out you can feel that stress slip away from your body.

Keep yourself focused and breathing until you are completely relaxed and can't think of any more stress that needs to be released. Remember that you have your arms wrapped around this gorgeous ruby that carries healing grounding energy from the earth. Remember that you are totally safe and that you can release even the deepest and oldest tensions if and when they come into your mind. When you feel you have completed this part of the meditation, stay holding the crystal for a few minutes and refocus on your breathing again. Feel yourself enjoy your body without stress, feel the difference.

The next part of the meditation is to continue holding the ruby crystal, keep breathing and think about the blessings in your life.

The love you feel for yourself and for others. The gratefulness for the good in your life and the appreciation you feel and think for the year gone by. Reflect on the past year in your mind's eye and all that has occurred. The changes you have undergone and the appreciations you feel for these changes. Even if you have had a tough year, this process in meditation can help change perspective and enlighten you to the good things in your life.

The final part of the meditation is to say a prayer of peace and gratefulness for the environment, people and animals on the planet and also for health and well-being. This can be simple. Just a few words in your mind that reflect how you feel and what you think on these issues.

Now look around the beautiful place where you are, take a few more deep breaths and transport yourself in your mind's eye back to the present. Open your eyes and savour the feeling. Often after a meditation it's good to have a shower, bath or cool swim. Water is a fabulous tool for changing energy. You will feel enlivened and revitalised after this meditation. You may also be more conscious of the stress you have released and be more able to enjoy each new day with gratefulness and appreciation.

Repeat the meditation as regularly as required. You may start the day feeling fully refreshed if you allow yourself the time to let go of the old and allow the new energies to enter and revitalise your body, mind and soul.

Energy healing

The essence of energy healing is breath, visualisation and the ability to mentally release and transcend any illnesses, pains or limitations that you have in your body or mind. This is a relatively easy concept once you have grasped the idea that energy healing is literally about allowing the flow of energy in your body to be consistent and optimal for cellular regeneration and balanced physical health.

There are some very old and tested techniques for energy healing. The common practice of reiki is one such way, whereby you shift energy through your body via breathing and visualisation. Other methods include the chakra system and the use of that system to help you regain balance and good health. Rebirthing and personal transitional techniques are other options.

There are many forms of energy healing, learn to be able to invoke these healings with a little trust, relaxation, appropriate breathing, visualisations and giving your body the grace and respect it deserves to create good health.

The chakras and how to use them for your Wellness Zone

In ancient cultural healing practices, the system of the chakras has withstood the test of time and is used as an access porthole into the deeper realms of healing. According to tradition, we are all born with this deeper awareness of the chakra system, and we are all able to tap into its magnificent healing potential as needed.

There are many exercises when it comes to thinking about chakras, and what they do for your body; you can play around and even create your own special techniques. There's nothing that evokes good health as quickly as self-healing and the feeling of being empowered by your own systems and methods.

These are the magical elements to your Wellness Zone, and magic is certainly a good thing when it is lighting your path with wellness.

What are the chakras?

There are seven chakras that go from the crown of your head to the base of your torso. Although there have been many texts written about this system that state there are more than seven chakras, most people have found success with only focusing on the main seven and using each one to help a certain aspect of health or certain areas of the body.

According to Indian tradition, chakras are a complete set of energy pathways that open and close a person to energies, from both the physical and the spiritual realms. They are your porthole to other dimensions and to bringing certain qualities that you may require. Once again this is related to your energy patterns and how you use them. Each chakra can open up so many possibilities that it's an awesome experience just working on one at a time.

Like your aura, or any aspect of you that is not seen clearly in the physical realm, it's a case of visualising the existence of the chakras, and they will become clear to you over time. After all, a chakra is not a visible entity.

They are effective catalysts to healing. People who are very sick physically become lighter, more joyous and heal faster when they regularly work on their chakras, along with being given the appropriate herbal medicine and nutritional support. You can lift negativity and bounce into a new attitude to life, by regularly cleansing and working on your chakras.

Use your breathing for chakra visualisations

The secret in chakra breathing is that you literally forget the nose. Imagine that you are breathing oxygen into the specific chakras that you choose to focus on at that time. You breathe into each chakra and then breathe out again through another chakra (or the same chakra if you prefer).

There are seven chakras. The top one is located on the crown of your head. The colour usually representing this chakra is either white or violet. This represents the energy coming down to you from the universe. It is ideally referred to as higher awareness energy that enhances your spiritual awareness and connection to the divine.

The second chakra is located between your eyes. This is the 'third eye' chakra. It is usually represented as a deep indigo purple colour and ideally connects you with your deeper self, your intuitive self.

The next chakra down is in your throat. This is represented by turquoise blue and is about your ability to express yourself and use your voice appropriately.

Below this is the heart chakra, represented by the colour green, and it is located in the sternum between your breasts. Ideally, this chakra is your capacity to love and be loved in the world. It represents emotions and your heartfelt self.

Following this is the chakra located directly over your solar plexus, this is yellow in colour and ideally represents your energy levels and your capacity to create and use energy well.

Just below your navel is the sixth chakra, represented by the colour orange. This ideally represents physical health and capacity for healing the body.

The seventh chakra is located in women on the cervix opening and in men between the penis and anus. This chakra is represented by the colour red and ideally represents your personal drive and sexuality. This is the grounding chakra, the one that keeps you connected to the earth.

As you can see, the top chakra opens you to the influences of the universe, whilst the bottom chakra keeps your feet firmly planted on the earth. The chakras in between work their way from intuitive to mental to the emotional and physical aspects of your life. This is where you can use your visualisations, intuition and personal healing abilities to incorporate your physical wellness with your intuitive wellness.

It's a complete visualisation in your mind throughout the whole process. The Wellness Zone of each and every one of us can be enhanced when you are open to looking at the chakras and this aspect of yourself which is unseen and unknown. We are all spirit, with human experience, so perhaps the chakras are a bridge between these two realms.

Chakra breathing and the wonderful healing it invokes

The cleansing chakra breathing technique

This technique incorporates each chakra. You will start from the top and slowly breathe in through one and out through the next one down. In this exercise, you will work your way through each chakra until you have completed all seven, breathing slowly in and out.

If you find this a little complicated to start with, simply breathe in and out of the same chakra until you can clearly see the colour and imagine the qualities that each one evokes. Once you know the colours and can clearly see in your mind's eye what you are doing, then breathing through the complete set of chakras in one go will be a joyful experience.

Imagine that the colours are becoming clearer and brighter with each breath in and out. If the colours are murky, then make them clear and crisp. Imagine your energy being balanced and old stale energy within each chakra being cleared out with each breath. This is called chakra clearing or cleansing, and many people do it regularly as part of their Wellness Zone.

Take a deep breath in, when you do this visualise that breath coming in through the crown of your head instead of your nose. (Of course you are breathing through your nose on the physical level, but you need to forget this and just picture that the breath is coming in through your crown chakra straight to your body.) When you exhale, visualise it leaving your body through your third eye chakra. Do this a few times then imagine the breath coming in through your third eye chakra and breathing out through your throat chakra.

Next, visualise it coming in through the throat and going out through the heart chakra, then in through the heart and out through the solar plexus chakra. Next, breathe in through your solar plexus and out through your belly chakra, and finally in through the belly and out through the basal chakra.

This should keep you concentrating purely on your breath for a while. It gets easier as you practice more. You can choose any chakra to breathe into and any to breathe out of again. It's a purely personal choice and of course depends on what you want to achieve through the process.

For example, if you have particular issues that you need to work through, you can focus on the chakras that surround those issues.

- For mental clarity, breathe in through the crown and out through the third eye
- Intuitive development, in through the third eye and out through solar plexus then in through the crown and out through the third eye
- Expression, in and out through the throat
- Love and anger, heart issues, in through the heart and out through the base
- Health and energy, in through solar and out through the belly
- Sexuality, in through the base and out through the crown

It really depends upon how you associate yourself with your chakras. You will develop your own techniques over time and find that you will choose the chakras you need to use each time. For example, if you're feeling stressed in a meeting where you feel out of control, you may choose to breathe in through your crown chakra and out through your base chakra. This will allow you the awareness of higher levels of consciousness whilst grounding you to the situation. Therefore you will feel more in control of yourself.

If you are feeling unmotivated and de-energised, then it may well help your focus and energy levels if you breathe in through your solar plexus chakra and out through your third eye. This will allow you to bring in the energy required to get motivated and connect your physical energy levels to your mental capacity, hopefully motivating you to do what's needed.

Consider that your master secretory glands are located in your head, so it is therefore of great importance to have a healthy mental state and makes sense to spend time breathing in your crown chakra. You may need grounding, so the base chakra is a good place to connect to the earth.

Clearing bodily toxins through chakra breathing

You are able to process current toxins through the chakras, and this can be done on your own if you are relaxed and open minded. Lie down in a warm and comfortable place. Close your eyes and breathe in through your crown chakra. When you do this, think that you are breathing in a beautiful fluorescent violet colour, and try to visualise this in your mind.

Relax, keep it simple and don't push your mind to see; it will happen eventually. All you need is to have faith in self-healing and trust that you are capable of clearing toxins and uneasiness from your cells.

Now imagine that the chakra is a bell shape and that this bell has an opening at the top. Open it, and what do you see? Is it dark and greyish, or even black and with lots of gunk, or is it a brilliant violet colour, clear and eternal? Maybe something in between?

Now the aim is simple. Without delving mentally into any of your personal problems, you are going to keep breathing that gorgeous violet energy straight down into and then out of the crown chakra, expelling at the same time any of that toxic waste that you have been vibrating. Keep doing this until the chakra is clean and you are breathing in and also out, a beautiful fluorescent violet colour, focus on purification of the chakra and it will happen.

Even if you only breathe through one chakra a day, you will clear the gunk and free up your physical self to vibrate to a richer and higher energy. You may, at some point, experience the visualisation of a black cord. Start to pull on it and keep pulling until you think that you either need to snap it off or it dissipates under its own energy. These black cords can represent old or outdated modes of thinking, patterns of relationship destruction or negative energy that is blocking the health of the chakra. Just keep breathing through it until the colour becomes clear again.

You may like to leave each chakra pulsating and glowing with wonderful vibrant energy after your breathing exercises. If you choose to see them that way, then they will become that way. The clearer and cleaner your chakras are, the better you will cope, on a physical level, with daily life and the challenges it brings. This is living visualisation and brings the ability to enhance your Wellness Zone with your own thoughts and solutions. There is no right or wrong way to create your visualisations, so long as they are healing and heartfelt and for the betterment of your Wellness Zone.

Once you have worked on each chakra and the process of cleansing has been going on for a while, you may want to take it further and start to revitalise your cells with your chakra breathing. You can focus on any colour from any chakra, bring it into your body and focus on where you want to transfer that energy. This is especially good for healing illness and chronic disease.

You may even visualise a meditation where you focus on each part of your body separately within the same meditation, and you can re-energise yourself completely whilst breathing and creating a really solid connection between your cells and your chakras.

Just think about vibration, your vibration. How do you want it to be? It's all up to you. If you have been in a particularly low energy area or in a place where there is a lot of environmental toxicity, then you should be clearing your chakras through breathing whenever you get the opportunity. This can be done spontaneously and even in public. Just concentrate, breathe through your chosen chakra and clear the energy. Sometimes you can accelerate this clearing and cleansing process by jumping into the water, either for a swim or a shower. Nothing changes your energy as quickly as water will; it is a very good medium to use in conjunction with chakra breathing.

The colours for each chakra

The crown chakra is violet
The third eye chakra is deep indigo purple
The throat chakra is turquoise blue
The heart chakra is lime green
The solar plexus chakra is bright yellow
The belly chakra is rich mandarin
The base chakra is ruby red

These are all pure, clear and clean colours, the most glorious and awesome visualisation of each colour that you could ever possibly imagine. A burst of fluorescence. If there is discolouration, or you are unable to see a chakra clearly in your mind's eye, then you may be dealing with an energy block or illness that needs to be eliminated from that part of the body.

The colours of the chakras are very personal, for example, your heart may be an olive green colour; this would indicate that there is trouble in the heart region of your body, either physically or emotionally. Your throat may be dark blue; this says that you are compromised in your expressions. The clearer and brighter the colour, the healthier and more balanced is the chakra is associated with these emotions, thoughts and health.

When you look at your Wellness Zone, you can incorporate your own chakras and their health into the overall plan. It's important that we take the energy issue from the top, and this is our chakras. Learn to move the energy around your body and accept that all which is real is not always seen.

When you use this system of energy for personal health, you may notice some benefits as you feel healthy and well but when you ignore this system, you may become bogged down on the physical plane and become lost with who you really are. This system of colour visualisation and associating it with different parts of your body can be the difference between wellness and sickness as you search for new solutions to old health problems. It may not be appropriate for everyone to delve into the world of visualisation, but you are limiting your mental capacity and yourself empowerment in the art of healing if you completely close your mind to these options.

The more muddy or unclear a colour in your visualisation of a chakra, the more you may want to work on that area and try to make the colour as clear as possible in your own mind. There is no scale of physical proof that the chakra will be healed, healthy and beautiful, and there is no physical scientific evidence to say categorically that your visualisations and your chakra work will lead to wellness. However, in research that has been conducted and with the reading available, many people are convinced that the energy of the chakra and the balance of your external energetic system is a fundamental and essential ingredient to have true health and wellness.

Your Wellness Zone is dependent upon you taking the time, making the energy and believing in the unseen. It is the ability for each and every cell in your body to vibrate to another level of energy that is classically called the chakra system. If this sounds strange, then you may wish to try just breathing in through your nose and visualising a colour, any colour, then breathe out again, breathing out the colour. Keep doing this for five minutes or so, and see how you feel. Try another colour and see what effect that has on your body. There are many visualisations and meditations that you can do to help you change your energy and feel more comfortable and well.

Enhancing chakras

The herbs for each chakra are dependent upon the required outcome. It's important that you think about what you want to achieve before taking herbs and using essential oils when you are doing chakra meditations and visualisations.

For flower and plant essences, the essence would naturally change as you change; therefore, the idea is to randomly pick an essence out of your personal kit and take a very small dose (one drop) before each specific session or exercise that you want to do. Don't go literally picking out essences, let the essence find you. You need to trust your intuition and go with what feels right when it comes to flower and plant essences. They have such a lovely vibration, and they can add a new dimension to your day when they are added with randomness and subtlety.

Crystals are something that you can use as jewellery or decoration. If the crystal looks like the colour or resonates with you to the energy of a specific chakra, then relish the idea and adopt that crystal to that chakra.

Some ideas may be: quartz as the crown, amethyst as the third eye, turquoise as the throat, green fluorite as the heart, citrine as the solar plexus, carnelian as the belly and ruby as the base. These base colours and stones can also be adapted to whatever other stones come into your life. For example, you could say that diamond was the crown, lepidolite the third eye, aquamarine the throat, chrysocolla the heart, sunstone the solar plexus, tourmaline the belly and obsidian was the base crystal. There may be many other combinations, and it just depends upon how you resonate to a stone and how you feel and think when that stone is in close contact with your body.

The more you study stones, the more choices you will have for specific energies resonating with each other, and you can become more selective in the balancing of your body as required.

Some traditional cultural medicines consist of ground-up crystals mixed with herbs and essential oils. These cultures recognise that there is a specific relationship between the earth, water, wood, fire and air. You may choose to study these concepts and incorporate them into your healing regime.

Herbs and essential oils for each chakra

The crown chakra—violet

This chakra deserves the utmost respect. It is at the top of your head and therefore all things below this chakra, and all other aspects of your life are dependent upon the health of your mind in all ways. Remember that all of your master hormonal secretions come from your brain; it is the ruling centre for all body function in every way, including your nervous system. So all functioning is dependent upon your mind being clear, healthy and operating optimally.

The herbs for this have an effect on your complete balancing and also stimulate and encourage brain functioning. The brahmi herb combination of ginkgo biloba, gotu kola and bacopa is excellent as a daily tonic to help keep you in tip-top thinking condition. If you use lavender flower extract, you can literally drink the violet vibration and keep your nervous system in good condition whilst encouraging the vibration of the crown chakra. The herb astragalus has been shown in research to have an effect on master hormonal secretions, and so this is another good adaptogenic herb to take to enhance the energy of your crown chakra.

Sandalwood essential oil is excellent when taken in the morning to enhance mental capacity and is also used traditionally to wake up and tune the pituitary gland. Rosemary and lavender essential oils, combined together are wonderful for the crown chakra as they also help to relax and enhance mental powers. Having a clear mind is essential to good health, and if you can take daily measures to keep your mind clear, then you will probably feel better all over.

The third eye chakra—indigo purple

This chakra is located between your eyes and above your nose. When you think about the qualities that this chakra evokes, creating intuition and strengthening the mental capacities of the crown chakra, whilst bridging the gap between the body and the mind, it makes sense that you will want to work physically in this area. Interestingly, the herb bilberry mixed with eyebright is good for this. Master hormonal secretions are all controlled from the brain and once again you may want to use astragalus and the herbs mentioned for the crown chakra. Hypericum is another herb for this third eye area as it brings about serenity.

Valerian, kava and chamomile are also good relaxing herbals to calm the mind and melissa is a good nervine herb to help lift the spirits.

Any herb that lifts the spirit and helps the mind to stay positive is welcome here, and this includes cocoa extract. Even a nice cup of hot chocolate, perhaps some organic chocolate or a piece of chocolate mud cake are all good medicine for the third eye chakra, when you feel the need for some mental uplifting or mood elevation.

Panax ginseng is a favourite third eye chakra herb as it gives you the ability to really think clearly for extended periods of time, that crisp awake and alert feeling that is associated with good energy is certainly helpful.

Essential oils for this area are the ones that create alertness. Basil is a good oil to keep you mentally alert. Also, clove bud oil can be used to help resolve past issues and move them about so that they are easier to deal with. Lessor periwinkle can help increase your vibrancy on a mental level.

The throat chakra—turquoise blue

Your throat chakra is located about where your Adam's apple is or would be. The best herb for this area is liquorice root which is smooth and soothing for expression and sore throats; other helpful herbs are thyme, sage and white horehound. The throat is really a very sensitive area; have you ever noticed that when you think you are not expressing yourself correctly, or if there is something you need to say and are unable to say it, then you end up with a sore throat. This is very common, and if we take the time to think blue, concentrate on our throat chakra and look at where we need to express ourselves, then we can learn to be able to use our voice appropriately and hence not suffer from the illnesses related to this area of our body.

The herbs for the throat are onion, garlic, honey, lemon, grapefruit, olive leaf and lemon myrtle. Kelp is useful when you are unable to express yourself at the right time. Essential oils are once again citrus type oils, including lemon, grapefruit, and neroli. Lemongrass is another oil to associate with this chakra and with expression. When you think about the throat chakra, also think about the lungs and herbs that can heal them. Echinacea, purpurea root and nettle, plus cat's claw are strong herbs blended together to heal the lungs.

The heart chakra—lime green

This chakra is associated with your feelings of love, acceptance and self-worth, from the basics through to how you respond emotionally to the world around you. Green is the colour but often the rose quartz crystal, which is pink, is associated with this chakra. Herbs that protect the cardiovascular system and increase circulation are the best herbs for this heart chakra. These include ginkgo biloba, hawthorn, bilberry, turmeric, globe artichoke, as well as healing herbs for the spirit, such as chamomile, valerian, passionflower, hypericum and melissa. As you can see, there is a crossover here between herbs of the heart and herbs of the mind; this is because the heart and mind need to be in harmony for you to be fully in harmony with yourself.

Rose essential oil is really the number one oil for your heart chakra, and really nothing else can match it for loving balancing energy, it resonates even in the hardest heart. Lavender is renowned for heart balancing, that may be why it has always been so popular amongst the ladies and new mums. Wintergreen is heart chakra oil and is well combined with clove bud and flower oils such as the beautiful German chamomile and nasturtium for heart chakra health. Green foods and herbs rich in chlorophyll are necessary to help you have good heart health. These include green barley grass, spirulina and wheatgrass.

The solar plexus chakra—bright yellow

Imagine that the sun has a direct line into your body through your solar plexus and that this line brings in all the physical energy that you will need. This is the solar plexus chakra's job, to bring you energy.

The herbs that bring you energy are nettle (my favoured herb to increase cellular integrity), withania (which is a good energy pick-up herb) and all of the herbs that balance and heal the kidneys, liver and adrenal glands, including milk thistle, dandelion, corn silk, asparagus and Siberian and panax ginseng.

Herbs that help digestive enzymes are also beneficial here too, including pineapple and paw paw extracts. Maca is one favourite solar plexus chakra herb, and cat's claw is also good. As this chakra is close to the sternum where T-cells are produced in your body, immuno-modulatory herbs such as cat's claw and astragalus are beneficial. Essential oils for this chakra are cinnamon, cedarwood, neroli again, grapefruit again, lemon again and lemongrass.

Pungent oils are the oils of choice for this chakra, as well as those that increase cellular energy. Turmeric is beneficial here as it evokes good cholesterol levels and helps the detoxification pathways of oestrogen from your liver, it stops built-up oestrogen from forming in your breasts which can be a precursor to cancer. All herbs that keep the energy moving around in your body are beneficial for the solar plexus chakra. Many chronic illnesses are exacerbated by stagnant energy, and this chakra is important to keep your energy moving freely. Keep the energy flowing to help avoid cancer and chronic illness.

The belly chakra—rich mandarin

This chakra is all about your own physical health on every level. It's about how well you are today and what coding you have programmed into your cells for your health tomorrow. The herbs for this chakra start with very basic digestive herbs, such as marshmallow and fennel seeds. They also include black walnut and pau d'Arco, which are both renowned for getting rid of parasites and unwanted poisons from the body. Other herbs for this area are garlic, capsicum, turmeric, bay leaves, fenugreek and ginger, and also peppermint which is deodorising and soothing. Of course, you will want some mandarin to eat and some mandarin oil to smell to help remind you of the value of longevity and good physical health.

Peaches, nectarines and apricots, in fact all fruit and vegetables of this colour range are good for this chakra. Whether it is carrot, apricot or peach essential oil, you will feel your health becoming stronger. Your libido is connected to this chakra, and your kidneys rely on its clean functioning. All herbs that benefit your libido and/or balance your kidneys are beneficial here when you are having problems with your belly chakra.

The base chakra—ruby red

This is your drive, your grounding and of course the core of your sexuality. The herbs that help this area of the base chakra, must first be connected with the belly and the solar plexus chakras. If you have limited energy in other areas, then you will be low in energy in this basal area of your life.

The herbs for the base chakra are raspberry leaf, bilberry berries, ginkgo biloba, and all the adaptogenic herbs, such as panax and Siberian ginseng, withania and astragalus. You may also want to use tribulus, olive leaf, red clover, black cohosh, dong quai and other herbs that are grounding and that keep you connected to the earth. Root herbs such as maca and ginseng serve the double purpose of being balancing and grounding.

Essential oils for this chakra are geranium, ylang-ylang and patchouli. Old-fashioned oils such as myrrh, sandalwood and frankincense are also beneficial for this chakra.

Make up your own mind about the chakras

It's important that you keep your mind focused on creating and maintaining your own Wellness Zone at each stage of the exercises you choose, if you decide to use the chakras as part of your healing and health regime. There is a lot of information available from various old and modern texts where you can learn more about the specific actions and healing properties associated with this system of healing.

You can make up your own list of what herbs and oils you wish to use for each chakra and for each type of visualisation you are undertaking.

A really personal gift to yourself would be to buy some lovely glass bottles that are quite small and decorative. Keep them in the bedroom or bathroom and fill with your desired oil blends and herbs, thereby having a bottled mixture for each chakra. You could even try to source a separate and appropriate looking bottle for each chakra and fill with the blends of your choice. Then they will be at hand, special and celebratory, for whenever you want or need them.

Many choices for essential oils and herbs

There are many essential oil choices that you can experiment with when using them to enhance your Wellness Zone. Essential oils have a special place in creating atmosphere; they can evoke emotional responses through their individual smells and the feelings associated, either from past experience or a perceived vision.

Try the combination of melissa, sandalwood and rose for focused softness. Neroli can be blended with grapefruit for energy, enhancing and revitalising. Blend ylang-ylang with some patchouli and basil for awakening and a lively party mood or the pure crispness of lime oil to keep you awake and alert on a long night. Send yourself to sleep with a dose of clove bud and lavender mixed down with a tad of valerian and chamomile, and when it comes to serious study sessions, you can't go past some good old-fashioned rosemary oil to smell every now and then.

You just need imagination, visualisation and the desire to turn your visions into reality for the good of your Wellness Zone and then do whatever you need to maintain it for as long as possible. This may mean creating your own special signature blends of oils, perfumes and herbs.

The healing space visualisation

Imagine that there is a special place where you could go to think about your ultimate health. You may imagine a cave or a mysterious room in a special and secret place where you are miraculously healed and where all your problems are solved? You can create this place, and you can use visualisation to help you create a magical and personal healing space where, whilst you are there, all your ills are a past memory. This healing space can be real, you just have to imagine it, and you will have it there forever in your mind!

Your healing space is your refuge from the world, a place where you are able to vent your deepest thoughts, thereby enabling your body and soul to rest and restore energy and balance. Your home may be your best refuge, a place where you can retreat with your loved ones and become ready to face the world again. This may be a garden, a room, a small display of special items or even a whole home dedicated to healing and wellness.

The healing space visualisation can create a mental healing space for you that is separate from the physical healing space you may have created in your own home. You create it mentally, and you will then be able to go there in your mind whenever you need an inner sanctuary from the external world.

First, find a quiet corner and relax, close your eyes and be prepared to take yourself on a mentally stimulating visual journey. Think about a special place that you love to visit, maybe somewhere beautiful that you know of from the past or even an imaginary place that you think is ideal and beautiful. This place needs to be peaceful, somewhere you are able to really relax. It needs to be a totally safe place where there is no conflict or untoward noise.

Now imagine that you are at this place and you are completely well and healthy. Imagine your ills are being cured and you are releasing any blocks or negativity from your life. Breathe it, feel it, see it. The idea of creating this visualisation is so that you have somewhere in your mind to visit when you feel like your body and soul need a bit of loving restoration.

Your healing space visualisation can be used at any time when you are sick and want some serenity and peace with your illness. It's a place where you can go mentally when you are stressed and out of your Wellness Zone. Your healing space can be any beautiful place where you feel completely relaxed and able to heal, get your sense of balance back and de-stress.

The spinning top

This meditation is quick, light and able to be done virtually anywhere at any time. All you need is your presence of mind and the ability to close your eyes for a few minutes. Of course, this exercise is always better done in a quiet pristine environment, but you can also do it with great success on the bus, train, plane or even travelling in a car, provided you're not driving of course.

The whole idea is to get your visualisation clear with colour and have the chakra spinning around very fast like a spinning top; you may remember these from your childhood. Remember how the string is wound around the top, you then find a flat piece of ground, pull the string and let it spin. The top spins very fast for a minute or two before it comes to a complete standstill and then you repeat the process.

With the spinning top visualisation, you need to block out all noises around you and ignore any interruptions until the top has stopped spinning. This is possibly the ultimate meditation for chronically busy people. It's quick and able to be done in a noisy environment but is effective in clearing your energy for a minute so you can get on with being super busy again, feeling refreshed.

This meditation lightens up the energy and allows you to get present with the current environment and stay grounded when you are stressed. It is also a good exercise when you are not well or having some kind of surgery or dialysis, maybe when you're having blood tests or need a distraction at the dentists.

1. Take a deep breath in through your nose, then when you breathe out, close your eyes.
2. Keep your eyes closed and breathe in and out deeply and slowly for three breaths. While you are doing this, quickly scan your body with your mind's eye and make a note of any physical pain, stress and emotional or mental thoughts that may be trying to get your attention.
3. Pick a part of your body that requires the most attention at this moment.
   * Perhaps you are over-thinking, and your mind needs the attention. In this case, choose your second eye chakra with the beautiful purple colour as your target.
   * Perhaps you are worried and need guidance, in this case choose the crown chakra.
   * Maybe you need to express something, will be speaking publicly or have something of great importance that will be said shortly. In this case, choose your turquoise blue throat for the attention.
   * Maybe the issues of the heart, circulation, emotions and love are the issues, you then need to think the green of the heart chakra.
   * Maybe you require energy, lots of pure energy to be delivered to your life, or you have issues with any of the nerves that go off your spinal cord around the torso area. Then you need to think yellow and bring in the energy of the sun and the light from that area.
   * Or perhaps you are dealing with a creative issue or physical illness. In that case, you need to concentrate on the rich, mandarin coloured belly chakra.
   * Is your issue sex, drive, ambition or grounding? Then the base chakra is the place to focus.
     You just need to make your choice in your mind's eye and then keep breathing. Choose any mental, emotional or physical issue that beckons your call. Then choose a corresponding chakra and colour to concentrate on for this exercise.
4. Now, you have made your choice, you need to take your mind's eye to the area and then start to see the chakra with the next breath inwards. What does it look like? Can you see it? Is it spinning beautifully like a top or do you need to give it a push-start so that it starts working well for you? Is the colour clear, or do you have to struggle to see any colour at all? Now you need to just breathe in and out for a minute or so and set up in your mind's eye the spinning top.

5. To do this you will have to visualise your chosen chakra like it is a spinning top, then you get a piece of golden thread or string and tie it around the top. Wrap the string round and round until you have tied maybe a metre of golden thread around the top. Let's say for example you have chosen the base chakra to spin, you have an important meeting in an hour and you need to be grounded. You will now be seeing (or imagining), in your mind's eye, the golden string, held around a red fluorescent spinning top. It is poised and ready to be released across the large flat surface in front of you. Visualise a nice wooden floor or a similarly large flat area. The idea is that the spinning top will stay spinning for a minute or so.

6. Now, let the top go, pull on the string and let it spin away. Focus on the top, spinning away all the stress, hurt and worry, all those distractions, blockages or limitations associated with that chakra. Imagine the top spinning beautifully on the floor for a minute or so until the string has completely been left behind and it finally slows down and drops to the floor in sheer exhaustion. Now … what is left? Is there a beautiful and magical red spinning top, resting on the ground following its exhausting experience? Is it the right colour? Now you can place the spinning top back into your body where it belongs and feel the sheer joy of a small step in cleansing and energising yourself.

7. You can now move onto the next chakra if you have time, or jump off the bus, open your eyes and talk to the children, restart your work for the day or resume whatever it was you were doing.

If you are particularly worried about any aspect of your physical body, then you should 'spin' each chakra more than once. If you practise this spinning top visualisation regularly, wherever you are, and whenever you think of it, I'm sure, like me, you'll start to feel better within yourself about all sorts of things in your life that need dealing with.

Think high thoughts for wellness

It's easy to get caught up in the slog of life and forget to look after yourself properly. Sometimes we stay on a certain level and operate in a particular way for a while before we notice that things need to shift for us to be able to operate at a better level of health. For each of us this process can vary.

Many people may be unaware that they are operating on a certain plateau which can be frustrating and stressful. You may feel stuck and feel a need to make some changes. If we can consciously make mental changes and commitments to act in a certain way or to make certain changes in our diet, lifestyle, career or even home environment, things will start moving along again. This is the process of personal development.

This process, however, can be slower or faster depending on your ability and desire to make the changes necessary to make life more comfortable. Think about what is holding you back or bogging you down in your life today then think about what creative solutions you can come up with to unblock and free those areas where you feel stuck. When we think of high thoughts, we can transcend our own limitations. By thinking the very best thoughts about our lives and what we can be doing to help our own personal development, we can create visualisations for the future to be better than the present.

This is important for your Wellness Zone, don't allow yourself to stay stuck in any position that is uncomfortable or creates stress and conflict in your mind. Make your mind an oasis where you can think high thoughts.

The simple act of awareness is often enough to trigger change

Do you ever regurgitate the past and live in your yesterday? If so, you need to learn to let go of these old experiences and get on with today in a positive and graceful way. Whatever is blocking the path to your Wellness Zone needs to be eliminated so that you can get on with the job of having a healthy and joyful lifestyle.

The first and possibly the most successful way to release blocks is by simply being aware that a block exists. It's that simple, just be aware. Awareness is often enough for us to consciously make some subtle changes that will alter the way we view our lives and look at what positive choices we can make in the future to alter the present limitations and blocks that stop us from reaching our full potential.

Just be still in your mind and look at your life from an observers perspective. Don't be critical and negative with yourself; be objective. Look at the good attributes and the positive actions and patterns you have first. Look at each one and thank yourself for having these qualities. Take a moment to be grateful for the goodness and the positives that you have created in your life.

From this, move to the neutral aspects of your life and the things that you don't really notice on a daily level. These are the almost automatic actions of the day. Think about and observe any little oddities or idiosyncrasies that occur in your life. Take a moment when you think of these, to acknowledge your neglect, or simply ponder the automaticness of these acts.

Breathing is a good example because we spend our whole life breathing in oxygen and breathing out carbon dioxide. But how often do you think about it? Now think of ways that you may be able to make these automatic acts conscious and to be aware of how they affect your life. For example, think about your breathing again, if you breathe deeply, this is healthier than shallow breathing.

Once we truly and objectively look at the different aspects of our lives and how we can alter them to make us more comfortable in our Wellness Zone, we can then begin to make small changes that will improve our daily health. Things will start to fall into place more easily, in fact often effortlessly we will find that we are actually living the way we want to because we have made the effort to mentally analyse our own unique ways and have proactively made changes. These can often be precursors for even bigger and more beneficial changes. The simple act of awareness, just seeing where we are and what we are doing is often enough to shift us and nudge us gently onto the next level of our health as we begin to see more clearly the patterns and the changes that need to take place.

Live simply and enjoy the journey

To live simply or to simply live? What's the difference?

How often do you look at your daily life and think of the complications? Do you live simply and try to organise yourself so that there is minimal pressure, confusion and upheaval? Or do you just roll along with the journey and get caught in your web of over-busy-ness?

It's very easy to become over busy. As a matter of course, when we get busy, we tend to take on more and get busier, then we wonder what's going on and why we are becoming bogged down with stress and illness. We are all vibrating to a certain frequency at any point in time; interestingly though, we can tune into whatever frequency we choose.

Sometimes these frequencies can become addictive, and we end up in a whirlwind of stress and exhaustion. Or we can choose to be relaxed and in control. It's all about your personal response to any situation. Doesn't that sound ideal? Just choose your frequency and tune into the rhythm of life. Today I shall be relaxed, focused and completely free of stress. Zoom, there you are: relaxed, focused and free of stress. It's all a matter of attitude really. So, simply living and living simply is also a matter of attitude.

We can choose to live simply, and once we have that organised, we can simply live. It actually doesn't work the other way around. If we try to simply live and then try to live simply, we will carry all of our old habits and baggage with us, and it won't be long before we forget to live simply and are in the fast lane of complicated life again.

To live simply, we need to think about what we do with our time, what we do with our lives and how to take out the unnecessary clutter to create a joyful and simple existence where we can be healthy and have good stress that we thrive on instead of negative stress that is destructive to us on all levels.

Take a look at your diet firstly

What do you eat? Is the food you eat fresh and nourishing to help nurture your nervous system, feed your body and bring energy? Or are you gulping down fast foods that are lacking in nutrition and feeding your stresses more as the day goes on? Do you thrive on stimulants and get lazy and tired when these are not available?

Eating fresh, alive and vibrant foods is always a good option. To actually have a few days at home where you can relax and look at how to simplify your life, would go a long way towards improving your health. Looking after yourself is not being selfish.

A well-balanced, healthy person is an asset to all; they are able to make better decisions, are happier people and can create a climate of benevolence so that everyone that comes in contact with them, directly or indirectly, will ultimately benefit. We all have the personal responsibility to make the most of ourselves and to live healthier and more fulfilled lives.

Think about your life and what would happen
if you had no tomorrow

What would you do with your time?

What are the things that you really want to do, and how can you go about achieving these goals? Think about this idea. Are there simple changes that you can make to your life to fulfil your dreams and create the life you have always wanted? Make moves today to be the person you want to be tomorrow. Create simplicity and an open path to wellness in your life.

PART V

THE HERBAL MEDICINE ZONE

Herbal medicines are natural medicines

Many modern-day pharmaceuticals are based on these ancient and time-honoured plants. You can access most herbal medicines through your Health Care Practitioner. In the following pages I have listed the different ways that herbal medicines can be taken. I have also included a glossary of botanical names to common names so that you can easily identify the herbs you need.

Herbal extracts

What are they?

Herbal extracts are concentrated liquid herbal preparations that are generally made up by Health Care Practitioners exclusively for their own clients. The term 'extract', is used for herbal concentrations that are one part herb to one part liquid (1:1 extract) or one part herb to two parts liquid (1:2 extract). These extracts can be processed using cold liquids or they can be heated and reduced to the standard extract required.

Many commercial companies now make herbal extracts that are available through your Health Care Practitioner. Herbal tinctures are less concentrated than extracts and are often in concentrations of one part herb to five parts liquid (1:5 tincture) or up to one part herb to ten parts liquid (1:10 tincture). The terms extract and tincture can often be used in the same manner; however, as you can see, the extract is more concentrated.

The herbal extracts and tinctures that I use on the *medicineroom.net* are all made here on our certified organic farm using fresh spring water and pure 100% medicinal grade ethanol. I try to source organic herbs from growers here in the southern hemisphere when available, and the extracts take between three weeks and nine months to extract. I do not use heat processes in the extraction of the liquid herbs. The reason why I extract my own herbs for my clients is that I want them to have unusual and rare herbs which are not always accessible through the wholesalers. I also enjoy the process of extraction and endeavour to know exactly where each product comes from, from beginning to end, when I provide a client with a required extract.

Some active constituents are only able to be accessed through the addition of ethanol or glycerine to the herbs. Not all actives are water-soluble and therefore the addition of ethanol is important in some herbs to access the medicinal benefits of that herb. This is what makes extracts and tinctures the best overall way to gain the most healing property from the plant.

How do you use them?

Taking liquid extracts would vary from person to person. Sometimes you may only need a small dose of 1 to 2 ml per day, and other times you may need a large dose of up to 60 ml per day. This depends on the circumstances, your illness, strength of the herbs, other medications and personal choice. Some people are sensitive to ethanol, and you can steam some of this off the top of the herbal dose simply by adding boiling water. Add one tablespoon of boiling water for each teaspoon of herbal extract. This will help to diffuse some of the alcohol from the herbs but will not take away the taste nor remove all of the alcohol; however, it may ease the after-effects of the herbs when you have a sensitivity to the ethanol.

You can also take 15 ml of herbal extract and place in a pot with 100 ml of boiling water, keep the water boiling for five minutes and then drink the herbal liquid. This is a more effective way to take off the alcohol; however, it will compromise the status of the herb, and you may lose some of its healing qualities by using this cooking method.

What are the advantages and disadvantages?

The advantages of extracts and tinctures are that they are easily absorbed into your body, from the first taste in your mouth, right down to your stomach where they are absorbed and will mostly miss out on any digestive processes, other than diffusion.

Herbal extracts are alcohol-based, and the alcohol is freely absorbed across the stomach lining straight into your bloodstream. This is the main advantage with these herbs because even people who have digestive or absorption problems or difficulty swallowing pills are able to take the extracts and tinctures relatively easily and fairly quickly reap the benefits. There is usually about a 20 to 30 minute kick-in time with extracts and tinctures before the herbs start to do their work on your body.

Extracts and tinctures are often the base of many tablets, when you take this concentrated form of herb, you are getting larger amounts of the healing ingredients without the expensive processing of pills, you are also giving your body pure herbal fuel. Other advantages are that your Health Care Practitioner can blend your mixes to suit your own unique condition.

Extracts are economical when you have a blend of two or more herbs, the disadvantages really only lie in the flavour and they usually taste terrible. I have yet to meet a person who likes the taste, but they are, however, a fast and effective medicine. Alcoholics or people with liver disease would do well to avoid these extracts without the supervision of their Health Care Practitioner.

Decoctions

Decoctions are the traditional way to boil up herbs. The herbs are usually given in dried form and in measured doses to last you a week or longer. This is a personal or traditional formula that your practitioner will have blended from dried roots, seeds, leaves, flowers and stems for your use.

You take these dried herbs in a specific quantity and boil them in water for half an hour or longer, allow to cool and then drink the required dose at intervals throughout the day as requested. Decoctions are a popular way to get herbal medicines to the public in an accessible way. Often the hard parts of herbs, such as roots and stems, are decocted to gain access to the benefits. You need to add quite a lot of water to the herbs and boil to reduce the water into a concentrated blend which is then cooled and used as required.

How do you use them?

Decoctions are taken specifically as prescribed by your practitioner. Usually, you would have your little bag of herbs and boil up the measured daily dose each morning and take as requested. You can decoct any herbs that are wet or dry and use them in various ways. For example, you can drink the formula or you can mix with a cream base and use topically as a skin cream.

What are the advantages and disadvantages?

The advantages are once again the same as extracts and tinctures, in that you can have a very personal formula made to suit your needs.

Decoctions are non-alcoholic, and therefore some active constituents are not accessible through the decoction process. However, the lack of alcohol is also an advantage in that they are good for alcoholics and people with liver disease and those sensitive to alcohol. Decoctions are generally cheap, easily accessible and effective medicines. They are also easily absorbed in the body.

Tablets

What are they?

Tablets are concentrated herbs mixed with various caking agents and made into a standard formula. Tablets are often made from herbal extracts and tinctures mixed with powders to create a combination of specific nutrients and herbs for commercial purposes. Practitioners rarely make tablets. Tablets can also be made with dried raw herbs.

How do you use them?

Taken daily as required to supply your body with various herbs. Often you can measure the dose swallowed by the number of tablets taken, and this is a good way to measure quantity in a standardised way. Tablets are more standard than practitioner-made extracts, tinctures and decoctions because of the harsh manufacturing guidelines in GMP (Good Manufacturing Practice).

Many Health Care Practitioners will prescribe tablets purely because there is a simple measured dose, no bad taste, no work involved from the patient and progress is easily monitored.

What are the advantages and disadvantages?

The main advantage is standardisation of the dose. Tablets are very measured, and you know how much you are getting of each herb. They are neutral in taste, so you don't get the herbal taste in your mouth. They are easy and convenient to travel with, and you can take them anywhere in your bag for use at any time in the day. Tablets are the non-messy way to have extracts and tinctures. However, they are more expensive as you are paying for the fillers, they are often in much smaller doses, so you need more to get the benefits, and they require the process of absorption.

Therefore, those who have absorption issues may well miss out on the benefits of taking the tablets as they can be excreted without absorption. Tablets made with dried raw herbs are even harder to absorb into your blood as they not only require the breakdown of the tablet but also the breakdown of the herb before you can utilise them in your body.

Capsules

What are they?

Capsules are raw dried herbs that have been placed into either gelatine or vegetable-based capsules, either by your practitioner or personally at home. Capsules are measured amounts of herbs, which when swallowed can be accessed by your body in the small intestine where you need to break them down for absorption.

How do you use them?

With a little machine or by hand, simply fill the capsule with your dried herbs and swallow. You can also purchase capsules from retail outlets and practitioners. Many Ayurvedic and Chinese practitioners prefer to make capsules for their patients as this is an easy way to take traditional medicines.

What are the advantages and disadvantages?

The main advantage here again is convenience, it's easy to swallow a pill and again, like the tablet, there is no taste involved. Capsules can be in single herb or blended combinations depending on your needs. The disadvantage of capsules is that they do not get absorbed into your digestive tract until the small intestine, which means that they require active digestion.

If you have malabsorption problems then capsules may be excreted without being absorbed. The gelatine capsule itself is often broken down in the stomach, and this means that some herbs can be processed here; however, they will get mixed in with foods and carried through to the small intestine. Taking capsules is risky business when you want to ensure that the dose consumed is the dose absorbed.

Infusions

What are they?

Herbal infusions are simply herbal teas. Any herb, fresh or dried, can be added to boiling water, allowed to sit and infuse for up to ten minutes and then sipped whilst hot for the soothing benefits and delicious aromas that many of these teas invoke.

Herbal teas are usually not the heavy-duty medicinal herbs; they are often made out of the nicer, tastier and good-smelling herbs that offer medicinal as well as enjoyment value. There is a ritual to tea drinking, and you can create your own rituals with herbal infusions.

How do you use them?

One teaspoon of dried herbs equals three teaspoons of fresh herbs. So, you would take one teaspoon of dried herbs, which equates to 3 to 5 grams of herb depending on your teaspoon measure, or three teaspoons of fresh garden herb (12 to 15 grams). Add to this 200 ml of boiling water and allow to sit for five to ten minutes. Place a cover over the cup or pot to keep it hot. Once the time is up, simply pour the herbal liquid through a strainer and drink the infusion.

Or you can cheat and add a ready-made teabag to a cup of boiling water and allow to sit for five to ten minutes before drinking, and you don't even need to take out the tea bag as the flavour becomes richer towards the bottom of the cup. You can also leave infusions to cool and drink them later.

What are the advantages and disadvantages?

Herbal infusions are quick, mostly delicious, usually enjoyable and medicinally beneficial. They can be taken at any time of the day and offer fairly quick results as they are easily absorbed into your body.

The disadvantages are that these teas are often not left long enough to become totally medicinal, and many of the properties of the herb are left in the pot. The longer you leave the tea to infuse, the better the medicinal value. One big advantage is the delicious aromas that come from herbal infusions; often this is medicine in itself.

Poultices and compresses

What are they?

Poultices are an external application that are usually freshly made for the skin at the time of the treatment. Poultices can be made from fresh or dried herbs mixed with a powder carrier such as slippery elm bark, marshmallow or oat bran combined with hot water and apple cider vinegar. The powders help mould the poultice to the body.

To make a poultice, mix equal parts of herb to liquid, and powder if needed. Usually, equal parts boiling water and apple cider vinegar, or you can add herbal tincture or extract to the water if preferred. Mix to a paste using your mortar and pestle or a strong spoon. Crush the herbs and make the paste as smooth as possible. You can also make a poultice out of herbal extract and powder if fresh or dried herbs are unavailable. Next, spread the mixture onto a clean piece of muslin or gauze and place over the affected area.

A compress usually comprises of liquid herbs mixed with hot water, then clean cotton or fabric is soaked in the liquid and placed directly over the wound or injury. For example, an arnica compress could be applied straight after injury to help reduce the possibility of inflammation as well as to reduce future bruising. A chamomile compress would help reduce the pain of burns but would be mixed with cold water instead of hot.

How do you use them?

Poultices are used whenever there is a chronic or acute skin condition or an underlying problem that may need healing from the outside. Often you will use a poultice to draw toxins or foreign objects to the surface where they can be eliminated. They can be used to help remove non-malignant growths from under the skin, also when muscles or tissues are damaged to help speed their repair. Poultices help to reduce inflammation and work very well on peripheral areas of the body such as ankles, legs, arms and hands.

You would use a poultice when external healing is necessary and when you want certain herbs and their qualities to be absorbed into the body at a specific place. Wrap bandages or place tape over the poultice to hold it in place and leave it on for 12 hours or longer. Sometimes poultices need to be left on the body for days on end, other times they only need to be left on overnight or for one dressing. You may need to give the skin a breathing space between poultices; it really depends on what the problem is and what results you desire.

Compresses are often applied directly after injury or used in the same way as a poultice. However, you need to replace the compress as it cools down as often these are most effective when hot and warm on the skin, unless you are trying to relieve a hot condition such as fever or burning, then you will need to use cool compresses.

What are the advantages and disadvantages?

The main advantage of a poultice is its direct effect on the body from an external perspective. You are able to leave the herbs in place for a time frame that allows drawing or absorption of the herbs to the affected areas. The disadvantage is the bulk of the poultice; the smell can also be very 'herby'. Poultices can really help speed the healing time of many ailments such as muscle and tendon damage, sprained ankles, toxins under the skin, foreign bodies lodged in the skin, rashes, burns, itches and other underlying conditions, such as acute pain from arthritis in the knees or hips. The advantages and disadvantages of compresses are similar to poultices; however, compresses are often lighter due to the liquid format and not so bulky. A compress is easier to prepare; however, it needs frequent changing throughout the day.

Creams and ointments

What are they?

Creams and ointments are used for the topical, external application of herbs in a medicinal and therapeutic way. These are usually either the fresh or dried herb, or a herbal extract mixed in with a carrier such as an ointment or cream base. Good creams are basically some form of plant oil that is emulsified (mixed and thickened), and then herbs are added. Often the percentage of herb is as high as 30%, which makes a strong medicinal cream. Ointments are usually plant oils, mixed with beeswax and herbs to make the ointment, which has a greasier feel than cream, and cream tends to soak into the skin faster. Generally, you would use a cream for absorption and an ointment to sit closer to the surface of the skin. Ointments do soak into the skin, but take longer.

How do you use them?

Creams and ointments are convenient. You can apply these on your skin at regular intervals throughout the day. The advantages of these applications are that they get straight to the place where you want the benefits. For example, you can place an arthritis cream or herbal ointment for itching directly on the skin and feel relief fairly fast. They can be used in conjunction with medicines and often help speed the healing process.

What are the advantages and disadvantages?

The advantage is instant access to the affected area. Creams and ointments are also preventative medicines as you can apply them to prevent bites, rashes, bruises, irritations, wind burn and other problems, including wrinkles! It's easy to carry around a pot of cream or ointment and apply regularly through the day as required.

Botanical and common names

This list has the common name first with the botanical name in italics beside it. There are endless herbs; however, the ones listed here are all fairly common.

Agrimony – *Agrimonia eupatoria*
Alfalfa – *Medicago sativa*
Allspice – *Pimenta dioica*
Almond – *Prunus amydalus*
Aloe vera – *Aloe barbadensis*
Andrographis – *Andrographis paniculata*
Angelica – *Angelica archagelica*
Anise seed – *Pimpinella anisum*
Apple – *Malus spp*
Asafetida – *Ferula assa-foetida*
AshwagandHa – *Withania somnifera*
Asparagus – *Asparagus racemosa*
Astragalus – *Astragalus membranaceus*
Arnica – *Arnica montana*
Avocado – *Persea americana*

Brahmi Bacopa – *Bacopa monnieri*
Barley – *Hordeum vulgare*
Basil, Large leaf, sweet – *Ocimum basilicum*
Beetroot – *Beta vulgaris*
Bergamot – *Monarda fistalosa*
Benzoin tree – *Styrax benzoin*
Bilberry – *Vaccinium myrtillus*
Birch – *Betula genus*
Bitter melon – *Momordica charantia*
Bladderwrack – *Fucus vesiculosis*
Black cohosh – *Cimicifuga racemosa*
Black pepper – *Piper nigrum*
Black Walnut – *Juglans nigra*
Blackberry – *Rubus fruticosus*
Blue flag – *Iris versicolor*
Boneset – *Eupatorium perfoliatum*
Borage – *Borage officinalis*
Brindleberry – *Garcinia quaesita*
Burdock – *Arctium lappa*
Butternut – *Juglans cinerea*
Calendula – *Calendula genera*
Calabar bean – *Physostigma venenosum*
Cactus – *Cactus grandiflorus*
Cancer bush – *Sutherandria frutescens*
Caraway seed – *Carum carvi*
Cardamom – *Elearia cardamomum*
Carob – *Ceratonia siliqua*
Carrots – *Daucus carota sativa*
Cascara sagrada – *Rhamnus purshiana*
Castor bean – *Ricinus communis*
Catnip – *Nepeta cataria*
Cats claw – *Uncaria tomentosa*
Cayenne – *Capsicum frutescens*
Celery – *Apium graveolens*
Centaury – *Centaurea genera*
Chamomile – *Matricaria recutita*
Chervil – *Anthriscus cerefolium*
Chaste tree berry – *Vitex agnus-castus*
Chickweed – *Stellaria media*

Chicory root – *Cichorium chicoree*
Chinese blackberry – *Rubus suavissimus*
Chinese wormwood – *Artemisia annua*
Cinnamon – *Cinamomum Cassia*
Cleavors – *Galium aparine*
Cloves – *Syzygium aromaticum*
Coltsfoot – *Tussilago farfara*
Comfrey – *Symphytum officinale*
Coriander seed – *Coriandrum sativum*
Cornsilk – *Zea mays*
Cranberry – *Vaccinium oxycoccos*
Cumin – *Cuminum cyminum*
Damiana – *Turnera diffusa*
Dandelion – *Taraxacum officinale*
Dates – *Phoenix dactylifera*
Devils claw – *Harpagophytum procumbens*
Dill – *Anethum graveolens*
Dong quai – *Angelica polymorphia*
Dwarf periwinkle – *Vinca minor*
Echinacea – *Echinacea augustifolia, E. purpurea*
Elderflower – *Sambucus nigra*
Elecampane – *Inula helenium*
Eucalyptus – *Eucalyptus globulus*
Evening primrose – *Primulus vulgaris*
Eyebright – *Euphrasia officinalis*
False unicorn – *Chamaelirium luteum*
Fennel – *Foeniculum vulgarae*
Fenugreek – *Trigonella foenum graecum*
Feverfew – *Tanacetum parthenium*
Fig – *Ficus carica*
Flaxseed – *Linum usitatissimum*
Greater Galangal – *Curcuma xanthorrhiza*
Garcinia – *Garcinia cambogia*
Garlic – *Allium sativum*
Gentian – *Gentiana catesbaei*
Ginger – *Zingiber officinalis*
Ginkgo – *Ginkgo biloba*
Ginseng (Oriental/Korean) – *Panax ginseng*
Ginseng (Chinese) – *Panax schinseng*

Ginseng (American/Wisconsin) – *Panax quinquefolius*
Ginseng (Siberian) – *Eleutherococcus senticosus*
Globe artichoke – *Cynara scolymus*
Goats rue – *Galenga officinale*
Goldenseal – *Hydrastis canadensis*
Goldenrod – *Solidago virga-aurea*
Gotu kola – *Centella asiatica*
Grapefruit – *Citrus paradisi*
Grapeseed – *Vitis vinifera*
Gravelroot – *Eupatorium purpureum*
Green barley – *Hordeum vulgare*
Guarana – *Paullinia cupara*
Gymnema – *Gymnema sylvestre*
Hawthorn – *Crataegus monogyna*
Heartease – *Viola tricolour*
Herb Robert – *Geranium robertianum*
Hibiscus flower – *Hibiscus genera*
Honeysuckle – *Lonicera caprifolium*
Hops – *Humulus lupulus*
Horehound – *Marrubium vulgare*
Horse chestnut – *Aesculus hippocstanum*
Horseradish – *Armoracia rusticana*
Horsetail – *Equisetum arvense*
Hydrangea – *Hydrangea genera*
Indian Barberry – *Berberis aristata*
Japanese horseradish – *Wasabi japonica*
Jasmine – *Jasmininum sambac*
Jerusalem artichoke – *Helianthus tuberosa*
Jewel weed – *Impatiens biflora*
Jojoba – *Simmondsia californica*
Juniper – *Juniperus scopularum, J. communis*
Kaffir lime – *Citrus hystrix*
Kava – *Piper methysticum*
Kola nut – *Cola nitida, C. acuminata*
Kudzu – *Pueraria thunbergiana*
Lady's mantle – *Alchemilla vulgaris*
Lavender – *Lavandula officinalis*
Lemon – *Citrus Limonia*
Lemon balm – *Melissa officinale*

Lemongrass – *Cymbopogon citrates*
Lemon scented myrtle – *Backhousia citrodora*
Lemon Tea tree – *Leptospermun petersonii*
Licorice – *Glycyrrhiza glabra*
Lime flower – *Tilea europea*
Lobelia – *Lobelia inflata*
Lungwort – *Lobaria pulmonaceae*
Maca – *Lepidium mayenii*
Ma-huang – *Ephedra sinica*
Marshmallow – *Althaea officinalis*
Meadowsweet – *Filipendula ulmaria*
Milk thistle – *Silybum marianum*
Mistletoe – *Viscum album*
Mother of herbs – *Coleus amboinicus*
Motherwort – *Leonurus cardiaca*
Mugwort – *artemisia vulgaris*
Mulberry – *Morus alba Linn*
Mullein – *Verbascum thapsus*
Myrrh – *Commiphora mol-mol*
Neem – *Azadirachta indica*
Noni – *Morinda citrifolia Linn*
Nutmeg – *Myristica fragrans*
Oats – *Avena sativa*
Olive – *Olea europaea*
Onion – *Allium cepa*
Orange – *Citrus sinensis*
Oregano – *Organum vulgare*
Papaya – *Carica papaya*
Parsley – *Petroselinum crispum*
Passionflower – *Passiflora incarnata*
Pau d'arco – *Tabebuia avellanedae*
Peach – *Prunus persica*
Pellitory off the wall – *Parietaria officinalis*
Pepper – *Piper nigrum*
Peppermint – *Mentha piperita*
Plantain – *Plantago major*
Pleurisy root – *Asclepias tuberosa*
Poke root – *Phytolacca decandra*
Prickly ash – *Zanthoxylum americana*

Psyllium seed – *Plantago psyllium*
Pumpkin – *Cucurbita maxima*
Quince – *Cydonia oblongata*
Quinoa – *Chenopodium quinoa*
Red clover – *Trifolium pratense*
Red raspberry – *Rubus idaeus*
Red root buckwheat – *Eriogonum racemosum*
Rehmannia – *Rehmannia glutinosa*
Reishi – *Ganoderma Lucidum*
Rhubarb – *Rheum officinale*
Rocket – *Eruca vesicaria sativa*
Rooibos – *Aspalathus linearis*
Rosehips – *Rosaceae genus*
Rosemary – *Rosmarinus officinalis*
Rue – *Ruta graveolens*
Saffron – *Crocus sativa*
Sage – *Salvia officinalis*
Sarsaparilla – *Smilax aristolochioefolia*
Sassafras – *Sassafras albidum*
Saw palmetto – *Serenoa repens*
Schisandra – *Schisandra chinsis*
Scullcap – *Scutellaria laterifolia*
Scurvy grass – *Cochlearia officinalis*
Self-heal – *Prunella vulgaris*
Senna – *Cassia senna*
Sesame – *Sesamum indicum*
Shepherd's purse – *Capsella bursa-pastoris*
Sheep sorrel – *Rumex acetosella*
Skullcap – *Scutellaria lateriflora*
Slippery elm – *Ulmus fulva*
Small leaf willow – *Epilobium parviflorum*
Sunflower – *Helianthus annuus*
Soy (soybean) – *Glycine max*
Spearmint – *Mentha spicata*
Speedwell (Figwort) – *Veronica officinalis*
SPIRULINA – *Arthrospira Platensis*
Star anise – *Illicum verum*
St. John's wort – *Hypericum perforatum*
Stevia – *Stevia rebaudiana*

Stinging nettle – *Urtica dioica*
Tamerind – *Tamarindus indica*
Tea, black – *Camellia sinensis*
Tea, green – *Camellia sinensis*
Tea tree – *Melaleuca alternifolia*
Thuja – *Thuja occidentalis*
Thyme – *Thymus vulgaris*
Tribulus – *Tribulus terrestris*
Turmeric – *Curcuma longa*
Uva-ursi – *Arctostaphylos uva-ursi*
Valerian – *Valeriana officinalis*
Vanilla – *Vanilla aromatica, V. planifolia*
Vervain – *Verbena officinalis*
White kidney bean – *Phaseolus vulgaris*
White oak – *Quercus & Lithocarpus genera*
White Peony – *Paeonia lactiflora*
Wild cherry – *Prunus serotina*
Wild yam – *Dioscorea villosa*
White willow – *Salix alba, Salix nigra*
Wintergreen – *Gaultheria procumbens*
Witch hazel – *Hamamelis virginiana*
Wood betony – *Pedicularis canadensis*
Wormwood – *Artemisia absinthium*
Yarrow – *Achillea millifolium*
Yellow dock – *Rumex crispus*
Yerba mate – *Iiex aquifolium*
Yucca – *Yucca genus*

INDEX

Printed by Printforce, United Kingdom